AF413321

MCQs in
Human
Anatomy and
Physiology

MCQs in Human Anatomy and Physiology

Pushpendra Patel

Founder of India's top pharmacy YouTube channel "Solution Pharmacy"

Vandana Janghel

Co-founder of India's top pharmacy YouTube channel "Solution Pharmacy"

Kavita Parate

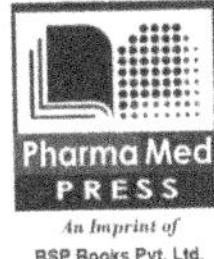

PharmaMed Press

An imprint of BSP Books pvt. Ltd

4-4-309/316, Giriraj Lane,

Sultan Bazar, Hyderabad - 500 095.

MCQs in Human Anatomy and Physiology
by Pushpendra Patel, Vandana Janghel and Kavita Parate

© 2023, *by Publisher*

All rights reserved. No part of this book or parts thereof may be reproduced, stored in a retrieval system or transmitted in any language or by any means, electronic, mechanical, photocopying, recording or otherwise without the prior written permission of the author.

Disclaimer: The authors and the publishers have taken due care to provide the authentic, reliable and up to date information related to the subject. However, neither the authors nor the publisher shall be responsible for any liability for any damage caused as a result of use of this book. The respective user must check the accuracy from other sources too.

Published by:

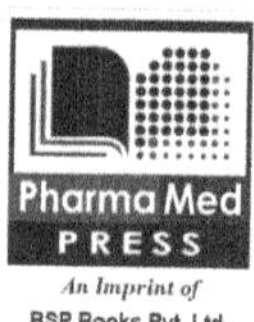

PharmaMed Press

An imprint of BSP Books Pvt. Ltd.

4-4-309/316, Giriraj Lane, Sultan Bazar, Hyderabad - 500 095.
Phone: 040-23445688; Fax: 91+40-23445611
e-mail: info@pharmamedpress.com
www.pharmamedpress.com/pharmamedpress.net

ISBN: 978-93-95039-69-7 (Hardback)

Contents

Introduction to the Book Pattern

Dear Students

Thank you for making a right decision by selecting this book as your preparative companion for the subject "Human Anatomy and Physiology". This book is designed in such a way that you will get maximum out of the subject via both online and offline mode. This book is an extract of complete "Human Anatomy and Physiology" as we have made this book by including maximum possible questions in the form of multiple-choice pattern which is being now followed by all most every discipline. We do understand student psychology that's why this multiple-choice book is made in such a way that you will never get tired and bored while solving because we have divided topics according to their importance, weightage and probability of questions being asked in many examinations.

This book contains 10 units as per the maximum followed syllabus of many semester and competitive examinations.

Tips to solve the questions –

1. Every unit is divided into many parts and as per its importance and tried to form many questions as many as possible so that you need not to follow any other books

2. After studying theory start practicing these questions starting from the unit 01, skipping the units and jumping to next unit will not help you in effective manner as further units are based on initial units

3. Each part of the unit contains 50 multiple choice questions and their answer Keyes

4. Start attempting questions right from the beginning of unit and by their 1st part and move further

5. Set a goal to solve these 50 questions of each part in 60 minutes in beginning

6. Take a rough page and start attempting every part and note down the answer of question as per your opinion

7. After attempting every part of 50 questions, check your answers from the answer keyes given just after the questions

8. Reattempt those questions which you have made wrong and then solve all the questions in 30 minutes or less than that

9. Once you have done with complete unit then reattempt these questions in online mode by downloading solution pharmacy mobile app from play store and a join solution's best ever course

10. Repeat the same process with all single units or parts, that means practice it from book and evaluate your knowledge and time by attempting it from app.

Introduction to Human Body, Cellular Levels of Structural Organization, Tissue Level of Organization

Part-01

1. Study of the structure of human body is called

   (A) Anatomy

   (C) Pharmacology

   (B) Physiology

   (D) Geology

2. Study of the function of the organ is called

   (A) Anatomy

   (C) Pharmacology

   (B) Physiology

   (D) None of the above

3. Who introduced the term Physiology?

   (A) Jean Fernel

   (C) Robert Hooke

   (B) Andrease Vesalius

   (D) None of the above

4. Who introduced the term Anatomy?

   (A) Andrease Vesalius

   (C) Xavier Bichat

   (B) Robert Hooke

   (D) None of the above

5. Study of human body part and organ is called

   (A) Gross anatomy

   (C) Histology

   (B) Cytology

   (D) None of the above

6. Gross anatomy is also known as

   (A) Microscopic Anatomy

   (C) Cytology

   (B) Macroscopic Anatomy

   (D) None of the above

7. Microscopic anatomy is also called as

   (A) Cytology

   (C) Gross anatomy

   (B) Histology

   (D) None of the above

8. The science of the origin and development of the individual from fertilization is termed as

   (A) Histology

   (B) Embryology

   (C) Cytology

   (D) None of the above

9. The branch of physiology which concerned with endocrine glands is called

   (A) Endocrinology

   (B) Cytology

   (C) Pathophysiology

   (D) None of the above

10. The study of the anatomy of tissue which is based on their visualization on X-ray films is

    (A) Pathophysiology

    (B) Immunology

    (C) Radiographic anatomy

    (D) None of the above

11. The study of anatomy of diseased tissues is called as

    (A) Pathological anatomy

    (B) Embryology

    (C) Radiographic anatomy

    (D) None of the above

12. The study of the circulatory system is called as

    (A) Renal physiology

    (B) Cardiovascular physiology

    (C) Immunology

    (D) None of the above

13. The study of the body's immune system is termed as

    (A) Immunology

    (B) Respiratory physiology

    (C) Renal physiology

    (D) Endocrinology

14. The branch of human physiology focusing on respiration is studied under

    (A) Endocrinology

    (B) Immunology

    (C) Renal physiology

    (D) Respiratory physiology

15. The branch of science associated with a disease or an injury is studied under

    (A) Pathophysiology

    (B) Embryology

    (C) Histology

    (D) None of the above

16. The study of the function of the human body during various acute and chronic exercise condition is known as

    (A) Pathophysiology

    (B) Exercise physiology

    (C) Histology

    (D) None of the above

17. The study of physiology of kidney in included under
    - (A) Renal physiology
    - (B) Pathophysiology
    - (C) Respiratory physiology
    - (D) Exercise physiology

18. The fluid outside the cell is called
    - (A) Interstitial fluid
    - (B) Extracellular fluid
    - (C) Intracellular fluid
    - (D) None of the above

19. Liquid contains inside the cell membranes is
    - (A) Intracellular fluid
    - (B) Extracellular fluid
    - (C) Interstitial fluid
    - (D) None of the above

20. Liquid found between the cells of the body is termed as
    - (A) Extracellular fluid
    - (B) Interstitial fluid
    - (C) Intracellular fluid
    - (D) None of the above

21. The position is used in all anatomical description to ensure accuracy and consistency are called
    - (A) Anatomical position
    - (B) Directional terms
    - (C) Regional terms
    - (D) None of the above

22. Nearer to the midline is called as
    - (A) Medial
    - (B) Lateral
    - (C) Distal
    - (D) Proximal

23. Further (Away) from the midline is called as
    - (A) Medial
    - (B) Proximal
    - (C) Lateral
    - (D) None of the above

24. The directional term "Superior" means
    - (A) Nearer the head
    - (B) Nearer the front of the body
    - (C) Nearer the back of the body
    - (D) None of the above

25. Nearer to the front of the body is termed as
    - (A) Lateral
    - (B) Anterior
    - (C) Posterior
    - (D) Inferior

26. The paired terms are used to describes the locomotion of the body in relation to other

    (A) Directional terms   (B) Anatomical terms

    (C) Regional terms   (D) None of the above

27. The skull is superior to the scapulae is an example of which directional terms

    (A) Lateral   (B) Superior

    (C) Inferior   (D) None of the above

28. Foot is inferior to the ankle is an example of

    (A) Inferior   (B) Anterior

    (C) Superior   (D) None of the above

29. Which of the following is a type of body plane?

    (A) Median plane   (B) Frontal plane

    (C) Transverse plane   (D) All of the above

30. When the body is divided longitudinally through the midline into right and left halves then this division is called as

    (A) Median plane   (B) Frontal plane

    (C) Transverse plane   (D) None of the above

31. Which plane is also called as coronal plane?

    (A) Median plane   (B) Frontal plane

    (C) Transverse plane   (D) None of the above

32. Which plane divide the body longitudinally into anterior and posterior section?

    (A) Frontal plane   (B) Median plane

    (C) Transverse plane   (D) None of the above

33. The section provides a cross – section dividing the body or body part into upper and lower part is known as

    (A) Median plane   (B) Transverse plane

    (C) Frontal plane   (D) None of the above

34. Which is refers to the back aspects of the body?

    (A) Median plane   (B) Lateral plane

    (C) Posterior plane   (D) None of the above

35. Which plane divide the body into two equal symmetrical halves?
    - (A) Transverse plane
    - (B) Median plane
    - (C) Frontal plane
    - (D) None of the above

36. Any vertical plane that is parallel to the median plane is known as
    - (A) Sagittal plane
    - (B) Median plane
    - (C) Frontal plane
    - (D) None of the above

37. Opposite of proximal position is known as
    - (A) Distal
    - (B) Lateral
    - (C) Median
    - (D) None of the above

38. Inferior directional terms represent
    - (A) Nearer the head
    - (B) Further from the head
    - (C) Nearer the front of the body
    - (D) None of the above

39. Cervical vertebrae are anatomically
    - (A) Superior to the rib cage
    - (B) Inferior to the thoracic vertebrae
    - (C) Located between the thoracic and sacral vertebrae
    - (D) None of the above

40. Adrenal gland located at
    - (A) Superior to the kidney
    - (B) Inferior to the kidney
    - (C) Frontal to the kidney
    - (D) None of the above

41. Thigh, leg, ankle and foot comes under
    - (A) Lower limb
    - (B) Upper limb
    - (C) Trunk
    - (D) Neck

42. Shoulder, armpit, arm, wrist and hand comes under
    - (A) Trunk
    - (B) Upper limb
    - (C) Lower limb
    - (D) Neck

43. Trunk consists of
    - (A) Face
    - (B) Pelvis
    - (C) Head
    - (D) Leg

44. Head consist of
    - (A) Face and skull
    - (B) Chest and pelvis
    - (C) Arm and hand
    - (D) Leg and foot

45. Major body cavity is/are
    (A) Dorsal cavity
    (B) Ventral cavity
    (C) Both (A) and (B)
    (D) None of the above

46. Which cavity contains organs of the nervous system that coordinate the body's function
    (A) Dorsal cavity
    (B) Ventral cavity
    (C) Pelvic cavity
    (D) Abdominal cavity

47. Dorsal cavity includes
    (A) Cranial cavity
    (B) Spinal cavity
    (C) Both (A) and (B)
    (D) None of the above

48. Cranial cavity contains
    (A) Spinal cord
    (B) Brain
    (C) Stomach
    (D) Spleen

49. Spinal cord is included under
    (A) Vertebral cavity
    (B) Cranial cavity
    (C) Thoracic cavity
    (D) None of the above

50. Which cavity contains organs that maintain the internal environment of the body
    (A) Ventral cavity
    (B) Dorsal cavity
    (C) Cranial cavity
    (D) None of the above

Answer Key

Introduction to Human Body, Cellular Levels of Structural Organization, Tissue Level of Organization (Part-01)

Question	Answer	Question	Answer
01	A = Anatomy	26	A = Directional Terms
02	B = Physiology	27	B = Superior
03	A = Jean Fernel	28	A = Inferior
04	A = Andrease Vesalium	29	D = All of the Above
05	A = Gross Anatomy	30	A = Median Plane
06	B = Macroscopic Anatomy	31	B = Frontal Plane
07	B = Histology	32	A = Frontal Plane
08	B = Embryology	33	B = Transverse Plane
09	A = Endocrinology	34	C = Posterior Plane
10	C = Radiographic Anatomy	35	B = Median Plane
11	A = Pathological Anatomy	36	A = Sagittal Plane
12	B = Cardiovascular Physiology	37	A = Distal
13	A = Immunology	38	B = Further from the Head
14	D = Respiratory Physiology	39	A = Superior to the Rib Cage
15	A = Pathophysiology	40	A = Superior to the Kidney
16	B = Exercise Physiology	41	A = Lower Limb
17	A = Renal Physiology	42	B = Upper Limb
18	B = Extracellular Fluid	43	B = Pelvis
19	A = Intracellular Fluids	44	A = Face and Skull
20	B = Intestinal Fluids	45	C = Both A and B
21	A = Anatomical Position	46	A = Dorsal cavity
22	A = Medial	47	C = Both A and B
23	C = Lateral	48	B = Brain
24	A = Nearer to the Head	49	A = Vertebral Cavity
25	B = Anterior	50	A = Ventral Cavity

Part-02

1. Which of the following cavity is surrounding by the rib cage?
   (A) Pelvic cavity
   (B) Abdominal cavity
   (C) Thoracic cavity
   (D) Cranial cavity

2. Thoracic cavity consists of
   (A) Pericardial cavity
   (B) Mediastinum
   (C) Two pleural cavities
   (D) All of the above

3. The lungs are consisting in which of the following cavity
   (A) Two pleural cavities
   (B) Pericardial cavity
   (C) Abdominal cavity
   (D) None of the above

4. Which cavity contains fluid filled space that surrounds the heart
   (A) Pericardial cavity
   (B) Abdominal cavity
   (C) Two pleural cavities
   (D) None of the above

5. Which cavity is central part of the thoracic?
   (A) Pericardial cavity
   (B) Mediastinum
   (C) Two pleural cavities
   (D) None of the above

6. Which cavity consist of oesophagus
   (A) Mediastinum
   (B) Pericardial cavity
   (C) Pelvic cavity
   (D) None of the above

7. Abdominopelvic cavity includes
   (A) Abdominal cavity
   (B) Pelvic cavity
   (C) Both (A) and (B)
   (D) None of the above

8. Which cavity contains stomach and spleen
   (A) Pelvic cavity
   (B) Abdominal cavity
   (C) Pericardial cavity
   (D) Mediastinum

9. Which cavity contains urinary bladder
   (A) Pelvic cavity
   (B) Mediastinum
   (C) Pericardial cavity
   (D) None of the above

10. At rest the heart contracts, or beats at which of the following rate
    - (A) 72 times per minute
    - (B) 56 times per minute
    - (C) 97 times per minute
    - (D) 104 times per minute

11. The main organ of circulatory system is
    - (A) Heart
    - (B) Lungs
    - (C) Liver
    - (D) Brain

12. Lymphatic system consists of
    - (A) Lymph node
    - (B) Lymph vessels
    - (C) Thymus
    - (D) All of the above

13. The main function of lymphatic system is/are
    - (A) Removal of excess fluid from body tissue
    - (B) Production of immune cells
    - (C) Transports fats from digestive system
    - (D) All of the above

14. Central nervous system consists of which of the following organ
    - (A) Brain
    - (B) Spinal cord
    - (C) Both (A) and (B)
    - (D) None of the above

15. The peripheral nervous system is a network of nerve fibres which include
    - (A) Sensory or afferent nerves
    - (B) Motor or efferent nerves
    - (C) Both (A) and (B)
    - (D) None of the above

16. Somatic senses include which of the following sensation
    - (A) Pain
    - (B) Touch
    - (C) Heat and cold
    - (D) All of the above

17. Nerves impulses can travel at speeds of
    - (A) 30 metres per second
    - (B) 100 metres per second
    - (C) 300 metres per second
    - (D) 500 metres per second

18. Reflex action involves which of the following action
    - (A) Withdrawal of a finger from a very hot surface
    - (B) Constriction of pupil in response to bright light
    - (C) Control of blood pressure
    - (D) All of the above

19. Synapse is the junction between two
    (A) Muscles   (B) Neurons
    (C) Cells   (D) Tissue

20. The site where communication takes place is called
    (A) Synapse   (B) Muscles
    (C) Cells   (D) Tissue

21. Nerve communicates with each other by releasing
    (A) Neurotransmitter   (B) Hormones
    (C) Fluids   (D) None of the above

22. Sensory receptors control vital functions which are
    (A) Heart rate   (B) Respiratory rate
    (C) Blood pressure   (D) All the above

23. The smallest independent units of living matter are
    (A) Cells   (B) Tissue
    (C) Organ   (D) None of the above

24. The specialised function of nerves is
    (A) To transmit electrical signal
    (B) These are integrated and coordinated
    (C) To provide a rapid and sophisticated communication system
    (D) All of the above

25. Organs is made up of number of different types of
    (A) Cells   (B) Tissues
    (C) Nerve cells   (D) None of the above

26. Stomach is made up of
    (A) Layer of smooth muscle tissue   (B) Layer of epithelial tissue
    (C) Both (A) and (B)   (D) None of the above

27. Which of the following is an example of accessory organ?
    (A) Pancreas   (B) Salivary glands
    (C) Liver   (D) All of the above

28. Which of the following is an example of body system?
    (A) Digestive system
    (B) Circulatory system
    (C) Nervous system
    (D) All of the above

29. Digestive system contributes in the process of
    (A) Ingestion
    (B) Digestion
    (C) Absorption
    (D) All of the above

30. Communication is a transport system that include
    (A) Blood
    (B) Cardiovascular system
    (C) Lymphatic system
    (D) All of the above

31. Which of the following is a type of communication?
    (A) Internal communication
    (B) External communication
    (C) Both (A) and (B)
    (D) None of the above

32. Internal communication is important in the maintenance of
    (A) Homeostasis
    (B) Regulation of vital body functions
    (C) Both (A) and (B)
    (D) None of the above

33. Communication with external environment involves
    (A) Special senses
    (B) Verbal activities
    (C) Non – verbal activities
    (D) All of the above

34. Survival for the life needs which of the following activity
    (A) Communication
    (B) Intake of raw material
    (C) Protection of the body
    (D) All of the above

35. The main function of blood is/are
    (A) Transport
    (B) Protection
    (C) Regulation
    (D) All of the above

36. Red blood cellsis alsotermed as
    (A) Erythrocytes
    (B) Leukocytes
    (C) Thrombocytes
    (D) None of the above

37. Leukocytes also known as
    (A) Red blood cells
    (B) White blood cells
    (C) Platelets
    (D) None of the above

38. In adults' body the amount of blood is
    - (A) 2-3 litres
    - (B) 1-2 litres
    - (C) 5-6 litres
    - (D) None of the above

39. The amount of water contains in plasma is
    - (A) 90 %
    - (B) 50 %
    - (C) 40 %
    - (D) None of the above

40. Plasma contains
    - (A) Nutrients
    - (B) Oxygen
    - (C) Hormones
    - (D) All of the above

41. Which of the following is a type of blood vessels?
    - (A) Arteries
    - (B) Veins
    - (C) Capillaries
    - (D) All of the above

42. Which blood vessel carry blood away from the heart
    - (A) Arteries
    - (B) Veins
    - (C) Capillaries
    - (D) None of the above

43. Which of the following is very tiny blood vessels?
    - (A) Veins
    - (B) Capillaries
    - (C) Arteries
    - (D) None of the above

44. Which of the following is pulmonary circulation?
    - (A) Kidney
    - (B) Liver
    - (C) Lungs
    - (D) None of the above

45. Which gland secrete hormones directly into the bloodstream
    - (A) Endocrine glands
    - (B) Exocrine
    - (C) Both (A) and (B)
    - (D) None of the above

46. Hormones stimulate
    - (A) Target glands or tissue
    - (B) Influence metabolism
    - (C) Regulate body growth
    - (D) All of the above

47. Special senses include
    - (A) Sight
    - (B) Hearing
    - (C) Smell
    - (D) All of the above

48. Production of sound in the larynx is comes under which communication
  - (A) Verbal communication
  - (B) Non - verbal communication
  - (C) Both (A) and (B)
  - (D) None of the above

49. Posture and movements are often associated with
  - (A) Verbal communication
  - (B) Non - verbal communication
  - (C) Both (A) and (B)
  - (D) None of the above

50. Which of the following example comes under non - verbal communication
  - (A) Nodding the head
  - (B) Shrugging the shoulder
  - (C) Both (A) and (B)
  - (D) None of the above

Answer Key

Introduction to Human Body, Cellular Levels of Structural Organization, Tissue Level of Organization (Part-02)

Question	Answer	Question	Answer
01	C = Thoracic Cavity	26	C = Both A and B
02	D = All of the Above	27	D = All of the above
03	A = Two Pleural Cavities	28	D = All of the above
04	A = Pericardial Cavity	29	D = All of the Above
05	B = Mediastinum	30	D = All of the Above
06	A = Mediastinum	31	C = Both A and B
07	C = Both A and B	32	C = Both A and B
08	B = Abdominal Cavity	33	D = All of the above
09	A = Pelvic Cavity	34	D = All of the Above
10	A = 72 Time Per Minute	35	D = All of the above
11	A = Heart	36	A = Erythrocytes
12	D = All of the Above	37	B = White Blood Cells
13	D = All of the Above	38	C = 5 to 06 Litres
14	C = Both A and B	39	A = 90%
15	C = Both A and B	40	D = All of the Above
16	D = All of the Above	41	D = All of the Above
17	B = 100 meters per second	42	A = Arteries
18	D = All of the Above	43	B = Capillaries
19	B = Neurons	44	C = Lungs
20	A = Synapse	45	A = Endocrine Glands
21	A = Neurotransmitters	46	D = All of the Above
22	D = All of the above	47	D = All of the Above
23	A = Cells	48	A = Verbal Communication
24	D = All of the Above	49	B = Nonverbal Commination
25	B = Tissues	50	C = Both A and B

Part-03

1. The excretory system involves
   (A) Respiratory system
   (B) Digestive system
   (C) Urinary system
   (D) All of the above

2. The substance which is excreted from the body is/are
   (A) Carbon dioxide
   (B) Urine
   (C) Feces
   (D) All of the above

3. The atmospheric air contains which amount of oxygen gas
   (A) 21 %
   (B) 75 %
   (C) 9 %
   (D) 46 %

4. In which part of respiratory system exchange of gases occurs or take place
   (A) Larynx
   (B) Pharynx
   (C) Alveoli
   (D) Trachea

5. A million of tiny air sacs are present in
   (A) Bronchi
   (B) Alveoli
   (C) Trachea
   (D) Pharynx

6. The atmospheric air contains which percentage of nitrogen
   (A) 21 %
   (B) 80 %
   (C) 14 %
   (D) 11 %

7. A balance diet is important for health because
   (A) They provide nutrients
   (B) They promote body function
   (C) They promote body growth
   (D) All of the above

8. Nutrient includes
   (A) Carbohydrates
   (B) Proteins
   (C) Vitamins
   (D) All of the above

9. The process in which complex food material break down into smallest material is called as
   - (A) Digestion
   - (B) Respiration
   - (C) Circulation
   - (D) None of the above

10. Digestive system consists of
   - (A) Alimentary canal
   - (B) Accessory organ
   - (C) Both (A) and (B)
   - (D) None of the above

11. Which of the following is not a part of alimentary canal?
   - (A) Pharynx
   - (B) Esophagus
   - (C) Stomach
   - (D) Pancreas

12. Which of the following is an accessory organ?
   - (A) Salivary gland
   - (B) Liver
   - (C) Pancreas
   - (D) All of the above

13. Digestive enzyme is synthesized by
   - (A) Salivary gland
   - (B) Pancreas
   - (C) Both (A) and (B)
   - (D) None of the above

14. Bile is secreted by
   - (A) Liver
   - (B) Pancreas
   - (C) Salivary gland
   - (D) Kidney

15. Metabolic reaction is classified into
   - (A) Anabolism
   - (B) Catabolism
   - (C) Both (A) and (B)
   - (D) None to the above

16. Most carbon dioxide excreted through the lungs during
   - (A) Expiration
   - (B) Inspiration
   - (C) Both (A) and (B)
   - (D) None of the above

17. The function of kidney is/are
   - (A) Removal of waste material
   - (B) Regulate water balance
   - (C) Maintain body pH
   - (D) All of the above

18. Urine contains which of the following constituents as their contents
   - (A) Water
   - (B) Urea
   - (C) Ammonia
   - (D) All of the above

19. The function of defensive system is/are
    (A) Protection against the environment
    (B) Defense against infection
    (C) Movement and survival of the species
    (D) All of the above

20. Superficial layer of skin is called as
    (A) Epidermis   (B) Dermis
    (C) Hypodermis   (D) Myocytes

21. Which layer of skin consists of dead flattened cells
    (A) Hypodermis   (B) Epidermis
    (C) Dermis   (D) Basal cells

22. The function of skin is/are
    (A) Protection against microbes
    (B) Protection against chemicals
    (C) Prevent dehydration
    (D) All of the above

23. Which layer of skin contains tiny sweat gland
    (A) Dermis   (B) Epidermis
    (C) Hypodermis   (D) Myocytes

24. Which layer of skin is rich in sensory nerve ending?
    (A) Hypodermis   (B) Dermis
    (C) Epidermis   (D) Melanocyte

25. Sensory nerve endings of skin are sensitive to
    (A) Pain   (B) Temperature
    (C) Touch   (D) All of the above

26. The defense mechanism of body is
    (A) Specific defense mechanism
    (B) Non- specific defense mechanism
    (C) Both (A) and (B)
    (D) None of the above

27. The musculoskeletal system includes the
    - (A) Bone of skeleton
    - (B) Skeletal muscles
    - (C) Joint
    - (D) All of the above

28. The function of skeleton is/are
    - (A) Provide rigid body framework
    - (B) Movement
    - (C) Protect organs
    - (D) All of the above

29. Function of skeletal muscles is/are
    - (A) Control of the voluntary nervous system
    - (B) Maintain posture and balance
    - (C) Move the skeleton
    - (D) All of the above

30. Growth is characterized by
    - (A) Increase in body
    - (B) Increase in cell size
    - (C) Increase in cell number
    - (D) All of the above

31. The process of development of specialized cell from unspecialized is called
    - (A) Differentiation
    - (B) Growth
    - (C) Reproduction
    - (D) None of the above

32. The condition of equilibrium that is maintained by keeping the body's internal environment care called as
    - (A) Homeostasis
    - (B) Hemostasis
    - (C) Both (A) and (B)
    - (D) None of the above

33. The basic component of homeostasis
    - (A) Detector
    - (B) Control center
    - (C) Effector
    - (D) All of the above

34. The term 'homeostasis' was coined by
    - (A) Walter B. cannon
    - (B) Chris Crick
    - (C) John Mathew
    - (D) Francis Crick

35. The significance of homeostasis in the survival of an organism was first discussed by
    - (A) Chris Crick
    - (B) Claude Bernard
    - (C) John Mathew
    - (D) Robert Hooke

36. The feedback mechanism of homeostasis includes
    (A) Positive feedback mechanism
    (B) Negative feedback mechanism
    (C) Both (A) and (B)
    (D) None of the above

37. Which system monitors the changes in the internal environment
    (A) Detector   (B) Control center
    (C) Effector   (D) None of the above

38. Which of the following system sends input in the form of nerve impulse to the control center?
    (A) Effector   (B) Detector
    (C) Both (A) and (B)   (D) None of the above

39. The function of control center is/are
    (A) Evaluate the input coming from detector
    (B) Generate the output in the form of nerve impulse
    (C) Send nerve impulse to the effector
    (D) All of the above

40. Which of the following system receives output from control center
    (A) Effector   (B) Detector
    (C) Both (A) and (B)   (D) None of the above

41. In negative feedback system, the response generated by the
    (A) Effector reverse or opposes the stimulus
    (B) Effector enhance or intensifies the stimulus
    (C) Bothe (A) and (B)
    (D) None of the above

42. In positive feedback system, the response is generated by the
    (A) Effector reverse or opposes the stimulus
    (B) Effector enhance or intensifies the stimulus
    (C) Both (A) and (B)
    (D) None of the above

43. Body temperature is one of the examples of a physiological variable which is controls by
    (A) Negative feedback system
    (B) Positive feedback system
    (C) Both (A) and (B)
    (D) None of the above

44. Body temperature is controlled by
    (A) Cerebrum
    (B) Hypothalamus
    (C) Cerebellum
    (D) Medulla oblongata

45. When body temperature rises, the hypothalamus activates and give symptom, that is/are
    (A) Stimulation of skeletal muscles causing shivering
    (B) Narrowing the blood vessels
    (C) Behavioral changes
    (D) All of the above

46. Blood pressure is regulated by
    (A) Negative feedback mechanism
    (B) Positive feedback mechanism
    (C) Alpha feedback mechanism
    (D) Gamma feedback mechanism

47. Change in blood pressure is detected by
    (A) Baroreceptor
    (B) Chemoreceptor
    (C) Thermoreceptor
    (D) Hydro receptor

48. Release of oxytocin hormone during child birth is an example of
    (A) Negative feedback mechanism
    (B) Positive feedback mechanism
    (C) Both (A) and (B)
    (D) None of the above

49. Oxytocin hormone enhances the process of
    (A) Contractions of uterus muscle
    (B) Relaxation of uterus muscle
    (C) Both (A) and (B)
    (D) None of the above

50. When homeostatic system getimbalanced, then body give sign and symptom which is /are
    (A) Headache
    (B) Nausea
    (C) Anxiety
    (D) All of the above

Answer Key

Introduction to Human Body, Cellular Levels of Structural Organization, Tissue Level of Organization (Part-03)

Question	Answer	Question	Answer
01	D = All of the Above	26	C = Both A and B
02	D = All of the Above	27	D = All of the Above
03	A = 21%	28	D = All of the above
04	C = Alveoli	29	D = All of the Above
05	B = Alveoli	30	D = All of the Above
06	B = 80%	31	A = Differentiation
07	D = All of the Above	32	A = Homeostasis
08	D = All of the Above	33	D = All of the Above
09	A = Digestion	34	A = Walter B. Cannon
10	C = Both A and B	35	B = Claude Bernard
11	D = Pancreas	36	C = Both A and B
12	D = All of the above	37	A = Detector
13	C = Both A and B	38	B = Detector
14	A = Liver	39	D = All of the Above
15	C = Both A and B	40	A = Effector
16	A = Expiration	41	A = Effector Reverse or Oppose the Stimulus
17	D = All of the Above	42	B = Effector Enhance or Intensify the Stimulus
18	D = All of the Above	43	A = Negative Feedback System
19	D = All of the Above	44	B = Hypothalamus
20	A = Epidermis	45	D = All of the Above
21	B = Epidermis	46	A = Negative Feedback Mechanism
22	D = All of the Above	47	A = Baroreceptor
23	A = Dermis	48	B = Positive Feedback Mechanism
24	B = Dermis	49	A = Contraction of Uterus Muscle
25	D = All of the Above	50	D = All of the Above

Part-04

1. Body's smallest functional unit is
   - (A) Cells
   - (B) Tissues
   - (C) Organs
   - (D) Organ system

2. Cell is grouped together to formed
   - (A) Tissue
   - (B) Organ
   - (C) Organ system
   - (D) None of the above

3. Cell is discovered by
   - (A) Robert Koch
   - (B) Robert Hooke
   - (C) Robert Brown
   - (D) Louis Pasteur

4. The study of the structure and function of the cell is called
   - (A) Histology
   - (B) Pathophysiology
   - (C) Cytology
   - (D) Immunology

5. The main part of cells is
   - (A) Plasma membrane
   - (B) Nucleus
   - (C) Cytoplasm
   - (D) All of the above

6. Human body developed from single cell which is termed as
   - (A) Zygote
   - (B) Nerve cell
   - (C) Blood cell
   - (D) Bone cell

7. Which of the following cell formed after fusion of ovum and spermatozoa
   - (A) Embryo
   - (B) Zygote
   - (C) Foetus
   - (D) Oocyte

8. A single cell performs all function of body in
   - (A) Unicellular organism
   - (B) Multicellular organism
   - (C) Tricellular organism
   - (D) Bicellular organism

9. Cell is surrounded by
   - (A) Plasma membrane
   - (B) Mucous membrane
   - (C) Epithelial membrane
   - (D) Serous membrane

10. Thickness of plasma membrane is
    (A) 7-10 nm
    (B) 2-3 nm
    (C) 11-12 nm
    (D) 14-15 nm

11. Function of plasma membrane includes
    (A) Protect the organelles of cell
    (B) Separates the extracellular fluid and intracellular fluid
    (C) Maintain the cells internal environment
    (D) All of the above

12. Which part of cell consist phospholipid bilayer
    (A) Plasma membrane
    (B) Nucleus
    (C) Ribosomes
    (D) Nucleolus

13. Phospholipid bilayer consist of following types of layers
    (A) Hydrophilic (water loving)
    (B) Hydrophobic (water hating)
    (C) Both (A) and (B)
    (D) None of the above

14. The phospholipid bilayer is made up of
    (A) Phospholipid
    (B) Cholesterol
    (C) Glycolipid
    (D) All of the above

15. The percent of phospholipid present in lipid bilayer is
    (A) 75%
    (B) 20%
    (C) 51%
    (D) 10%

16. The percent of glycolipid present in lipid bilayer is
    (A) 20%
    (B) 45%
    (C) 5%
    (D) 26%

17. The percent of cholesterol present in lipid bilayer is
    (A) 20%
    (B) 60%
    (C) 46%
    (D) 6%

18. The structure of the plasma membrane is best described using a structural model called
    (A) Fluid mosaic model
    (B) Watson and Crick model
    (C) Stiff flat model
    (D) Torso model

19. Fluid mosaic model of plasma membrane was proposed by
    (A) Singer and Nicolson
    (B) Watson and crick
    (C) George Mendel
    (D) David Robertson

20. Function of membrane protein is/are
    (A) They act as receptor
    (B) Transport substance across the membrane
    (C) Some protein act as enzymes
    (D) All of the above

21. The head present in phospholipid molecule is termed as
    (A) Polar
    (B) Non polar
    (C) Neutral
    (D) amphiphilic

22. The tail present in phospholipid molecule is called
    (A) Non polar
    (B) Polar
    (C) Neutral
    (D) Amphiphilic

23. Which of the following is lipid soluble molecules which is freely passes through plasma membrane?
    (A) Glucose
    (B) Steroids
    (C) Electrolyte
    (D) Urea

24. Which of the following is an example of water-soluble substance which is not freely passes through plasma membrane?
    (A) Glucose
    (B) Carbon dioxide
    (C) Steroids
    (D) Oxygen

25. An example of fat-soluble substance is/are
    (A) Oxygen
    (B) Carbon dioxide
    (C) Steroid
    (D) All of the above

26. The head part of phospholipid is of following nature
    (A) Hydrophilic
    (B) Hydrophobic
    (C) Amphiphilic
    (D) None of the above

27. The tail part of phospholipid is of following nature
    (A) Hydrophobic
    (B) Hydrophilic
    (C) Amphiphilic
    (D) None of the above

28. The hydrophilic layer is water loving and are polar in nature
    (A) True   (B) False

29. The hydrophobic layer is water hating and are nonpolar in nature
    (A) True   (B) False

30. Which of the following is not an example of water-soluble substance?
    (A) Glucose   (B) Urea
    (C) Steroid   (D) Electrolyte

31. The glycolipid means
    (A) The lipid attached with carbohydrate group
    (B) The lipid attached with protein group
    (C) The lipid attached with amino acid group
    (D) The protein attached with carbohydrate

32. Which part of a cell act as barrier and allow only selected substance can pass through it
    (A) Plasma membrane   (B) Cytoplasm
    (C) Nucleus   (D) Ribosomes

33. Ion channels are located in
    (A) Ribosomes   (B) Nucleus
    (C) Mitochondria   (D) Plasma membrane

34. Which channel is present in plasma membrane?
    (A) Potassium channel   (B) Calcium channel
    (C) Sodium channel   (D) All of the above

35. Receptor is composed of
    (A) Lipid   (B) Protein
    (C) Carbohydrate   (D) Fat

36. The substance moves inside the cell to support the cell's metabolic reaction
    (A) Nutrients   (B) Water
    (C) Electrolytes   (D) All of the above

37. An example of unwanted substance which move out of the cell is/are
    (A) Carbon dioxide   (B) Urea
    (C) Nitrogenous compounds   (D) All of the above

38. The transport mechanism can be classified into

    (A) Passive transport   (B) Active transport
    (C) Both (A) and (B)   (D) None of the above

39. The movement of substances along the concentration gradient from the region of higher concentration to lower concentration without using energy is called

    (A) Passive transport   (B) Osmosis
    (C) Active transport   (D) Endocytosis

40. Which of the following is a type of diffusion?

    (A) Simple diffusion   (B) Facilitated diffusion
    (C) Both (A) and (B)   (D) None of the above

41. Which transport mechanism follows concentration gradient phenomenon

    (A) Passive transport   (B) Active transport
    (C) Endocytosis   (D) Pinocytosis

42. The process of movement of chemical substance from an area of higher concentration to an area of lower concentration until it reaches equilibrium is called

    (A) Simple diffusion   (B) Facilitated diffusion
    (C) Osmosis   (D) Phagocytosis

43. Simple diffusion occurs mainly in

    (A) Gases   (B) Liquid
    (C) Solution   (D) All of the above

44. Transfer of oxygen from lungs into body is an example of

    (A) Facilitated diffusion   (B) Osmosis
    (C) Simple diffusion   (D) None of the above

45. The substance which is transfer through simple diffusion is/are

    (A) Oxygen   (B) Carbon dioxide
    (C) Alcohol   (D) All of the above

46. The electrolytes diffusion through the protein layer of the plasma membrane as some integral protein channel

    (A) K^+ (B) Na^+
    (C) Cl^- (D) All of the above

47. Which of the following is water - soluble material and can cross the membrane by passing through water - filled channels?

    (A) Oxygen
    (B) Sodium
    (C) Fatty acid
    (D) Steroids

48. Which of the following is lipid - soluble material and can cross the membrane by dissolving in the lipid part of the membrane?

    (A) Sodium
    (B) Potassium
    (C) Calcium
    (D) Fatty acid

49. The passive process is used by the substance that are unable to diffuse through the semipermeable membrane is

    (A) Facilitated diffusion
    (B) Osmosis
    (C) Bulk transport
    (D) Endocytosis

50. Passive transport mechanism is

    (A) Osmosis
    (B) Facilitated diffusion
    (C) Simple diffusion
    (D) All of the above

Answer Key

Introduction to Human Body, Cellular Levels of Structural Organization, Tissue Level of Organization (Part-04)

Question	Answer	Question	Answer
01	A = Cells	26	A = Hydrophilic
02	A = Tissue	27	A = Hydrophobic
03	B = Robert Hooke	28	A = True
04	C = Cytology	29	A = True
05	D = All of the Above	30	C = Steroids
06	A = Zygote	31	A = The Lipid Attached with carbohydrate group
07	B = Zygote	32	A = Plasma membrane
08	A = Unicellular Organism	33	D = Plasma Membrane
09	A = Plasma Membrane	34	D = All of the Above
10	A = 07 to 10nm	35	B = Proteins
11	D = All of the Above	36	D = All of the Above
12	A = Plasma Membrane	37	D = All of the Above
13	C = Both A and B	38	C = Both A and B
14	D = All of the Above	39	A = Passive Transport
15	A = 75 %	40	C = Both A and B
16	C = 5%	41	A = Passive Transport
17	A = 20%	42	A = Simple Diffusion
18	A = Fluid Mosaic Model	43	D = All of the Above
19	A = Singer and Nicolson	44	C = Simple Diffusion
20	D = All of the Above	45	D = All of the Above
21	A = Polar	46	D = All of the Above
22	A = non-Polar	47	B = Sodium
23	B = Steroids	48	D = Fatty Acids
24	A = Glucose	49	A = Facilitated Diffusion
25	D = All of the Above	50	D = All of the Above

Part-05

1. The movement of solvent from an area of lower concentration to higher concentration through semipermeable membrane is called
   - (A) Osmosis
   - (B) Diffusion
   - (C) Facilitated diffusion
   - (D) Bulk transport

2. Osmosis is a type of
   - (A) Passive transport
   - (B) Active transport
   - (C) Endocytosis
   - (D) Exocytosis

3. Osmotic pressure of solution is directly proportional to
   - (A) Concentration of solution
   - (B) Temperature
   - (C) Lowering of vapour pressure
   - (D) All of the above

4. If RBC is placed in a solution, where the salt concentration outside the RBC is equals to the salt concentration inside the RBC then the solution is called as
   - (A) Isotonic solution
   - (B) Hypertonic solution
   - (C) Hypotonic solution
   - (D) Monotonic solution

5. RBC is placed in a solution in which no change observed in the shape of RBC is called
   - (A) Hypertonic solution
   - (B) Hypotonic solution
   - (C) Isotonic solution
   - (D) Monotonic solution

6. The concentration of sodium chloride in isotonic solution is
   - (A) 0.9 % w/v
   - (B) 0.09 % w/v
   - (C) 0.1 % w/v
   - (D) 1.9 % w/v

7. When RBC is placed in hypotonic solution, which changes is occurred
   - (A) Swelling of RBC
   - (B) Shrinking of RBC
   - (C) No change observed in RBC
   - (D) None of the above

8. If RBC is placed in a solution where the water molecules are in higher concentration outside the RBC, then the solution is called
   - (A) Hypertonic solution
   - (B) Hypotonic solution
   - (C) Isotonic solution
   - (D) Monotonic solution

9. When RBC is placed in hypertonic solution which changes will occur
    (A) Swelling of RBC
    (B) Shrinking of RBC
    (C) No change observed in RBC
    (D) None of the above

10. If RBC is placed in a solution where water molecules are in lower concentration outside the RBC, then the solution is called
    (A) Hypertonic solution
    (B) Hypotonic solution
    (C) Isotonic solution
    (D) Monotonic solution

11. Factor affecting the rate of diffusion is/are
    (A) Concentration gradient
    (B) Temperature
    (C) Surface area
    (D) All of the above

12. The greater the concentration gradient the rate of diffusion become
    (A) Higher
    (B) Lower
    (C) No change
    (D) None of the above

13. The higher the temperature the rate of diffusion become
    (A) Decrease
    (B) Increase
    (C) No change
    (D) None of the above

14. Rate of diffusion is inversely proportional to the
    (A) Concentration gradient
    (B) Size of molecule
    (C) Temperature
    (D) Surface area

15. The movement of the substance against the concentration gradient from lower concentration to higher concentration is called
    (A) Passive transport
    (B) Active transport
    (C) Osmosis
    (D) Facilitated transport

16. Which process require energy to move the solutes across the membrane against the concentration gradient
    (A) Active transport
    (B) Passive transport
    (C) Osmosis
    (D) Facilitated diffusion

17. Type of active transport
    (A) Primary active transport
    (B) Secondary active transport
    (C) Both (A) and (B)
    (D) None of the above

18. Ions that are actively transported across the plasma membrane

    (A) Na^+

    (B) H^+

    (C) K^+

    (D) All of the above

19. In which transport system energy is obtained directly from the hydrolysis of ATP

    (A) Primary active transport

    (B) Secondary active transport

    (C) Pinocytosis

    (D) Phagocytosis

20. The pump responsible for the distribution of Na^+ and K^+ ions across the plasma membrane is

    (A) Calcium ATPase pump

    (B) Sodium potassium ATPase pump

    (C) Hydrogen potassium ATPase pump

    (D) Chloride ATPase pump

21. The mechanism maintains the anequal concentration of sodium and potassium ions on either side of the plasma membrane is

    (A) Active transport mechanism

    (B) Passive transport mechanism

    (C) Pinocytosis

    (D) Phagocytosis

22. Major intracellular cation is

    (A) Potassium

    (B) Sodium

    (C) Calcium

    (D) Chloride

23. Major extracellular cation is

    (A) Sodium

    (B) Calcium

    (C) Chloride

    (D) Potassium

24. The ions much higher inside the cell than out side

    (A) Sodium

    (B) Potassium

    (C) Calcium

    (D) Chloride

25. The ions much higher out the cell then inside

    (A) Sodium

    (B) Calcium

    (C) Potassium

    (D) Chloride

26. In sodium potassium pump how much ATP energy required
   - (A) 10%
   - (B) 30%
   - (C) 80%
   - (D) 5%

27. How many sodium ions can pump towards the out of the cell?
   - (A) Two
   - (B) Three
   - (C) Four
   - (D) One

28. How many potassium ions pumps towards the inside the cell?
   - (A) Two
   - (B) One
   - (C) Three
   - (D) Four

29. Which enzyme activate the binding of Na^+ and K^+ ions which trigger the hydrolysis of ATP into ADP
   - (A) ATPase
   - (B) Transferase
   - (C) Lyase
   - (D) Ligase

30. The transport in which the transporter protein simultaneously binds to substance and transports the other substance against its concentration gradient is
   - (A) Secondary active transport
   - (B) Primary active transport
   - (C) Pinocytosis
   - (D) Passive diffusion

31. Type of secondary active transport
   - (A) Sodium cotransport
   - (B) Sodium counter transport
   - (C) Both (A) and (B)
   - (D) None of the above

32. In which prosses the transporter moves Na^+ and another substance in the same direction
   - (A) Sodium counter transport
   - (B) Sodium cotransport
   - (C) Facilitated diffusion
   - (D) Osmosis

33. Symporter involve in
   - (A) Sodium cotransport
   - (B) Sodium counter transport
   - (C) Endocytosis
   - (D) Osmosis

34. $Na^+/$ glucose and $Na^+/$ amino acid transporter is an example of
   - (A) Secondary active transport
   - (B) Primary active transport
   - (C) Facilitated diffusion
   - (D) Simple diffusion

35. Na^+/H^+ antiporter is an example of
    (A) Primary active transport
    (B) Secondary active transport
    (C) Facilitated diffusion
    (D) Simple diffusion

36. The process in which the transporter moves Na^+ and another substance in the opposite direction across the membrane is called
    (A) Sodium counter transport
    (B) Sodium cotransport
    (C) Osmosis
    (D) Facilitated

37. Antiporters involve in
    (A) Sodium cotransport
    (B) Sodium counter transport
    (C) Simple diffusion
    (D) Phagocytosis

38. Which transporter regulates the pH of the cytoplasm
    (A) Na^+/H^+ counter - transport
    (B) Na^+/Ca^{2+} counter - transport
    (C) $Na^+/$ glucose symporter
    (D) $Na^+/$ amino acid symporter

39. Na^+/Ca^{2+} transporter is an example of
    (A) Sodium cotransporter
    (B) Sodium counter transporter
    (C) Facilitate diffusion
    (D) Osmosis

40. Which substance transported by bulk transport mechanism
    (A) Bacteria
    (B) Red blood cells
    (C) Macromolecule
    (D) All of the above

41. The process in which large molecules enter into cells
    (A) Simple diffusion
    (B) Endocytosis
    (C) Osmosis
    (D) Facilitated diffusion

42. The macromolecules that cannot cross the plasma membrane and are transported by
    (A) Pinocytosis
    (B) Phagocytosis
    (C) Both (A) and (B)
    (D) None of the above

43. Which of the following is types of endocytosis?
    (A) Pinocytosis
    (B) Phagocytosis
    (C) Receptor mediated endocytosis
    (D) All of the above

44. Which process is also called "cell drinking"?
    (A) Pinocytosis
    (B) Phagocytosis
    (C) Osmosis
    (D) Receptor mediated endocytosis

45. Which process involves the uptake of tiny droplets of solutes dissolved in the extracellular fluid
    (A) Phagocytosis
    (B) Pinocytosis
    (C) Receptor mediated endocytosis
    (D) Exocytosis

46. Which process is also called "cell eating"?
    (A) Pinocytosis
    (B) Phagocytosis
    (C) Receptor mediated endocytosis
    (D) Simple diffusion

47. Phagocytes includes
    (A) Neutrophils
    (B) Monocytes
    (C) Tissue macrophages
    (D) All of the above

48. The area of the plasma membrane folds inwards around the droplets to form a vesicle the vesicle is called
    (A) Endosome
    (B) Liposome
    (C) Noisome
    (D) Centrosome

49. The cells in the body show phagocytosis and the cells is termed as
    (A) Phagocytes
    (B) Lipocyte
    (C) Adipocyte
    (D) Osteocyte

50. Process mainly engulf and destroy foreign substances and protect the body from disease
    (A) Pinocytosis
    (B) Phagocytosis
    (C) Facilitate diffusion
    (D) Receptor – mediated endocytosis

Answer Key

Introduction to Human Body, Cellular Levels of Structural Organization, Tissue Level of Organization (Part-05)

Question	Answer	Question	Answer
01	A = Osmosis	26	B = 30%
02	A = Passive Transport	27	B = Three
03	D = All of the Above	28	A = Two
04	A = Isotonic Solution	29	A = ATPase
05	C = Isotonic Solution	30	A = Secondary Active Transport
06	A = 0.9 %W/V	31	C = Both A and B
07	A = Swelling of RBC	32	B = Sodium Co-transport
08	B = Hypotonic Solution	33	A = Sodium Co-transport
09	B = Shrinking of RBC	34	A = Secondary Active Transport
10	A = Hypertonic Solution	35	B = Secondary Active Transport
11	D = All of the Above	36	A = Sodium Counter Transport
12	A = Higher	37	B = Sodium Counter Transport
13	B = Increase	38	A = Na^+/H^+ Counter Transport
14	B = Size of Molecule	39	B = Sodium Counter Transport
15	B = Active Transport	40	D = All of the Above
16	A = Active Transport	41	B = Endocytosis
17	C = Both A and B	42	C = Both A and B
18	D = All of the above	43	D = All of the Above
19	A = Primary Active Transport	44	A = Pinocytosis
20	B = Sodium Potassium ATPase Pump	45	B = Pinocytosis
21	A = Active Transport Mechanism	46	B = Phagocytosis
22	A = Potassium	47	D = All of the Above
23	A = Sodium	48	A = Endosome
24	B = Potassium	49	A = Phagocytes
25	A = Sodium	50	B = Phagocytosis

Part-06

1. In phagocytosis process which particle are taken into the cell
   - (A) Cell fragments
   - (B) Foreign material
   - (C) Microbes
   - (D) All of the above

2. The process by which the ligands bind to the receptors present on the plasma membrane and are taken inside the cell is called
   - (A) Receptor mediated endocytosis
   - (B) Receptor mediated exocytosis
   - (C) Pinocytosis
   - (D) Phagocytosis

3. By which process hormones and vitamins uptake into the cell take place
   - (A) Pinocytosis
   - (B) Phagocytosis
   - (C) Receptor mediated endocytosis
   - (D) Exocytosis

4. Clathrin is a receptor protein which involved in
   - (A) Receptor mediated endocytosis
   - (B) Pinocytosis
   - (C) Exocytosis
   - (D) Phagocytosis

5. The process in which ligand receptor complexes move across the cell inside the vesicles and ejected on the opposite side is
   - (A) Transcytosis
   - (B) Exocytosis
   - (C) Pinocytosis
   - (D) Phagocytosis

6. The process by which substance move out of a cell
   - (A) Exocytosis
   - (B) Endocytosis
   - (C) Pinocytosis
   - (D) Phagocytosis

7. Exocytosis involved the release of secretory substance like
   - (A) Hormones
   - (B) Digestive enzyme
   - (C) Neurotransmitter
   - (D) All of the above

8. The substance secreted and are store in membrane - enclosed vesicles called
    (A) Transport vesicle
    (B) Secretory vesicle
    (C) Inhibitory vesicle
    (D) Excitatory vesicle

9. The fluid portion present inside the cell is called
    (A) Cytoplasm
    (B) Mitochondria
    (C) Nucleus
    (D) Lysosome

10. Cytoplasm is divided into which of the following components
    (A) Cytosol
    (B) Organelles
    (C) Both (A) and (B)
    (D) None of the above

11. Cytosol is the watery fluid present in
    (A) Cytoplasm
    (B) Mitochondria
    (C) Plasma membrane
    (D) Lysosome

12. The amount of water present in cytosol is
    (A) 10-20%
    (B) 75-90%
    (C) 35-50%
    (D) 50-70%

13. Cytosol contains suspended substance such as
    (A) Ions
    (B) glucose
    (C) amino acid
    (D) All of the above

14. Which of the following is organelle of cell?
    (A) Golgi apparatus
    (B) Lysosome
    (C) Mitochondria
    (D) All of the above

15. The type of organelle presents in cytoplasm
    (A) Non membranous organelles
    (B) Membranous organelles
    (C) Both (A) and (B)
    (D) None of the above

16. The organelles lack of membrane and are in direct contact with the cytosol is called
    (A) Non membranous organelles
    (B) Membranous organelles
    (C) Filamentous organelles
    (D) None of the above

17. Which of the following is an example of non membranous organelle?
    (A) Ribosomes
    (B) Mitochondria
    (C) Lysosomes
    (D) Golgi apparatus

18. Which of the following is not an organelle of membranous organelles?
    - (A) Mitochondria
    - (B) Cytoskeleton
    - (C) Lysosome
    - (D) Golgi apparatus

19. The organelles are surrounded by the lipid bilayer membrane is called
    - (A) Membranous organelles
    - (B) Non membranous organelles
    - (C) Filamentous organelles
    - (D) None of the above

20. An example of membranous organelles is/are
    - (A) Lysosomes
    - (B) Mitochondria
    - (C) Golgi apparatus
    - (D) All of the above

21. Aerobic respiration take place in
    - (A) Mitochondria
    - (B) Ribosome
    - (C) Lysosome
    - (D) Golgi apparatus

22. Which organelle produces energy in the form of ATP
    - (A) Lysosome
    - (B) Mitochondria
    - (C) Ribosome
    - (D) Endoplasmic reticulum

23. Cristae present in
    - (A) Cytoplasm
    - (B) Mitochondria
    - (C) Lysosome
    - (D) Ribosome

24. Most of the ATP generate in which organelle of cell
    - (A) Cytoplasm
    - (B) Endoplasmic reticulum
    - (C) Lysosomes
    - (D) Mitochondria

25. Which of the following is ATP generation process occurs in mitochondria?
    - (A) Citric acid cycle
    - (B) Electron transport system
    - (C) Both (A) and (B)
    - (D) None of the above

26. The "Power house of the cell" is
    - (A) Mitochondria
    - (B) Lysosome
    - (C) Ribosome
    - (D) Cytoplasm

27. Larger number of mitochondria are present in
    - (A) Muscles
    - (B) Liver
    - (C) Kidneys
    - (D) All of the above

28. Lysosomes are formed by
    (A) Golgi apparatus
    (B) Ribosome
    (C) Endoplasmic reticulum
    (D) Cytoplasm

29. Which enzymeis found in lysosomes
    (A) Lipases
    (B) Nucleases
    (C) Proteases
    (D) All of the above

30. The molecule breakdown by the lysosomes is
    (a) DNA
    (b) RNA
    (c) Protein
    (d) All of the above

31. Lysosomal enzymes are also called
    (A) Lysozymes
    (B) Lipozymes
    (C) Ribozymes
    (D) Liozymes

32. Autophagy is the process of
    (A) Self - eating
    (B) Self - drinking
    (C) Self - repairing
    (D) Self - death

33. Which of the following is the function of lysosomes?
    (A) Autolysis
    (B) Digestion
    (C) Autophagy
    (D) All of the above

34. Which organelle is called "suicidal bag" of cell?
    (A) Ribosome
    (B) Mitochondria
    (C) Lysosome
    (D) Cytoplasm

35. Which of the following is hydrolytic enzyme?
    (A) Phosphatase
    (B) Lipase
    (C) Protease
    (D) All of the above

36. Lysosomes that have not entered into the digestive event are called
    (A) Primary lysosomes
    (B) Secondary lysosomes
    (C) Tertiary lysosomes
    (D) None of the above

37. Lysosomes undergo digestion is called
    (A) Secondary lysosomes
    (B) Primary lysosomes
    (C) Tertiary lysosomes
    (D) None of the above

38. Which organelle contain enzymes which involved in lipid metabolism
    (A) Peroxisomes
    (B) Cytoplasm
    (C) Nucleus
    (D) Endoplasmic reticulum

39. Peroxisomes contain oxidative enzymes that are capable of oxidising of various organic substance such as
    (A) Amino acids
    (B) Fatty acids
    (C) Alcohol
    (D) All of the above

40. Which by product is generated in the oxidation reaction in peroxisomes
    (A) Dihydrogen trioxide
    (B) Hydrogen peroxide
    (C) Nitrogen dioxide
    (D) Carbon trioxide

41. The series of interconnecting membranous canals in the cytoplasm is called
    (A) Endoplasmic reticulum
    (B) Mitochondria
    (C) Lysosome
    (D) Ribosome

42. Cisternae is a flattened sacs or tubules which is found in
    (A) Ribosomes
    (B) Endoplasmic reticulum
    (C) Cytoplasm
    (D) Nucleus

43. Which of the following forms a link between the nucleus and plasma membrane?
    (A) Golgi apparatus
    (B) Ribosomes
    (C) Lysosomes
    (D) Endoplasmic reticulum

44. Which of the following is the type of endoplasmic reticulum?
    (A) Rough endoplasmic reticulum
    (B) Smooth endoplasmic reticulum
    (C) Both (A) and (B)
    (D) None of the above

45. The outer surface of rough endoplasmic reticulum is studded with
    (A) Ribosomes
    (B) Lysosomes
    (C) Peroxisomes
    (D) Mitochondria

46. Function of endoplasmic reticulum is/are
    (A) Synthesis of lipid
    (B) Synthesis of steroid hormones
    (C) Detoxification of some drug
    (D) All of the above

47. In which endoplasmic reticulum protein is synthesized
    (A) Rough endoplasmic reticulum
    (B) Smooth endoplasmic reticulum
    (C) Both (A) and (B)
    (D) None of the above

48. Smooth endoplasmic reticulum does not have ....on the outer surface of its membrane
    (A) Ribosome   (B) Lysosome
    (C) Nucleolus   (D) Peroxisome

49. Smooth endoplasmic reticulum synthesis the
    (A) Lipid   (B) Estrogens
    (C) Testosterone   (D) All of the above

50. Which of the following is associated with the detoxification of certain toxic substances and drugs?
    (A) Smooth endoplasmic reticulum
    (B) Rough endoplasmic reticulum
    (C) Nucleus
    (D) Ribosome

Answer Key

Introduction to Human Body, Cellular Levels of Structural Organization, Tissue Level of Organization (Part-06)

Question	Answer	Question	Answer
01	D = All of the Above	26	A = Mitochondria
02	A = Receptor mediated Endocytosis	27	D = All of the Above
03	C = Receptor mediated Endocytosis	28	A = Golgi Apparatus
04	A = Receptor mediated Endocytosis	29	D = All of the Above
05	A = Transcytosis	30	D = All of the Above
06	A = Exocytosis	31	A = Lysozyme
07	D = All of the Above	32	A = Self Eating
08	B = Secretory Vesicle	33	D = All of the Above
09	A = Cytoplasm	34	C = Lysosome
10	C = Both A and B	35	D = All of the Above
11	A = Cytoplasm	36	A = Primary Lysosome
12	B = 75-90%	37	A = Secondary Lysosome
13	D = All of the Above	38	A = Peroxisome
14	D = All of the Above	39	D = All of the Above
15	C = Both A and B	40	B = Hydrogen Peroxide
16	A = Non-Membranous Organelles	41	A = Endoplasmic Reticulum
17	A = Ribosome	42	B = Endoplasmic Reticulum
18	B = Cytoskeleton	43	D = Endoplasmic Reticulum
19	A = Membranous Organelles	44	C = Both A and B
20	D = All of the above	45	A = Ribosomes
21	A = Mitochondria	46	D = All of the Above
22	B = Mitochondria	47	A = Rough Endoplasmic Reticulum
23	B = Mitochondria	48	A = Ribosome
24	D = Mitochondria	49	D = All of the Above
25	C = Both A and B	50	A = Smooth Endoplasmic Reticulum

Part-07

1. Ribosomes is composed of which type of RNA
   (A) rRNA
   (B) mRNA
   (C) tRNA
   (D) none of the above

2. Ribosomes is the site of synthesis for
   (A) Protein
   (B) Lipid
   (C) Fat
   (D) Vitamin

3. Which organelle is called "Protein Factories" of the cell?
   (A) Ribosomes
   (B) Lysosomes
   (C) Mitochondria
   (D) Nucleus

4. Golgi apparatus is also called as
   (A) Golgi body
   (B) Golgi complex
   (C) Both (A) and (B)
   (D) None of the above

5. Golgi apparatus consist of flattened membranous sacs called
   (A) Cisternae
   (B) Sisternae
   (C) Cristae
   (D) Syristae

6. The major function of Golgi apparatus is/are
   (A) Processing of protein
   (B) Packaging of protein
   (C) Delivering of protein to different part of the cell
   (D) All of the above

7. The cytoskeleton is composed of protein fibers which are
   (A) Microfilaments
   (B) Intermediate filaments
   (C) Microtubules
   (D) All of the above

8. Thinnest fibers of cytoskeleton are
   (A) Microfilaments
   (B) Intermediate filaments
   (C) Microtubules
   (D) Macrotubules

9. The microfilaments provide
   (A) Structural support
   (B) Maintain shape of cell
   (C) Responsible for cellular movements
   (D) All of the above

10. Which cytoskeleton is thicker than microtubules?
    (A) Microfilaments
    (B) Intermediate filaments
    (C) Macrotubules
    (D) None of the above

11. Most of the microfilaments are composed of the protein which is
    (A) Actin
    (B) Elastin
    (C) Collagen
    (D) Keratin

12. Largest cytoskeletal component is
    (A) Microtubules
    (B) Microfilament
    (C) Intermediate filaments
    (D) Macrotubules

13. Microtubules mainly composed of protein, which is called as
    (A) Tubulin
    (B) Collagen
    (C) Keratin
    (D) Elastin

14. Function of microtubules is/are
    (A) They give structural strength to cell
    (B) Responsible for movement of the organelles within the cell
    (C) Chromosomes during cell division
    (D) All of the above

15. Centrosomes located near the
    (A) Nucleus
    (B) Ribosomes
    (C) Mitochondria
    (D) Golgi apparatus

16. Centrosome consists of which of the following component
    (A) Pericentriolar area
    (B) Centrioles
    (C) Both (A) and (B)
    (D) None of the above

17. During cell division pericentriolar area is responsible for the formation of
    (A) Mitotic spindle
    (B) Meiotic spindle
    (C) Bipolar spindle
    (D) Mother centriole

18. How many groups of tubules consist in each centrosome?

    (A) Nine

    (B) Seven

    (C) Eleven

    (D) Five

19. The motile projections of the plasma membrane that consists of microtubules called

    (A) Cell extension

    (B) Cell expansion

    (C) Cell division

    (D) Cell separation

20. The small, hair – like projections that extend from the cell surface is called

    (A) Cilia

    (B) Flagella

    (C) Microvilli

    (D) Pili

21. Mostly cilia are present in

    (A) Lungs

    (B) Heart

    (C) Kidney

    (D) Liver

22. The long, whip- like projections that move an entire cell called

    (A) Flagella

    (B) Cilia

    (C) Microvilli

    (D) Pili

23. Microvilli is the absorptive cells that found in the line of

    (A) Small intestine

    (B) Lungs

    (C) Liver

    (D) Kidney

24. Function of microvilli in small intestine is/are

    (A) Increase surface area

    (B) Make structure of the cells

    (C) Maximizing the absorption of nutrient

    (D) All of the above

25. Tail of spermatozoa is an example of

    (A) Flagella

    (B) Cilia

    (C) Microvilli

    (D) None of the above

26. Which organelle present in the center of the cell

    (A) Mitochondria

    (B) Ribosomes

    (C) Lysosome

    (D) Nucleus

27. The cell which does not contain nucleus
    (A) WBC
    (B) Nerve cell
    (C) Mature RBC
    (D) Muscle cell

28. Which of the following is the largest organelle of cell?
    (A) Nucleus
    (B) Mitochondria
    (C) Golgi apparatus
    (D) Ribosome

29. The nucleus is covered by a double layered membrane called
    (A) Nuclear membrane
    (B) Serous membrane
    (C) Synovial membrane
    (D) Mucous membrane

30. The outer layer of nuclear membrane is continuous with the
    (A) Endoplasmic reticulum
    (B) Golgi apparatus
    (C) Ribosome
    (D) Mitochondria

31. The movement of substance between nucleus and cytoplasm is regulated by
    (A) Nuclear pore
    (B) Chromatin
    (C) Nucleoplasm
    (D) Chromosome

32. Which organelle contain genetic materials contain in form of DNA
    (A) Nucleus
    (B) Cytoplasm
    (C) Golgi apparatus
    (D) Endoplasmic reticulum

33. The nucleus membrane encloses various structure which include
    (A) Nucleoplasm
    (B) Nucleoli
    (C) Both (A) and (B)
    (D) None of the above

34. The fluid medium of nucleus is
    (A) Nucleoplasm
    (B) Nucleoli
    (C) Nuclear membrane
    (D) Nuclear pore

35. The spherical bodies present inside the nucleus is called
    (A) Nucleoli
    (B) Nucleoplasm
    (C) Chromatin
    (D) Nuclear pore

36. Nucleoli are composed of clusters of
    (A) DNA
    (B) RNA
    (C) Proteins
    (D) All of the above

37. Which of the following is not a component of nucleus?
    (A) Chromosomes
    (B) Nuclear membrane
    (C) Nucleolus
    (D) Mitochondria

38. Hereditary units of cell are called
    (A) Genes
    (B) Chromosomes
    (C) DNA
    (D) RNA

39. Thread - like linear strand of DNA is called
    (A) Chromosomes
    (B) Genes
    (C) RNA
    (D) Protein

40. How many numbers of chromosomes contain in the cells of human body?
    (A) 46
    (B) 40
    (C) 42
    (D) 48

41. How many pair of chromosomes contain in the cells of human body?
    (A) 21 pair
    (B) 23 pair
    (C) 12 pair
    (D) 26 pair

42. Function of nucleus is/ are
    (A) Control activities of the cell
    (B) Contains hereditary material that is pass from one generation to next
    (C) Facilitate protein synthesis
    (D) All of the above

43. The process by which cell divides into two and duplicate its genetic material is called
    (A) Cell division
    (B) Cell separation
    (C) Cell extension
    (D) Cell expansion

44. Types of cell division are
    (A) Somatic cell division
    (B) Reproductive cell division
    (C) Both (A) and (B)
    (D) None of the above

45. In somatic cell division, cell undergoes a nuclear division called
    (A) Mitosis
    (B) Meiosis
    (C) Binary fission
    (D) Cytosis

46. The special kind of two – step division is called
    (A) Meiosis
    (B) Mitosis
    (C) Binary fission
    (D) Cytosis

47. Which cell division is responsible for the formation of gametes?
    (A) Somatic cell division
    (B) Reproductive cell division
    (C) Both (A) and (B)
    (D) None of the above

48. The main stage in somatic cell division is
    (A) Interphase
    (B) Mitosis
    (C) Cytokinesis
    (D) All of the above

49. Which of the following is not subphase of interphase?
    (A) G_1 phase
    (B) S phase
    (C) G_2 phase
    (D) Telophase II

50. Primary growth phase of cell division is
    (A) S phase
    (B) G_1 phase
    (C) G_2 phase
    (D) Prophase II

Answer Key

Introduction to Human Body, Cellular Levels of Structural Organization, Tissue Level of Organization (Part-07)

Question	Answer	Question	Answer
01	A = r-RNA	26	D = Nucleus
02	A = Protein	27	C = Mature RBC
03	A = Ribosome	28	A = Nucleus
04	C = Both A and B	29	A = Nuclear Membrane
05	A = Cisternae	30	A = Endoplasmic Reticulum
06	D = All of the Above	31	A = Nuclear Pore
07	D = All of the Above	32	A = Nucleus
08	A = Microfilaments	33	C = Both A and B
09	D = All of the Above	34	A = Nucleoplasm
10	B = Intermediate Filaments	35	A = Nucleoli
11	A = Actin	36	D = All of the Above
12	A = Microtubules	37	D = Mitochondria
13	A = Tubulin	38	A = Genes
14	D = All of the Above	39	A = Chromosome
15	A = Nucleus	40	A = 46
16	C = Both A and B	41	B = 23 Pair
17	A = Mitotic Spindle	42	D = All of the Above
18	A = Nine	43	A = Cell Division
19	A = Cell Extension	44	C = Both A and B
20	A = Cilia	45	A = Mitosis
21	A = Lungs	46	A = Meiosis
22	A = Flagella	47	B = Reproductive Cell Division
23	A = Small Intestine	48	D = All of the Above
24	D = All of the Above	49	D = Telophase II
25	A = Flagella	50	B = G_1 Phase

Part-08

1. The interval between the G1 and G2 phase is
   (A) S phase
   (B) Anaphase
   (C) Telophase
   (D) Cytokinesis

2. The chromosome resembles a fine network of dark thread called
   (A) Chromatin
   (B) Cristae
   (C) Cisternae
   (D) Cytoskeleton

3. G1 phase is also known as
   (A) First gap phase
   (B) Second gap phase
   (C) Third gap phase
   (D) Fourth gap phase

4. In which phase replication of centrosome begin
   (A) G2 phase
   (B) S- phase
   (C) Telophase
   (D) Anaphase

5. In which phase the chromosomes replicate and forms two identical copies of DNA
   (A) S-phase
   (B) G2 phase
   (C) G1 phase
   (D) None of the above

6. Which of the following is the final phase for the preparation of cell division?
   (A) G2 phase
   (B) S phase
   (C) G1 phase
   (D) Telophase

7. In which phase the centrosome finishes its replication
   (A) S- phase
   (B) G1 phase
   (C) G2 phase
   (D) Anaphase

8. How many identical nuclei is formed as a result of mitosis?
   (A) Two
   (B) Three
   (C) One
   (D) Four

9. Which of the following is not stage of mitosis?
   (A) Prophase
   (B) Metaphase
   (C) Anaphase
   (D) G1 phase

10. Longer phase of cell cycle is
    (A) Interphase
    (B) Anaphase
    (C) Telophase
    (D) Metaphase

11. In prophase the two chromatids are joined to each other at
    (A) Centromere
    (B) Centrosome
    (C) Spindle fibres
    (D) Cytoskeleton

12. In prophase the mitotic apparatus appears and consists
    (A) Three centriole
    (B) Two centrioles
    (C) Four centrioles
    (D) One centriole

13. In which phase nuclear envelope disappears
    (A) Prophase
    (B) Anaphase
    (C) Metaphase
    (D) Telophase

14. Mitotic spindle disappears in which of the following phase
    (A) Prophase
    (B) Telophase
    (C) Anaphase
    (D) Metaphase

15. In which phase chromatids align on the centre of the spindle, attached by their centromere
    (A) Metaphase
    (B) Telophase
    (C) Anaphase
    (D) Prophase

16. In telophase which of the following activities occurs
    (A) Mitotic spindle disappears
    (B) The chromosomes uncoil
    (C) Nuclear envelope reforms
    (D) All of the above

17. Which of the following is shortest stage of mitosis?
    (A) Anaphase
    (B) Telophase
    (C) Prophase
    (D) Metaphase

18. In which phase the actual separation of the cell into two new daughter cell takes place
    (A) Cytokinesis
    (B) S-phase
    (C) Prophase
    (D) Anaphase

19. In which organ reproductive cell division by meiosis occurs
    (A) Female gonads or ovaries
    (B) Male gonads or testis
    (C) Both (A) and (B)
    (D) None of the above

20. Reproductive cell division result in the production of gametes that contain half of genetic material i.e.

    (A) 23 chromosomes   (B) 21 chromosomes

    (C) 20 chromosomes   (D) 26 chromosomes

21. During meiosis the chromosomes reduced in number is called

    (A) Haploid   (B) Diploid

    (C) Triploid   (D) Biploid

22. Which of the following is somatic cells which contain 23 pair of chromosomes?

    (A) Brain cells   (B) Stomach cells

    (C) Kidney cells   (D) All of the above

23. The chromosomes that make up each pair and they contain similar genes arranged in the same order is called

    (A) Homologous chromosomes   (B) Haploid

    (C) Autosome   (D) Chromosome

24. Sex chromosomes is designated as

    (A) X   (B) Y

    (C) Both (A) and (B)   (D) None of the above

25. In female the homologous pair of sex chromosomes consist of

    (A) Two X chromosomes   (B) One X chromosomes

    (C) Two Y chromosomes   (D) Four Y chromosomes

26. In male the homologous pair of sex chromosomes consist of

    (A) One X and one Y chromosomes   (B) Two Y chromosomes

    (C) Two X chromosomes   (D) Four X chromosomes

27. The 22 pairs of chromosomes are called

    (A) Homologous chromosomes   (B) Haploid

    (C) Autosomes   (D) Centromere

28. The stage of meiosis includes

    (A) Meiosis I   (B) Meiosis II

    (C) Both (A) and (B)   (D) None of the above

29. Which of the following is phase of meiosis I?
    (A) Prophase I
    (B) Metaphase I
    (C) Anaphase I
    (D) All of the above

30. In which stage of meiosis-I, the replication of chromosomes shorten, coil, thicken and become visible.
    (A) Prophase I
    (B) Metaphase I
    (C) Anaphase I
    (D) Telophase I

31. In which stage the nuclear membrane and nucleoli disappear
    (A) Prophase I
    (B) Metaphase I
    (C) Telophase I
    (D) Anaphase I

32. The chromosomes pair up with their homologue and are brought so close together by a process called
    (A) Synapsis
    (B) Cytokinesis
    (C) Autosomes
    (D) Tetrad

33. The pair of homologous chromosomes in which each pair contains two sister chromatids is called
    (A) Tetrad
    (B) Haploid
    (C) Diploid
    (D) Autosomes

34. The process in which the sister chromatids are so close together that they may exchange genetic material is called
    (A) Binding
    (B) Pairing
    (C) Crossing over
    (D) Joining

35. Which of the following is not a stage of meiosis I
    (A) Prophase I
    (B) Telophase I
    (C) Anaphase I
    (D) Interphase

36. In metaphase I the centromeres of the two homologous chromosomes attached to the
    (A) Microtubules
    (B) Microfilament
    (C) Microfilament
    (D) Macrotubules

37. In which phase of meiosis-I, the homologous pairs of chromosomes line along the equatorial plate of the cell
    (A) Anaphase I
    (B) Telophase I
    (C) Metaphase I
    (D) Prophase I

38. In which phase of meiosis-I the pairs of homologous chromosomes spilt up

(A) Telophase I
(B) Anaphase I
(C) Prophase I
(D) Metaphase I

39. In which phase of meiosis-I the spindle disappears and new nuclear membrane forms around each cluster of chromosomes at opposite poles

(A) Anaphase I
(B) Telophase I
(C) Metaphase I
(D) Prophase I

40. Which of the following is phase of meiosis II?

(A) Prophase II
(B) Telophase II
(C) Anaphase II
(D) All of the above

41. In which phase of meiosis II, the nuclear membrane disappears but no duplication of DNA occurs

(A) Prophase II
(B) Metaphase II
(C) Telophase II
(D) Anaphase II

42. In which phase of meiosis II, the chromosomes line up on the equatorial plate

(A) Prophase II
(B) Metaphase II
(C) Anaphase II
(D) Telophase II

43. In which phase of meiosis II, the centromeres spilt and sister chromatids separates and move towards opposite poles of the cell

(A) Anaphase II
(B) Prophase II
(C) Telophase II
(D) Metaphase II

44. In which phase of meiosis II, the spindle disappears and a new nuclear membrane form around the separated chromatids

(A) Metaphase II
(B) Telophase II
(C) Anaphase II
(D) Prophase II

45. The formation and maintenance of specialized tissues of multicellular organisms depend on the coordinated regulation of

(A) Cell number
(B) Cell morphology
(C) Cell location
(D) All of the above

46. The cell has to communicate with each other, which accomplished by a process called
    - (A) Cell signalling
    - (B) Cell replication
    - (C) Cell division
    - (D) Cell metabolism

47. The communicate between two cells in called
    - (A) Intercellular signalling
    - (B) Intracellular signalling
    - (C) Extracellular signalling
    - (D) External signalling

48. Higher organisms have to coordinate a large number of physiological activities such as
    - (A) Intermediary metabolism
    - (B) Cell growth
    - (C) Cell morphology
    - (D) All of the above

49. Which of the following is an example of extracellular signalling molecule?
    - (A) Growth factors
    - (B) Hormones
    - (C) Neurotransmitters
    - (D) All of the above

50. Which of the following is an example of chemical signalling?
    - (A) Endocrine signalling
    - (B) Autocrine signalling
    - (C) Paracrine signalling
    - (D) All of the above

Answer Key

Introduction to Human Body, Cellular Levels of Structural Organization, Tissue Level of Organization (Part-08)

Question	Answer	Question	Answer
01	A = S Phase	26	A = One X and One Y Chromosome
02	A = Chromatin	27	C = Autosomes
03	A = First Gap Phase	28	C = Both A and B
04	B = S-Phase	29	D = All of the Above
05	A = S-Phase	30	A = Prophase I
06	A = G_2 Phase	31	A = Prophase I
07	C = G_2 Phase	32	A = Synapsis
08	A = Two	33	A = Tetrad
09	D = G_1 Phase	34	C = Crossing Over
10	A = Interphase	35	D = Interphase
11	A = Centromere	36	A = Microtubules
12	B = Two centrioles	37	C = Metaphase I
13	A = Prophase	38	B = Anaphase I
14	B = Telophase	39	B = Telophase I
15	A = Metaphase	40	D = All of the Above
16	D = All of the Above	41	A = Prophase II
17	A = Anaphase	42	B = Metaphase II
18	A = Cytokinesis	43	A = Anaphase II
19	C = Both A and B	44	B = Telophase II
20	A = 23 Chromosome	45	D = All of the Above
21	A = Haploid	46	A = Cell Signalling
22	D = All of the Above	47	A = Intracellular Signalling
23	A = Homologous Chromosome	48	D = All of the Above
24	C = Both A and B	49	D = All of the Above
25	A = Two X Chromosome	50	D = All of the Above

Part-09

1. The signaling in which the cell that is producing the messenger will expresses receptors on its surface so that can respond to that messenger is called
   (A) Paracrine signaling
   (B) Autocrine signaling
   (C) Endocrine signaling
   (D) Exocrine signaling

2. In which signaling the messenger molecules travel only to a short distance through the extracellular space to cells that are close proximity to the cell that is generating the message
   (A) Paracrine signaling
   (B) Endocrine signaling
   (C) Autocrine signaling
   (D) Exocrine signaling

3. The signaling in which messenger molecules reach their target cells via passage through bloodstream is called
   (A) Endocrine signaling
   (B) Paracrine signaling
   (C) Autocrine signaling
   (D) Exocrine signaling

4. How many types of cells signaling are?
   (A) Four
   (B) Five
   (C) Seven
   (D) Nine

5. Intercellular signaling controls
   (A) Growth
   (B) Cell division
   (C) Metabolic fluxes
   (D) All of the above

6. Which signaling is "self – targeting"
   (A) Autocrine signaling
   (B) Endocrine signaling
   (C) Paracrine signaling
   (D) Exocrine signaling

7. The signaling which is responsible for cells infected with virus
   (A) Endocrine signaling
   (B) Paracrine signaling
   (C) Autocrine signaling
   (D) Exocrine signaling

8. In breast cancer the progesterone has been found to act as
   (A) Endocrine signaling
   (B) Autocrine signaling
   (C) Paracrine signaling
   (D) Exocrine signaling

9. The nerve cells communicate with each other at synapses through neurotransmitter is called

   (A) Synaptic signaling
   (B) Autocrine signaling
   (C) Endocrine signaling
   (D) Direct contact signaling

10. Synaptic sign is a type of

    (A) Endocrine signaling
    (B) Paracrine signaling
    (C) Autocrine signaling
    (D) Direct contact signaling

11. Autocrine hormones or cell signal are

    (A) Growth factor
    (B) Cytokines
    (C) Both (A) and (B)
    (D) None of the above

12. The gland that produces hormones that act on their own glandular cell is called

    (A) Autocrine gland
    (B) Endocrine gland
    (C) Exocrine gland
    (D) Paracrine gland

13. Which of the following is a long-distance cell signaling?

    (A) Endocrine signaling
    (B) Autocrine signaling
    (C) Paracrine signaling
    (D) Direct contact signaling

14. In which signaling the signals travel to distant cell through circulatory system

    (A) Paracrine signaling
    (B) Autocrine signaling
    (C) Direct contact signaling
    (D) Endocrine signaling

15. Direct contact signaling is also referred as

    (A) Cell to cell signaling
    (B) Endocrine signaling
    (C) paracrine signaling
    (D) Autocrine signaling

16. The autocrine signaling involve in

    (A) Fibroblast growth factors
    (B) Heparin – binding epidermal growth factor
    (C) Angiopoietin – like protein
    (D) All of the above

17. Blood platelets secrete eicosanoids which influence their own activity is an example of

    (A) Autocrine signaling
    (B) Endocrine signaling
    (C) Direct contact signaling
    (D) Paracrine signaling

18. The release of chemokines by neutrophils which attract other cells is an example of
    (A) Paracrine signaling
    (B) Autocrine signaling
    (C) Exocrine signaling
    (D) Endocrine signaling

19. Which of the following is types of receptors?
    (A) Internal receptors
    (B) Cell surface receptors
    (C) Both (A) and (B)
    (D) None of the above

20. Internal receptors also known as
    (A) Intracellular receptors
    (B) Extracellular receptors
    (C) Intercellular receptors
    (D) Cell surface receptors

21. Internal receptors are found in
    (A) Cell surface
    (B) Cytoplasm
    (C) Extracellular fluids
    (D) Interstitial space

22. Cell surface receptors are found in
    (A) Surface of the cell
    (B) Cytoplasm
    (C) Extracellular fluids
    (D) Interstitial space

23. Cell surface receptors are also known as
    (A) Transmembrane receptor
    (B) Transdermal receptor
    (C) Transcellular receptor
    (D) Intracellular receptor

24. The self – sustaining growth of cancer cells is attributed to
    (A) Paracrine signaling
    (B) Autocrine signaling
    (C) Endocrine signaling
    (D) Exocrine signaling

25. Which of the following is correct for growth factors?
    (A) Fats
    (B) Polypeptides
    (C) Vitamins
    (D) Carbohydrates

26. The ligand may be
    (A) Drugs
    (B) Neurotransmitters
    (C) Hormones
    (D) All of the above

27. The channel that connects two neighboring cells and help in communication is
    (A) Gap junction
    (B) Space junction
    (C) Neighbor junction
    (D) Side junction

28. Function of gap junction is/ are
    (A) Allow a direct exchange of metabolites
    (B) Signaling molecules between the cells
    (C) Both (A) and (B)
    (D) None of the above

29. Gap junction are coated by
    (A) Proteins
    (B) Lipids
    (C) Fats
    (D) Carbohydrates

30. Cell communicates via
    (A) Messenger substance
    (B) Gap junction
    (C) Surface proteins
    (D) All of the above

31. The chemical signals which are proteins or other molecules are produced by
    (A) Sending cell
    (B) Target cell
    (C) Non – target cell
    (D) Gap junction

32. The molecules secreted from the signaling cell and released into
    (A) Extracellular space
    (B) Intracellular space
    (C) Cytoplasm
    (D) Nucleus

33. The signals released by a cell are detected by
    (A) Target cell
    (B) Non – target cell
    (C) Sending cell
    (D) Gap junction

34. Which of the following signal molecules does not interact with cell surface receptors?
    (A) Glucagon
    (B) Testosterone
    (C) Gastrin
    (D) Insulin

35. Hormones signaling is mainly regulated via
    (A) External trigger signals
    (B) Feedback loops
    (C) Amount of receptor
    (D) All of the above

36. The transmission of a signal from a sending cell to a receiving cell is called
    (A) Tissue – tissue signaling
    (B) Organ – organ signaling
    (C) Cell - cell signaling
    (D) Cell interaction

37. The junction between two nerve cells where signal transmission occurs is called
    - (A) Synapse
    - (B) Muscle
    - (C) Nucleus
    - (D) Cell body

38. When the impulse reaches the synapse, it triggers the release of ligands called
    - (A) Neurotransmitters
    - (B) Hormones
    - (C) Pheromones
    - (D) None of the above

39. Endocrine gland release hormones which include
    - (A) Thyroid
    - (B) Hypothalamus
    - (C) Pituitary
    - (D) All of the above

40. Pituitary gland release growth hormone, which is an example of
    - (A) Endocrine signaling
    - (B) Paracrine signaling
    - (C) Autocrine signaling
    - (D) Direct contact signaling

41. The water – filled channel directly connect neighboring cells and allow small signaling molecules called
    - (A) Extracellular mediators
    - (B) Intracellular mediators
    - (C) Intercellular mediators
    - (D) Interstitial mediators

42. Mechanism of activation of signaling proteins is via
    - (A) Binding of activators
    - (B) Covalent modifications
    - (C) Membrane association
    - (D) All of the above

43. Cell surface receptors are
    - (A) Hydrophilic
    - (B) Large
    - (C) Act as ligand
    - (D) All of the above

44. A cell – surface receptor has domain
    - (A) An extracellular ligand – binding domain
    - (B) A hydrophobic domain extended through the membrane
    - (C) Intracellular domain
    - (D) All of the above

45. The major signal transducers are
    - (A) Receptor
    - (B) Signaling enzyme
    - (C) Regulatory GTPases
    - (D) All of the above

46. The messenger enters into target cell and binds and activates the receptor localized in the

    (A) Cytosol   (B) Mitochondria

    (C) Ribosome   (D) Lysosome

47. Receipt of external signals occurs by

    (A) Transmembrane receptors

    (B) Cytosolic or nuclear localized receptors

    (C) Both (A) and (B)

    (D) None of the above

48. Small intracellular mediators are

    (A) cAMP   (B) Ca^{++}

    (C) Nitric oxide   (D) All of the above

49. Which of the following is type of signalingligands

    (A) Small hydrophobic ligand

    (B) Nitric oxide gas serves as ligand

    (C) Water soluble ligand

    (D) All of the above

50. The release of prostaglandins is an example of

    (A) Autocrine signaling   (B) Paracrine signaling

    (C) Endocrine signaling   (D) Direct contact signaling

Answer Key

Introduction to Human Body, Cellular Levels of Structural Organization, Tissue Level of Organization (Part-09)

Question	Answer	Question	Answer
01	B = Autocrine Signalling	26	D = All of the Above
02	A = Paracrine Signalling	27	A = Gap Junction
03	A = Endocrine Signalling	28	C = Both A and B
04	A = Four	29	A = Proteins
05	D = All of the above	30	D = All of the Above
06	A = Autocrine Signalling	31	A = Sending Cells
07	C = Autocrine Signalling	32	A = Extracellular Space
08	B = Autocrine Signalling	33	A = Target Cells
09	A = Synaptic Signalling	34	B = Testosterone
10	B = Paracrine Signalling	35	D = All of the Above
11	C = Both A and B	36	C = Cell-Cell Signalling
12	B = Endocrine Gland	37	A = Synapse
13	A = Endocrine Signalling	38	A = Neurotransmitters
14	D = Endocrine Signalling	39	D = All of the Above
15	A = Cell to cell Signalling	40	A = Endocrine Signalling
16	D = All of the Above	41	B = Intracellular Mediators
17	A = Autocrine Signalling	42	D = All of the Above
18	A = Paracrine Signalling	43	D = All of the Above
19	C = Both A and B	44	D = All of the Above
20	A = Intracellular Receptor	45	D = All of the Above
21	B = Cytoplasm	46	A = Cytosol
22	A = Surface of the Cell	47	C = Both A and B
23	A = Transmembrane Receptor	48	D = All of the Above
24	B = Autocrine Signalling	49	D = All of the Above
25	B = Polypeptides	50	A = Autocrine Signalling

Part-10

1. A group of similar cells that work together to perform a specialized function are called
   - (A) Tissue
   - (B) Organ
   - (C) Organ system
   - (D) Nerves

2. The science that deals with the study of tissues is called
   - (A) Cytology
   - (B) Pathophysiology
   - (C) Histology
   - (D) Immunology

3. Body tissues can be classified into
   - (A) Epithelial tissue
   - (B) Connective tissue
   - (C) Muscle tissue
   - (D) All of the above

4. Which tissue covers the body and lines cavities, hollow organs and tubes
   - (A) Connective tissue
   - (B) Muscle tissue
   - (C) Epithelial tissue
   - (D) Nervous tissue

5. Which of the following tissue is found in glands
   - (A) Epithelial tissue
   - (B) Connective tissue
   - (C) Muscle tissue
   - (D) Nervous tissue

6. Epithelial tissue performs function which include
   - (A) Protection of underlying tissues
   - (B) Secretion
   - (C) Absorption
   - (D) All of the above

7. Epithelial tissues are found in
   - (A) Outer layer of skin
   - (B) Lining of intestine
   - (C) Sweat gland
   - (D) All of the above

8. Protection of skin from dehydration and mechanical or chemical damage is an example of
   - (A) Epithelial tissue
   - (B) Connective tissue
   - (C) Muscle tissue
   - (D) Nervous tissue

9. All gland which are involved in secretion are made up of

   (A) Connective tissue   (B) Nervous tissue

   (C) Epithelial tissue   (D) Muscle tissue

10. Which tissue present in the lining of small intestine which absorbs nutrients from the digested food

   (A) Connective tissue   (B) Nervous tissue

   (C) Muscle tissue   (D) Epithelial tissue

11. Which of the following tissue present in lining of respiratory tract?

   (A) Connective tissue   (B) Epithelial tissue

   (C) Nervous tissue   (D) Muscle tissue

12. In epithelial tissue, cells usually lie on a

   (A) Basement membrane   (B) Synovial membrane

   (C) Cutaneous membrane   (D) Serous membrane

13. Function of basement membrane is/are

   (A) Support epithelium   (B) Serves as ultrafilter

   (C) Maintenance of epithelial integrity   (D) All of the above

14. Component of basement membrane is/are

   (A) Laminin   (B) Entactin

   (C) Heparan sulphate   (D) All of the above

15. Epithelial membrane is/are

   (A) Mucous membrane   (B) Serous membrane

   (C) Both (A) and (B)   (D) None of the above

16. Which junction keep the neighbouring tissues well cemented together

   (A) Adhering junction   (B) Gap junction

   (C) Tight junction   (D) Synapse

17. Which junction prevent leakage across tissues

   (A) Tight junction   (B) Adhering junction

   (C) Gap junction   (D) Synapse

18. Which of the following tissue are present in the lining of excretory tract?

   (A) Muscle tissue   (B) Epithelial tissue

   (C) Connective tissue   (D) Nervous tissue

19. Which junction facilitate the movement of ions and molecules across the tissue

     (A) Gap junction
     (B) Tight junction
     (C) Adhering junction
     (D) Synapse

20. The epithelial membrane consists of a layer of epithelial tissue and has underlying

     (A) Connective tissue
     (B) Nervous tissue
     (C) Muscle tissue
     (D) None of the above

21. Mucus is secreted by

     (A) Mast cells
     (B) Goblet cells
     (C) Nerve cells
     (D) Stem cells

22. Mucus helps in

     (A) Lubrication
     (B) Protection
     (C) Easy movement of materials
     (D) All of the above

23. In which tract mucus membrane lies

     (A) Respiratory tract
     (B) Digestive tract
     (C) Both (A) and (B)
     (D) None of the above

24. Sensory receptor is present in the epithelial tissue of

     (A) Nose
     (B) Eye
     (C) Test bud
     (D) All of the above

25. Various gland made up of epithelial cells which secrete

     (A) Hormones
     (B) Sweat
     (C) Enzyme
     (D) All of the above

26. Which membrane lines in the body cavities which do not open outside the body

     (A) Serous membrane
     (B) Mucous membrane
     (C) Synovial membrane
     (D) Cutaneous membrane

27. Which of the following epithelial forms the inner lining of lung alveoli and blood vessels?

     (A) Cuboidal epithelial
     (B) Columnar epithelial
     (C) Squamous epithelial
     (D) Ciliated columnar

28. Simple epithelium consists of
    (A) Single layer of identical cells
    (B) Double layer of identical cells
    (C) Triple layer of identical cells
    (D) Multiple layers of identical cells

29. Gap, tight and adhering junctions are found in
    (A) Epithelial tissue
    (B) Muscular tissue
    (C) Connective tissue
    (D) Nervous tissue

30. Epithelial tissue can be divided into
    (A) Covering and lining epithelium
    (B) Glandular epithelium
    (C) Both (A) and (B)
    (D) None of the above

31. On the basis of arrangement of cells epithelial cells can be divided into
    (A) Simple epithelium
    (B) Stratified epithelium
    (C) Pseudo stratified epithelium
    (D) All of the above

32. The epithelium which are flat and sheet link appearance are called
    (A) Squamous epithelium
    (B) Cuboidal epithelium
    (C) Columnar epithelium
    (D) Stratified squamous epithelium

33. Type of simple epithelium is/are
    (A) Simple squamous
    (B) Simple cuboidal
    (C) Simple columnar
    (D) All of the above

34. Simple squamous form the lining of
    (A) Heart
    (B) Blood vessels
    (C) Alveoli of lungs
    (D) All of the above

35. The line of heart, blood vessels and lymphatic vessels is also known as
    (A) Endothelium
    (B) Mesothelium
    (C) Exothelium
    (D) Metathelium

36. The major function of simple squamous epithelium is/are
    (A) Secretion
    (B) Diffusion
    (C) Absorption
    (D) All of the above

37. Which epithelium consist of single layer of cube- shaped cells
    (A) Simple cuboidal epithelium
    (B) Simple squamous epithelium
    (C) Simple columnar epithelium
    (D) Stratified squamous epithelium

38. Simple cuboidal epithelium forms the lining of
    (A) Kidney tubules
    (B) Smaller ducts of many gland
    (C) Surface of ovary
    (D) All of the above

39. Which epithelium consists of a single layer of cylindrical cells
    (A) Simple columnar epithelium
    (B) Simple squamous epithelium
    (C) Simple cuboidal epithelium
    (D) Stratified squamous epithelium

40. Simple columnar epithelium exists in the form of
    (A) Non ciliated simple columnar epithelium
    (B) Ciliated simple columnar epithelium
    (C) Both (A) and (B)
    (D) None of the above

41. Which tissue found in glomerular (Bowmen's) capsule of kidneys
    (A) Simple squamous epithelium
    (B) Simple cuboidal epithelium
    (C) Simple columnar epithelium
    (D) Stratified cuboidal epithelium

42. The free surface of the simple columnar epithelium lining of small intestine
    is covered with
    (A) Cilia   (B) Microvilli
    (C) Flagella   (D) Goblet cell

43. In trachea columnar epithelium is ciliated and also contains
    (A) Goblets cell   (B) Microvilli
    (C) Flagella   (D) None of the above

44. The non - ciliated simple columnar epithelium consist of cells with
   (A) Microvilli (finger like projection)
   (B) Goblet cell (secrete mucous)
   (C) Both (A) and (B)
   (D) None of the above

45. The ciliated simple columnar epithelium contains cells with
   (A) Cilia
   (B) Microvilli
   (C) Goblet cell
   (D) Flagella

46. Which of the following agent propel the ova present in uterine tubes towards the uterus?
   (A) Microvilli
   (B) Cilia
   (C) Mucous
   (D) Flagella

47. On the basis of shape of cells epithelium can be divided into
   (A) Squamous cells
   (B) Cuboidal cells
   (C) Columnar cells
   (D) All of the above

48. The cells change shape from cuboidal to flat, and beck, as the body part expand or stretch
   (A) Transitional cells
   (B) Cuboidal cells
   (C) Squamous cells
   (D) Columnar cells

49. Which epithelium consists of several layer of cells of various shapes
   (A) Simple epithelium
   (B) Cuboidal epithelium
   (C) Columnar epithelium
   (D) Stratified epithelium

50. Types of stratified epithelium
   (A) Stratified squamous epithelium
   (B) Stratified columnar epithelium
   (C) Stratified cuboidal epithelium
   (D) All of the above

Answer Key

Introduction to Human Body, Cellular Levels of Structural Organization, Tissue Level of Organization (Part-10)

Question	Answer	Question	Answer
01	A = Tissue	26	A = Serous Membrane
02	C = Histology	27	C = Squamous Epithelial
03	D = All of the Above	28	A = Single Layer Identical Cell
04	C = Epithelial Tissue	29	A = Epithelial Tissue
05	A = Epithelial Tissue	30	C = Both A and B
06	D = All of the Above	31	D = All of the Above
07	D = All of the Above	32	A = Squamous Epithelium
08	A = Epithelial Tissue	33	D = All of the Above
09	C = Epithelial Tissue	34	D = All of the Above
10	D = Epithelial Tissue	35	A = Endothelium
11	B = Epithelial Tissue	36	D = All of the Above
12	A = Basement membrane	37	A = Simple Cuboidal Epithelium
13	D = All of the Above	38	D = All of the above
14	D = All of the Above	39	A = Simple Columnar Epithelium
15	C = Both A and B	40	C = Both A and B
16	A = Adhering Junction	41	A = Simple Squamous Epithelium
17	A = Tight Junction	42	B = Microvilli
18	B = Epithelial Tissue	43	A = Goblet cells
19	A = Gap Junction	44	C = Both A and B
20	A = Connective Tissue	45	A = Cilia
21	B = Goblet Cells	46	B = Cilia
22	D = All of the Above	47	D = All of the Above
23	C = Both A and B	48	A = Transitional Cells
24	D = All of the Above	49	D = Stratified Epithelium
25	D = All of the Above	50	D = All of the Above

Part-11

1. In stratified epithelium tissue, cells exist in forms of
   (A) Keratinized
   (B) Non – keratinized
   (C) Both (A) and (B)
   (D) None of the above

2. Which protein contains over the surface of keratinized epithelial cells
   (A) Keratin
   (B) Albumin
   (C) Tubulin
   (D) Elastin

3. An example of keratinized stratified squamous epithelium is/are
   (A) Skin
   (B) Hair
   (C) Nails
   (D) All of the above

4. Which epithelium consists several layers of cells in which the superficial layer is of flattened cells arranged in layer upon a basal membrane
   (A) Stratified squamous epithelium
   (B) Simple squamous epithelium
   (C) Stratified columnar epithelium
   (D) Simple columnar epithelium

5. Which epithelium found on dry surfaces subjected to face wear and tear
   (A) Non – keratinized stratified squamous epithelium
   (B) Keratinized stratified squamous epithelium
   (C) Stratified cuboidal epithelium
   (D) Stratified columnar epithelium

6. An example of non – keratinized stratified squamous epithelium is/are
   (A) Mouth
   (B) Oesophagus
   (C) Tongue
   (D) All of the above

7. Which epithelial forms a tough, relatively waterproof protective layer that prevents drying of live cells underneath
   (A) Keratinized stratified squamous epithelium
   (B) Non – keratinized stratified squamous epithelium
   (C) Stratified cuboidal epithelium
   (D) Stratified columnar epithelium

8. Which epithelium consists of two or more layers of cube – shaped cells
   (A) Stratified cuboidal epithelium
   (B) Stratified columnar epithelium
   (C) Simple squamous epithelium
   (D) Stratified squamous epithelium

9. Stratified cuboidal epithelium present in
   (A) Male urethra
   (B) Ducts of sweat glands
   (C) Sweat glands
   (D) All of the above

10. Which epithelium consists of several layers of cylindrical cells
   (A) Stratified cuboidal epithelium
   (B) Stratified columnar epithelium
   (C) Stratified squamous epithelium
   (D) Simple squamous epithelium

11. Which epithelium composed of several layers of pear – shaped cells
   (A) Transitional epithelium
   (B) Columnar epithelium
   (C) Squamous epithelium
   (D) Cuboidal epithelium

12. The adjacent epithelial cells are held together by
   (A) Desmosomes
   (B) Liposomes
   (C) Microsomes
   (D) Macrosomes

13. Which epithelial consists of a group of highly specialized epithelial cells that secrete substances into ducts, into blood or in the surface
   (A) Glandular epithelium
   (B) Cuboidal epithelium
   (C) Squamous epithelium
   (D) Transitional epithelium

14. Type of glands are
   (A) Endocrine gland
   (B) Exocrine gland
   (C) Both (A) and (B)
   (D) None of the above

15. Which gland are also called "ductless gland"?
   (A) Endocrine gland
   (B) Exocrine gland
   (C) Merocrine gland
   (D) Holocrine gland

16. An example of unicellular exocrine gland is
   (A) Goblet cells
   (B) Sweat gland
   (C) Salivary gland
   (D) Pancreas

17. An example of multicellular exocrine glands is
    (A) Salivary gland
    (B) Pancreas
    (C) Sweat gland
    (D) All of the above

18. Which gland form the secretion and release it from the cells
    (A) Merocrine gland
    (B) Apocrine gland
    (C) Holocrine gland
    (D) Endocrine gland

19. An example of merocrine gland
    (A) Salivary gland
    (B) Sebaceous gland
    (C) Pituitary gland
    (D) Thyroid gland

20. Multicellular exocrine gland can be functionally classified into
    (A) Merocrine gland
    (B) Apocrine gland
    (C) Holocrine gland
    (D) All of the above

21. Which gland accumulate the secretion at the apical surface of the cell
    (A) Holocrine gland
    (B) Apocrine gland
    (C) Merocrine gland
    (D) Adrenal gland

22. Which gland accumulate the secretion in the cytosol of the skin
    (A) Holocrine gland
    (B) Apocrine gland
    (C) Merocrine gland
    (D) Pituitary gland

23. Sebaceous gland of skin is an example of
    (A) Apocrine gland
    (B) Merocrine gland
    (C) Holocrine gland
    (D) Pituitary gland

24. Which gland present as ducts at the surface of covering
    (A) Exocrine gland
    (B) Endocrine gland
    (C) Pituitary gland
    (D) Thyroid gland

25. Which of the following tissue is the most abundant and widely distributed tissue in the body?
    (A) Connective tissue
    (B) Muscle tissue
    (C) Nervous tissue
    (D) Epithelial tissue

26. Which of the following is function of connective tissue?
    (A) Structural support
    (B) Protection
    (C) Transportation
    (D) All of the above

27. Bones protect the vital organs of the body such as
    - (A) Heart
    - (B) Lungs
    - (C) Brain
    - (D) All of the above

28. Major transport system within the body is/are
    - (A) Blood
    - (B) Nutrient
    - (C) Hormones
    - (D) All of the above

29. Type of connective tissue include
    - (A) Bone
    - (B) Cartilage
    - (C) Fat
    - (D) All of the above

30. Connective tissues contain which type of fibres
    - (A) Collagen fibres
    - (B) Elastic fibres
    - (C) Reticulate fibres
    - (D) All of the above

31. The different type of cells presents in connective tissues include
    - (A) Fibroblast
    - (B) Mast cells
    - (C) Fat cell
    - (D) All of the above

32. The cells are the most numerous, large, flat, with irregular process is called
    - (A) Fibroblast
    - (B) Fat cells
    - (C) Plasma cell
    - (D) Mast cell

33. Fibroblasts makes
    - (A) Collage fibres
    - (B) Elastic fibres
    - (C) Both (A) and (B)
    - (D) None of the above

34. The cells store triglyceride (Fats) and are abundant in the adipose connective tissue
    - (A) Macrophage
    - (B) Fat cells
    - (C) Mast cells
    - (D) Plasma cells

35. Fat cells also known as
    - (A) Adipocytes
    - (B) Leukocyte
    - (C) Lymphocyte
    - (D) Hepatocyte

36. Which cells are irregular shaped that are capable of engulfing foreign matter by phagocytosis?
    - (A) Fat cells
    - (B) Plasma cells
    - (C) Mast cells
    - (D) Macrophages

37. Plasma cells developed from
    - (A) T- lymphocyte
    - (B) B- lymphocyte
    - (C) Fat cells
    - (D) Mast cells

38. Which cells secrete antibodies that attack and neutralize the foreign substance in the body
    - (A) Plasma cells
    - (B) Fat cells
    - (C) Fibroblast
    - (D) Nerve cells

39. Which cells mainly found in loose connective tissue and around blood vessels
    - (A) Fat cells
    - (B) Mast cells
    - (C) Plasma cells
    - (D) Macrophage

40. Which chemical is released by mast cell which involved in inflammatory response
    - (A) Histamine
    - (B) Serotonin
    - (C) Adrenaline
    - (D) Melanin

41. The matrix consists major component, including
    - (A) Ground substances
    - (B) Fibres
    - (C) Both (A) and (B)
    - (D) None of the above

42. Which of the following consist of collagen protein and provide strength to the connective tissue?
    - (A) Elastic fibres
    - (B) Collagen fibres
    - (C) Reticular fibres
    - (D) Spindle fibres

43. Which of the following consist of elastin protein and provide strength as well as elasticity?
    - (A) Elastic fibres
    - (B) Collagen fibres
    - (C) Reticular fibres
    - (D) Spindle fibres

44. Which of the following consist of collagen with a coating of glycoprotein and provide support and strength to the cell?
    - (A) Collagen fibres
    - (B) Reticular fibres
    - (C) Elastic fibres
    - (D) Spindle fibres

45. The connective tissue can be classified into
    - (A) Loose connective tissue
    - (B) Dense connective tissue
    - (C) Specialised connective tissue
    - (D) All of the above

46. Which tissue consist of a large number of cells and fibres that are loosely woven among them
   (A) Dense connective tissue
   (B) Loose connective tissue
   (C) Elastic connective tissue
   (D) Specialised connective tissue

47. Adipose tissue consists of
   (A) Fat cells
   (B) Plasma cells
   (C) Fibroblast
   (D) Mast cells

48. Which of the following prevents blood coagulation?
   (A) Histamine
   (B) Heparin
   (C) Serotonin
   (D) Melanin

49. Which connective tissue is mainly found in the epidermis of the skin and subcutaneous layer?
   (A) Areolar connective tissue
   (B) Reticular connective tissue
   (C) Dense connective tissue
   (D) Specialized connective tissue

50. Type of adipose tissue
   (A) White adipose tissue
   (B) Brown adipose tissue
   (C) Both (A) and (B)
   (D) None of the above

Answer Key

Introduction to Human Body, Cellular Levels of Structural Organization, Tissue Level of Organization (Part-11)

Question	Answer	Question	Answer
01	C = Both A and B	26	D = All of the above
02	A = Keratin	27	D = All of the Above
03	D = All of the Above	28	D = All of the Above
04	A = Stratified Squamous Epithelium	29	D = All of the Above
05	B = Keratinized Stratified Squamous Epithelium	30	D = All of the Above
06	D = All of the Above	31	D = All of the Above
07	A = Keratinized Stratified Squamous Epithelium	32	A = Fibroblast
08	A = Stratified Cuboidal Epithelium	33	C = Both A and B
09	D = All of the Above	34	B = Fat Cells
10	B = Stratified Columnar Epithelium	35	A = Adipocytes
11	A = Transitional Epithelium	36	D = Macrophage
12	A = Desmosomes	37	B = B-Lymphocytes
13	A = Glandular Epithelium	38	A = Plasma Cells
14	C = Both A and B	39	B = Mast Cells
15	A = Endocrine Gland	40	A = Histamines
16	A = Goblet Cells	41	C = Both A and B
17	D = All of the Above	42	B = Collagen Fibres
18	A = Merocrine Gland	43	A = Elastic Fibres
19	A = Salivary Glands	44	B = Reticular Fibres
20	D = All of the Above	45	D = All of the Above
21	B = Apocrine Gland	46	B = Loose Connective Tissue
22	A = Holocrine Gland	47	A= Fat Cells
23	C = holocrine Gland	48	B = Heparin
24	A = Exocrine Gland	49	A = Areolar Connective Tissue
25	A = Connective Tissue	50	C = Both A and B

Part-12

1. How much of white adipose tissue up body weight in adult
   - (A) 2-3%
   - (B) 20-25%
   - (C) 10-12%
   - (D) 70-80%

2. Which hormones is secreted by white adipose tissue?
   - (A) Leptin
   - (B) Insulin
   - (C) Cortisol
   - (D) Thyroid

3. Adipose tissue is distributed within
   - (A) Subcutaneous fat
   - (B) Visceral fat
   - (C) Bone marrow fat
   - (D) All of the above

4. The main function of white adipocytes is to store excess energy in the form of
   - (A) Fatty molecule
   - (B) Vitamin
   - (C) Protein
   - (D) Carbohydrate

5. Which tissue act as a thermal insulator and store energy
   - (A) Reticular tissue
   - (B) Adipose tissue
   - (C) Loose connective tissue
   - (D) Dense connective tissue

6. Transitional epithelium found in
   - (A) Pelvis
   - (B) Ureter
   - (C) Urinary bladder
   - (D) All of the above

7. Which cells produce collagen, reticular fibers and ground substance and are seen to be active during wound repair
   - (A) Fibroblast
   - (B) Mast cell
   - (C) Pigment cell
   - (D) Macrophage

8. Visceral fat is predominantly found around the organs in the abdominal cavity such as
   - (A) Liver
   - (B) Intestines
   - (C) Kidney
   - (D) All of the above

9. Melanin is produced by
   (A) Plasma cells
   (B) Pigment cells
   (C) Mast cells
   (D) Adipose cells

10. Pigment cells is also known as
    (A) Melanocyte
    (B) Adipocyte
    (C) Leukocyte
    (D) Histocytes

11. Pigment cells are present in
    (A) Skin
    (B) Choroid
    (C) Iris of eye ball
    (D) All of the above

12. Collagen fibers are produced by fibroblast and are present in
    (A) Bone
    (B) Cartilage
    (C) Tendons
    (D) All of the above

13. Mast cells is found in
    (A) Epithelial tissue
    (B) Connective tissue
    (C) Muscle tissue
    (D) Nervous tissue

14. Which tissue generates more heat on metabolism and thus maintains the body temperature in new born
    (A) Brown adipose tissue
    (B) Loose connective tissue
    (C) Dens connective tissue
    (D) Reticular connective tissue

15. Which connective tissue of a fine network of reticular fibers and reticular cells
    (A) Dense connective tissue
    (B) Loose connective tissue
    (C) Reticular connective tissue
    (D) Areolar connective tissue

16. The reticular connective tissue supports the organs such as
    (A) Liver
    (B) Bone marrow
    (C) Spleen
    (D) All of the above

17. Reticular tissue contains
    (A) Reticular cells
    (B) Monocytes
    (C) Lymphocytes
    (D) All of the above

18. Which tissue made up of closely packed bundles of collagen fibers with very little matrix
    - (A) Fibrous connective tissue
    - (B) Elastic connective tissue
    - (C) Reticular connective tissue
    - (D) Loose connective tissue

19. Which of the following present in fibrous connective tissue between the bundles of collagen fibers?
    - (A) Fibroblasts
    - (B) Mast cells
    - (C) Plasma cells
    - (D) Fat cells

20. Fibrous connective tissue is found in
    - (A) Tendons
    - (B) Ligament
    - (C) Periosteum of bone
    - (D) All of the above

21. Muscle to bones isattached by
    - (A) Ligament
    - (B) Tendons
    - (C) Cartilage
    - (D) Hyaline cartilage

22. Bone to boneareattached by
    - (A) Cartilage
    - (B) Tendon
    - (C) Ligaments
    - (D) Hyaline cartilage

23. In fibrous connective tissue which fibers are responsible for strength and help to attach various structures strongly
    - (A) Collagen fibers
    - (B) Elastic fibers
    - (C) Reticular fibers
    - (D) Spindle fibers

24. Which connective tissue is capable of considerable extension and recoil?
    - (A) Fibrous connective tissue
    - (B) Elastic connective tissue
    - (C) Loose connective tissue
    - (D) Reticular connective tissue

25. Which connective tissue found in organs where stretching or alteration of shape is required
    - (A) Elastic connective tissue
    - (B) Reticular connective tissue
    - (C) Dense connective tissue
    - (D) Adipose connective tissue

26. Elastic connective tissues are presents in
    (A) Trachea
    (B) Bronchi
    (C) Lungs
    (D) All of the above

27. Cells of cartilage is called
    (A) Chondrocytes
    (B) Adipocytes
    (C) Leukocytes
    (D) Monocytes

28. Which of the following is a type of cartilage?
    (A) Hyaline cartilage
    (B) Fibrocartilage
    (C) Elastic cartilage
    (D) All of the above

29. The most abundant cartilage in the body is
    (A) Hyaline cartilage
    (B) Elastic cartilage
    (C) Fibrocartilage
    (D) Reticular tissue

30. Which cartilage consists of small groups of chondrocytes within lacunae embedded in the matrix with fine collagen fibers
    (A) Elastic cartilage
    (B) Hyaline cartilage
    (C) Fibrocartilage
    (D) Reticular tissue

31. Hyaline cartilageare found in
    (A) On the end of long bones
    (B) Anterior ends of ribs
    (C) Forming part of the larynx, trachea and bronchi
    (D) All of the above

32. Which cartilage consists of a dense mass of collagen fibers embedded in the matrix with chondrocytes widely dispersed in it
    (A) Fibrocartilage
    (B) Hyaline cartilage
    (C) Elastic cartilage
    (D) Reticular tissue

33. Fibrocartilage found in
    (A) Intervertebral discs
    (B) Pubic symphysis
    (C) On the rim of the bony sockets of the hip and shoulder joints
    (D) All of the above

34. Which cartilage consists of chondrocytes embedded in the matrix consisting of elastic fibers
    (A) Fibrocartilage
    (B) Elastic cartilage
    (C) Hyaline cartilage
    (D) Reticular tissue

35. Elastic cartilage found in
    (A) Lobe of the ear
    (B) Epiglottis
    (C) Auditory tubes
    (D) All of the above

36. Bone cells are called
    (A) Osteocytes
    (B) Leukocytes
    (C) Adipocytes
    (D) Melanocytes

37. Which of the following are surrounded by a matrix of collagen fibers, strengthened by organic salts, especially calcium and phosphate?
    (A) Bone cells
    (B) Blood cells
    (C) Mast cells
    (D) Plasma cells

38. Bone matrix is rich in
    (A) Calcium and potassium
    (B) Calcium and phosphate
    (C) Sodium and potassium
    (D) Sodium and calcium

39. Bone is made up of
    (A) Compact bone
    (B) Spongy bone
    (C) Bone marrow
    (D) All of the above

40. Function of bone is/are
    (A) Allow movement
    (B) Makes blood cells
    (C) Provides protections of organs
    (D) All of the above

41. Types of bone can be identified by naked eye
    (A) Compact bone, having a solid or dense appearance
    (B) Spongy or cancellous bone, having a 'spongy' or fine honeycomb appearance
    (C) Both (A) and (B)
    (D) None of the above

42. Which of the following is fluid connective tissue?
    (A) Blood
    (B) Bone
    (C) Cartilage
    (D) Tendons

43. Which of the following is the component of blood?
    (A) Red blood cells   (B) White blood cells
    (C) Platelets   (D) All of the above

44. Red blood cells are also called as
    (A) Leukocytes   (B) Erythrocytes
    (C) Thrombocytes   (D) Osteocytes

45. Leukocytes are also called as
    (A) Red blood cells   (B) Platelets
    (C) White blood cells   (D) Bone cells

46. Platelets are also called as
    (A) Thrombocytes   (B) Osteocytes
    (C) Erythrocytes   (D) Leukocytes

47. Blood transports
    (A) Oxygen   (B) Carbon dioxide
    (C) Waste products   (D) All of the above

48. Lymphoid tissue found in
    (A) Lymph nodes   (B) Thymus
    (C) Spleen   (D) All of the above

49. The tissue consists of fibers that have ability to contract and relax
    (A) Muscle tissue   (B) Epithelial tissue
    (C) Nervous tissue   (D) Connective tissue

50. Muscle contraction requires a rich blood supply providing
    (A) Sufficient oxygen   (B) Calcium and nutrients
    (C) Removing waste products (D) All of the above

Answer Key

Introduction to Human Body, Cellular Levels of Structural Organization, Tissue Level of Organization (Part-12)

Question	Answer	Question	Answer
01	B = 20 -25 %	26	D = All of the Above
02	A = Leptin	27	A = Chondrocytes
03	D = All of the Above	28	D = All of the Above
04	A = Fatty Molecules	29	A = Hyaline Cartilage
05	B = Adipose Tissue	30	B = Hyaline Cartilage
06	D = All of the Above	31	D = All of the Above
07	A = Fibroblast	32	A = Fibrocartilage
08	D = All of the Above	33	D = All of the above
09	B = Pigment Cells	34	B = Elastic Cartilage
10	A = Melanocytes	35	D = All of the above
11	D = All of the Above	36	A = Osteocytes
12	D = All of the Above	37	A = Bone Cells
13	B = Connective Tissue	38	B = Calcium and Phosphate
14	A = Brown Adipose Tissue	39	D = All of the Above
15	C = Reticular Connective Tissue	40	D = All of the above
16	D = All of the Above	41	C = Both and B
17	D = All of the Above	42	A = Blood
18	A = Fibrous Connective Tissue	43	D = All of the Above
19	A = Fibroblast	44	B = Erythrocytes
20	D = All of the Above	45	C = White Blood Cells
21	B = Tendons	46	A = Thrombocytes
22	C = Ligaments	47	D = All of the Above
23	A = Collagen Fibres	48	D = All of the Above
24	B = Elastic Connective Tissue	49	A = Muscle Tissue
25	A = Elastic Connective Tissue	50	D = All of the Above

Part-13

1. What is the percent of globulins present in plasma protein?
   (A) 56 %
   (B) 38 %
   (C) 15 %
   (D) 10 %

2. What is the percent of albumins present in plasma protein?
   (A) 55 %
   (B) 30 %
   (C) 26%
   (D) 14 %

3. Types of muscle tissues is/are
   (A) Skeletal muscle tissue
   (B) Smooth muscle tissue
   (C) Cardiac muscle tissue
   (D) All of the above

4. Which of the following is contractile proteins in muscle fibers?
   (A) Actin and myosin
   (B) Albumin and globulin
   (C) Keratin and elastin
   (D) Collagen and albumin

5. Which of the following are cylindrical, multinucleated, striated and under voluntary control?
   (A) Skeletal muscle fibers
   (B) Smooth muscle cells
   (C) Cardiac muscle tissue
   (D) Hyaline cartilage

6. Which muscle are attached to the bones of the skeleton?
   (A) Smooth muscle tissue
   (B) Skeletal muscle tissue
   (C) Cardiac muscle tissue
   (D) Loose connective tissue

7. The outermost layer of bone is
   (A) Periosteum
   (B) Epidermis
   (C) Interstitial matrix
   (D) Dermis

8. The major function of skeletal muscle tissue is
   (A) Maintenance of posture
   (B) Movement of bones
   (C) Both (A) and (B)
   (D) None of the above

9. Which muscle tissue named as "striated muscle tissue"
   (A) Skeletal muscle tissue
   (B) Smooth muscle tissue
   (C) Reticular tissue
   (D) Nervous tissue

10. Which muscle tissue is non striated and involuntary because of lacks of striations?

    (A) Skeletal muscle tissue   (B) Loose connective tissue

    (C) Smooth muscle tissue   (D) Areolar connective tissue

11. Which muscle fibers is small, spindle shaped with only one central nucleus?

    (A) Smooth muscle fibers   (B) Skeletal muscle fibers

    (C) Cardiac muscle fibers   (D) Loose connective tissue

12. Smooth muscle tissue found in the walls of hollow organ such as

    (A) Blood vessel   (B) Stomach

    (C) Gallbladder   (D) All of the above

13. Voluntary muscle is found in

    (A) Lungs   (B) Liver

    (C) Heart   (D) Arms

14. Which tissue found only in the wall of heart

    (A) Skeletal muscle tissue   (B) Cardiac muscle tissue

    (C) Smooth muscle tissue   (D) Loose connective tissue

15. Which muscle fibers are cylindrical, branched and usually have only one nucleus?

    (A) Skeletal muscle fibers   (B) Cardiac muscle fibers

    (C) Smooth muscle fibers   (D) Areolar muscle fibers

16. In which muscle tissue intercalated disc are present

    (A) Smooth muscle tissue   (B) Cardiac muscle tissue

    (C) Skeletal muscle tissue   (D) Areolar muscle tissue

17. Harversian system is found in

    (A) Plasma cells   (B) Bone

    (C) Cartilage   (D) Nerve cells

18. How much of total body mass comprises skeletal muscle?

    (A) 30 – 40 %   (B) 5 – 10 %

    (C) 70 – 80 %   (D) 15 – 20 %

19. Which cell convert stimuli into nerve impulses

    (A) Fat cell   (B) Nerve cell

    (C) Bone cell   (D) Plasma cell

20. Type of tissue found in the nervous system

    (A) Excitable cells   (B) Non – excitable cells

    (C) Both (A) and (B)   (D) None of the above

21. Neurons are having following component in its body

    (A) Cell body   (B) Dendrites

    (C) Axons   (D) All of the above

22. Which part of neuron contains nucleus

    (A) Cell body   (B) Axon

    (C) Dendrites   (D) Axonal knobs

23. Which part of neuron receive stimuli and conduct them to cell body

    (A) Nucleus   (B) Dendrites

    (C) Axon   (D) Axonal knobs

24. Which part of neuron transmit the impulses towards another neuron or some other tissue

    (A) Axon   (B) Cell body

    (C) Nucleus   (D) Dendrites

25. Excitable cells are also known as

    (A) Neurons   (B) Glial cells

    (C) Fat cells   (D) Blood cells

26. Non - excitable cells are also known as

    (A) Glial cells   (B) Neurons

    (C) Fat cells   (D) Bone cells

27. Which neurons having single process

    (A) Bipolar   (B) Unipolar

    (C) Multipolar   (D) Tripolar

28. Which neuron found in the nervous system of embryo

    (A) Tripolar   (B) Bipolar

    (C) Unipolar   (D) Multipolar

29. Which neurons having one dendron and one axon

    (A) Bipolar   (B) Multipolar

    (C) Tripolar   (D) Unipolar

30. Which neuron found in the retina of eye

   (A) Unipolar   (B) Bipolar

   (C) Tripolar   (D) Multipolar

31. Which neuron having many dendron and one axon

   (A) Multipolar   (B) Unipolar

   (C) Tripolar   (D) Bipolar

32. The most common amino acid of collagen fibers is

   (A) Proline   (B) Glycine

   (C) Lysin   (D) Alanine

33. The most common cells of connective tissue

   (A) Nerve cell   (B) Osteoblast

   (C) Fibroblast   (D) Adipocyte

34. Heparin is produced by

   (A) Mast cells   (B) Osteocytes

   (C) Nerve cells   (D) Osteoblast

35. Bile is produced by which cells

   (A) Hepatocytes   (B) Osteocytes

   (C) Melanocytes   (D) Adipocytes

36. β - cells of pancreas produce

   (A) Glucagon   (B) Insulin

   (C) Oxytocin   (D) Thyroxin

37. The vagina is lined by which epithelium

   (A) Simple cuboidal epithelium

   (B) Stratified cuboidal epithelium

   (C) Simple squamous epithelium

   (D) Stratified squamous epithelium

38. Ameloblasts are derived from

   (A) Inner dental epithelium   (B) Dental sac

   (C) Dental papilla   (D) Outer dental epithelium

39. Endometrium is lined by which epithelium
    (A) Stratified cuboidal epithelium
    (B) Simple columnar epithelium
    (C) Transitional epithelium
    (D) Pseudostratified epithelium

40. Calcitonin is secreted by which gland
    (A) Thyroid gland
    (B) Salivary gland
    (C) Adrenal gland
    (D) Pineal gland

41. Which of the following epithelium found in gall bladder?
    (A) Simple columnar epithelium
    (B) Stratified cuboidal epithelium
    (C) Stratified squamous epithelium
    (D) Pseudostratified epithelium

42. α - cells of pancreas secretes
    (A) Insulin
    (B) Glucagon
    (C) Vasopressin
    (D) Oxytocin

43. Melatonin is secreted by which of the following gland
    (A) Pineal gland
    (B) Pituitary gland
    (C) Salivary gland
    (D) Thyroid gland

44. Which of the following hormone is secreted by pituitary gland?
    (A) Growth hormone
    (B) Oxytocin
    (C) Luteinizing hormone
    (D) All of the above

45. The group of cancer cell of epithelial cells are called
    (A) Carcinoma
    (B) Sarcoma
    (C) Melanoma
    (D) Leukemia

46. The tip of the nose and external ears have
    (A) Ligament
    (B) Cartilage
    (C) Bone
    (D) Areolar tissue

47. A disease of muscles in which fibers do not function resulting in muscular weakness
    (A) Myalgia
    (B) Myositis
    (C) Myopathy
    (D) Fibrositis

48. Sarcomas is a form of cancer of connective tissue occurs in
    (A) Muscles   (B) Bones
    (C) Cartilages   (D) All of the above

49. The gaps between two adjacent myelin sheaths are called
    (A) Nodes of Ranvier   (B) Dendrites
    (C) Nucleus   (D) Cell body

50. In which tissue rapid healing of wound is found
    (A) Epithelial tissue   (B) Muscular tissue
    (C) Connective tissue   (D) Nervous tissue

Answer Key

Introduction to Human Body, Cellular Levels of Structural Organization, Tissue Level of Organization (Part-13)

Question	Answer	Question	Answer
01	B = 38 %	26	A = Glial Cells
02	A = 55%	27	B = Unipolar
03	D = All of the above	28	C = Unipolar
04	A = Actin and Myosin	29	A = Bipolar
05	A = Skeletal Muscle Fibres	30	B = Bipolar
06	B = Skeletal Muscle Tissue	31	A = Multipolar
07	A = Periosteum	32	B = Skin
08	C = Both A and B	33	C = Skin
09	A = Skeletal Muscle Tissue	34	A = 1.5 to 02 Square Meter
10	C = Smooth Muscle Tissue	35	A = All of the Above
11	A = Smooth Muscle Fibres	36	B = All of the Above
12	D = All of the Above	37	D = Skin
13	D = Arms	38	A = Dermatology
14	B = Cardiac Muscle Tissue	39	B = Both A and B
15	B = Cardiac Muscle Fibres	40	A = Epidermis
16	B = Cardiac Muscle Tissue	41	A = Stratified Squamous Keratinized Epithelium
17	B = Bone	42	B = Dermis
18	A = 30 to 40 %	43	A = Hypodermis
19	B = Nerve Cells	44	D = Hypodermis
20	C = Both A and B	45	A = Dermis
21	D = All of the Above	46	B = Hypodermis
22	A = Cell Body	47	C = Hypodermis
23	B = Dendrites	48	D = All of the Above
24	A = Axon	49	A = Melanocytes
25	A = Neurons	50	A = Epidermis

Notes

Unit - II

Integumentary System, Skeletal System, Joints

Part-01

1. The outermost layer of epidermis is
   (A) Stratum corneum
   (B) Stratum Basale
   (C) Stratum spinosum
   (D) Stratum granulosum

2. How many layers of dead keratinized cells consist in Stratum corneum?
   (A) 5 – 10 layers
   (B) 70 – 80 layers
   (C) 25 – 30 layers
   (D) 60 – 70 layers

3. Dead keratinized cells are non – nucleated and are filled with
   (A) Keratin protein
   (B) Albumin protein
   (C) Tubulin protein
   (D) Collagen protein

4. Keratinized cells also covered with
   (A) Lipids
   (B) Glucose
   (C) Minerals
   (D) Carbohydrates

5. The keratinized cells make stratum corneum
   (A) Effective barrier
   (B) Abrasion resistance
   (C) Protect the deeper layer
   (D) All of the above

6. Which layer of epidermis lies directly beneath the Stratum corneum
   (A) Stratum granulosum
   (B) Stratum lucidum
   (C) Stratum spinosum
   (D) Stratum Basale

7. Which layer of epidermis consist 3 – 5 layers of flattened, transparent, dead keratinized cells
   (A) Stratum corneum
   (B) Stratum lucidum
   (C) Stratum granulosum
   (D) Stratum spinosum

8. Which layer situated just below the Stratum corneum
   - (A) Stratum spinosum
   - (B) Stratum granulosum
   - (C) Stratum Basale
   - (D) Stratum lucidum

9. Which of the following layer consist 2 – 5 layers of flattened keratinocytes?
   - (A) Stratum lucidum
   - (B) Stratum granulosum
   - (C) Stratum spinosum
   - (D) Stratum Basale

10. Keratinocytes contains
    - (A) Keratin
    - (B) Tubulin
    - (C) Collagen
    - (D) Melanin

11. The cytoplasm of keratinocytes contains
    - (A) Keratohyalin granules
    - (B) Albumin granules
    - (C) Collagen granules
    - (D) Tubulin granules

12. Which of the following granules convert tofilaments into keratin and lamellar granules?
    - (A) Nissl's granules
    - (B) Tubulohyalin granules
    - (C) Keratohyalin granules
    - (D) Zymogen granules

13. Which layer lies above the stratum germinativum
    - (A) Stratum corneum
    - (B) Stratum spinosum
    - (C) Stratum lucidum
    - (D) Stratum granulosum

14. Which layer consist 8 – 10 layers of spiny keratinocytes
    - (A) Stratum spinosum
    - (B) Stratum corneum
    - (C) Stratum lucidum
    - (D) Stratum granulosum

15. Which layer situated below the Stratum granulosum
    - (A) Stratum corneum
    - (B) Stratum lucidum
    - (C) Stratum spinosum
    - (D) Stratum Basale

16. Which of the following is innermost layer of epidermis?
    - (A) Stratum germinativum
    - (B) Stratum corneum
    - (C) Stratum lucidum
    - (D) Stratum granulosum

17. Which layer is responsible for the formation of all other upper epidermal layers?
    - (A) Stratum corneum
    - (B) Stratum germinativum
    - (C) Stratum lucidum
    - (D) Stratum spinosum

18. Which layer consist of a single row of cuboidal or columnar keratinocytes
    - (A) Stratum germinativum
    - (B) Stratum corneum
    - (C) Stratum lucidum
    - (D) Stratum granulosum

19. Where does mitotic cell division or replacement of skin take place
    - (A) Stratum lucidum
    - (B) Stratum corneum
    - (C) Stratum granulosum
    - (D) Stratum germinativum

20. Which of the following cell contain in Stratum germinativum and is responsible for producing skin colour?
    - (A) Melanocytes
    - (B) Adipocytes
    - (C) Leukocytes
    - (D) Osteocytes

21. Stratum germinativum also known as
    - (A) Stratum Basale
    - (B) Stratum corneum
    - (C) Stratum lucidum
    - (D) Stratum spinosum

22. Which of the following is the second and deeper layer of skin?
    - (A) Dermis
    - (B) Epidermis
    - (C) Hypodermis
    - (D) Subcutaneous layer

23. Which part lies directly beneath the epidermis
    - (A) Sebaceous gland
    - (B) Hypodermis
    - (C) Dermis
    - (D) Sweat glands

24. Which part of skin is composed of dense connective tissue with white collagen fibres and yellow elastin fibres?
    - (A) Hypodermis
    - (B) Dermis
    - (C) Epidermis
    - (D) Subcutaneous layer

25. The specialized nerve endings sensitive to touch, temperature, pressure and pain are widely distributed in the
    - (A) Dermis
    - (B) Epidermis
    - (C) Hypodermis
    - (D) Subcutaneous layer

26. The dermis layer made up of
    - (A) Papillary layer
    - (B) Reticular layer
    - (C) Both (A) and (B)
    - (D) None of the above

27. Which of the following layer of dermis adjacent to the epidermis and consist fine elastic fibres?

(A) Reticular layer
(B) Papillary layer
(C) Fatty layer
(D) Stratum corneum

28. The cells of papillary layer called

(A) Papillae
(B) Reticule
(C) Melanin
(D) Collagen

29. Which part of skin referred as "true skin"

(A) Dermis
(B) Stratum corneum
(C) Stratum spinosum
(D) Stratum lucidum

30. The projections from the dermis to the epidermis called

(A) Hypodermal ridges
(B) Epidermal ridges
(C) Dermal ridges
(D) Subcutaneous ridges

31. Which cells are mainly found in the dermis?

(A) Fibroblasts
(B) Macrophages
(C) Mast cells
(D) All of the above

32. Structure found in the dermis are

(A) Small blood and lymph vessels
(B) Sensory nerve endings
(C) Sweat glands and their ducts
(D) All of the above

33. Which of the following layer of dermis are watched in order to see the fingerprints?

(A) Papillary layer
(B) Stratum lucidum
(C) Stratum spinosum
(D) Reticular layer

34. The papillary layer of dermis is most closely with which layer of epidermis

(A) Stratum spinosum
(B) Stratum Basale
(C) Stratum lucidum
(D) Stratum corneum

35. Langerhans cells are commonly found in the

(A) Stratum spinosum
(B) Stratum basale
(C) Stratum lucidum
(D) Stratum corneum

36. Upper layer of dermis is

(A) Papillary layer
(B) Reticular layer
(C) Stratum corneum
(D) Stratum lucidum

37. Lower layer of dermis is
    (A) Papillary layer
    (B) Reticular layer
    (C) Stratum corneum
    (D) Stratum Basale

38. Which layer of dermis consists of bundles of tough collagen fibres, fibroblasts and some elastic fibres
    (A) Stratum spinosum
    (B) Reticular layer
    (C) Stratum lucidum
    (D) Stratum corneum

39. The collagen and elastic fibres in the reticular layer are responsible for
    (A) Extensibility
    (B) Elasticity
    (C) Strength of skin
    (D) All of the above

40. Sweat glands are most numerous in the
    (A) Palms of the hands
    (B) Soles of the feet
    (C) Axillae and groins
    (D) All of the above

41. Type of sweat gland found in skin is/are
    (A) Eccrine sweat gland
    (B) Apocrine sweat gland
    (C) Both (A) and (B)
    (D) None of the above

42. Which sweat gland open on the skin surface through tiny pores
    (A) Eccrine sweat gland
    (B) Apocrine sweat gland
    (C) Holocrine sweat gland
    (D) Endocrine sweat gland

43. Which sweat gland open into hair follicles
    (A) Apocrine sweat gland
    (B) Eccrine sweat gland
    (C) Holocrine sweat gland
    (D) Endocrine sweat gland

44. Which sweat gland found in genital area
    (A) Eccrine sweat gland
    (B) Apocrine sweat gland
    (C) Endocrine sweat gland
    (D) Holocrine sweat gland

45. Eccrine sweat gland consists of which segment
    (A) Secretory segment
    (B) Duct segment
    (C) Both (A) and (B)
    (D) None of the above

46. The secretory segment consist which type of cells that lies on the basal lamina
    (A) Clear cells
    (B) Dark cells
    (C) Myoepithelial
    (D) All of the above

47. The clear cells contain large amount of
    (A) Glycogen
    (B) Numerous smooth endoplasmic reticulum
    (C) Mitochondria
    (D) All of the above

48. Which gland of skin is responsible for thermoregulatory sweating?
    (A) Eccrine sweat gland   (B) Apocrine sweat gland
    (C) Holocrine sweat gland   (D) Endocrine sweat gland

49. Apocrine sweat gland is found in the skin of
    (A) Axilla   (B) Areola
    (C) Perianal skin   (D) All of the above

50. Which gland is also known as sudoriferous glands?
    (A) Sweat glands   (B) Pituitary glands
    (C) Thyroid glands   (D) Adrenal glands

Answer Key

Integumentary System, Skeletal System, Joints (Part-01)

Question	Answer	Question	Answer
01	A = Stratum Corneum	26	C = Both A and B
02	C = 25 to 30 Layers	27	B = Papillary Layer
03	A = Keratin Protein	28	A = Papillae
04	A = Lipids	29	A = Dermis
05	D = All of the Above	30	B = Epidermal Ridge
06	B = Stratum Lucidum	31	D = All of the Above
07	B = Stratum Lucidum	32	D = All of the Above
08	D = Stratum Lucidum	33	A = Papillary Layer
09	B = Stratum Granulosum	34	B = Stratum Basale
10	A = Keratin	35	A = Stratum Spinosum
11	A = Keratohyalin Granules	36	A = Papillary layer
12	C = Keratohyalin Granules	37	B = Reticular Layer
13	B = Stratum Spinosum	38	B = Reticular Layer
14	A = Stratum Spinosum	39	D = All of the Above
15	C = Stratum Spinosum	40	D = All of the Above
16	A = Stratum Germinativum	41	C = Both A and B
17	B = Stratum Germinativum	42	A = Eccrine Sweat Gland
18	A = Stratum Germinativum	43	A = Apocrine Sweat Gland
19	D = Stratum Germinativum	44	B = Apocrine Sweat Gland
20	A = Melanocytes	45	C = Both A and B
21	A = Stratum Basale	46	D = All of the Above
22	A = Dermis	47	D = All of the Above
23	C = Dermis	48	A = Eccrine Sweat Gland
24	B = Dermis	49	D = All of the Above
25	A = Dermis	50	A = Sweat Gland

Part-02

1. At base of the hair follicle there is a cluster of cells which is called
   - (A) Hair papilla
   - (B) Hair reticula
   - (C) Hair shaft
   - (D) Hair root

2. The part of hair above the skin is called
   - (A) Hair shaft
   - (B) Hair papilla
   - (C) Hair root
   - (D) Hair follicle

3. The root of hair surrounded by epithelial tube is called
   - (A) Hair shaft
   - (B) Hair papilla
   - (C) Hair follicle
   - (D) Hair reticula

4. Which of the following is the function of hairs?
   - (A) Excretion
   - (B) Protection
   - (C) Secretion
   - (D) All of the above

5. Which of the following is the site of mitotic cell division in hair?
   - (A) Hair shaft
   - (B) Hair follicle
   - (C) Hair bulb
   - (D) Hair root

6. The shaft and root of hair consist the concentric layers of cells are
   - (A) Cuticle
   - (B) Cortex
   - (C) Medulla
   - (D) All of the above

7. The outermost part of hair shaft is
   - (A) Medulla
   - (B) Cuticle
   - (C) Cortex
   - (D) Reticula

8. Which part is located between the hair cuticle and hair medulla?
   - (A) Cortex
   - (B) Reticula
   - (C) Hair root
   - (D) Hair follicle

9. Innermost layer of hair shaft is called
   - (A) Cuticle
   - (B) Medulla
   - (C) Cortex
   - (D) Reticula

10. Which layer of hair consists highly keratinized single layer of thin, flat cells

 (A) Medulla   (B) Cortex

 (C) Cuticle   (D) Reticula

11. Which layer of hair forms the major part of the shaft and consists of the elongated cells

 (A) Cortex   (B) Medulla

 (C) Cuticle   (D) Reticula

12. Which layer of hair is composed of two or three rows of irregularly shaped cells?

 (A) Cuticle   (B) Medulla

 (C) Cortex   (D) Reticula

13. The bundles of smooth muscle fibres attached to the hair follicle called

 (A) Arrector pili   (B) Sebaceous gland

 (C) Hair shaft   (D) Hair root

14. What happens when the melanin produced by the hair follicle stops?

 (A) Hair turns white   (B) Hair fall

 (C) Dandruff   (D) Hair turns black

15. Hair growth cycle consists of following stages

 (A) Growth stage   (B) Resting stage

 (C) Both (A) and (B)   (D) None of the above

16. In which of the hair growth stage, the epithelial cells in the bulb of the hair follicle divide by mitosis cell division.

 (A) Resting stage   (B) Growth stage

 (C) Decline stage   (D) Saturation stage

17. In which hair growth stage, the hair follicle rests and the growth of hair stops

 (A) Resting stage   (B) Growth stage

 (C) Decline stage   (D) Maturation stage

18. Which of the following part consists of rapidly proliferating keratinocytes that move upward to produce the hair shaft?

 (A) Hair matrix   (B) Infundibulum

 (C) Bulge   (D) Hair root

19. The lower portion of upper part of hair follicle between the opening of the sebaceous gland and insertion of arrector pili is

   (A) Infundibulum   (B) Isthmus
   (C) Hair shaft   (D) Hair root

20. The uppermost portion of hair follicle extending from the opening of the sebaceous gland to the surface of the skin is

   (A) Hair matrix   (B) Infundibulum
   (C) Hair shaft   (D) Hair root

21. Growth stage of hair follicle cycle is called

   (A) Anagen   (B) Catagen
   (C) Exogen   (D) Kenogen

22. Resting stage of hair follicle cycle is called

   (A) Catagen   (B) Telogen
   (C) Exogen   (D) Kerogen

23. Normal hair loss in an adult per day is about

   (A) 70-100 hair per day   (B) 300-400 hair per day
   (C) 10-20 hair per day   (D) 400-500 hair per day

24. The plates of tightly packed, hard, dead keratinized epidermal cells called

   (A) Hair   (B) Nails
   (C) Gland   (D) Skin

25. Nail consists of the following parts

   (A) Nail body   (B) Free edge
   (C) Nail root   (D) All of the above

26. Which of the following is visible part of the nail and appears pinkish because of blood flowing capillaries in underlying dermis?

   (A) Nail body   (B) Nail root
   (C) Cuticle   (D) Nail fold

27. The finger nails grow at an average rate of

   (A) 1mm / week   (B) 4mm / week
   (C) 5mm / week   (D) 6mm / week

28. Sebaceous glands are also known as
   - (A) Sweat gland
   - (B) Oil gland
   - (C) Adrenal gland
   - (D) Pineal gland

29. The sebaceous gland produces an oily substance called
   - (A) Serum
   - (B) Fluids
   - (C) Sebum
   - (D) Water

30. The sebum is secreted into the hair follicles and on the skin of parts of the body except
   - (A) Palms of hand
   - (B) Soles of feet
   - (C) Both (A) and (B)
   - (D) None of the above

31. Function of sebum
   - (A) Lubricates the surface of skin and hair
   - (B) Act as bacterial and fungicidal agent
   - (C) Present the drying of skin
   - (D) All of the above

32. Component of sebum are
   - (A) Triglycerides
   - (B) Wax esters
   - (C) Squalene
   - (D) All of the above

33. Sebaceous glands are the example of
   - (A) Holocrine gland
   - (B) Apocrine gland
   - (C) Merocrine gland
   - (D) Endocrine gland

34. Which layer of epidermis receives the most nutrients from the dermal blood vessels
   - (A) Stratum corneum
   - (B) Stratum basale
   - (C) Stratum granulosum
   - (D) Stratum spinosum

35. Meissner's corpuscles located in the dermal papillae, and are responsible of sensing of
   - (A) Pain
   - (B) Bacteria
   - (C) Temperature
   - (D) Pressure

36. The subcutaneous tissue of skin is mostly made up of
   - (A) Melanin
   - (B) Fatty cells
   - (C) Muscle
   - (D) Keratin

37. Function of subcutaneous layer is/are

(A) Insulation
(B) Thermoregulation
(C) Energy reserve
(D) All of the above

38. Subcutaneous layer is thickest in the area of body such as

(A) Buttocks
(B) Palms
(C) Soles
(D) All of the above

39. which cell found in hypodermis

(A) Osteocytes
(B) Adipocytes
(C) Oocytes
(D) Gametocyte

40. The skin plays an important role in the regulation of body temperature, which is maintained at

(A) 31°C
(B) 37 °C
(C) 35°C
(D) 40°C

41. Skin regulates body temperature by

(A) Liberating sweat
(B) Adjusting flow of blood in the dermis
(C) Both (A) and (B)
(D) None of the above

42. Which of the following protects the skin from the sun's ultraviolet rays?

(A) Melanin
(B) Adipocytes
(C) Nerve cells
(D) Bone cells

43. Skin is a minor excretory organ of some substance like small amount of

(A) Salts
(B) Ammonia
(C) Urea
(D) All of the above

44. The substance that are absorbed through the skin is/are

(A) Vitamin A
(B) Vitamin D
(C) Nicotine
(D) All of the above

45. Which substance present in the skin, converted to vitamin D by the action of UV rays

(A) 7 – dehydrocholesterol
(B) Amino acid tyrosine
(C) Uridine diphosphate
(D) Deoxyribose

46. Inflammation of the skin is called

   (A) Hepatitis   (B) Dermatitis

   (C) Bronchitis   (D) Gastritis

47. Which of the following is the cause of dermatitis?

   (A) Industrial chemicals   (B) Strong acids or alkalis

   (C) Hypersensitivity reaction   (D) All of the above

48. A type of skin cancer that begins in the basal cells

   (A) Squamous cell carcinoma

   (B) Basal cell carcinoma

   (C) Malignant carcinoma

   (D) Columnar cell carcinoma

49. Which cancer produces nodular tumour and can spread to dermis, metastasize and may cause death

   (A) Squamous cell carcinoma

   (B) Basal cell carcinoma

   (C) Malignant carcinoma

   (D) Columnar cell carcinoma

50. Cutaneous receptors of skin includes

   (A) Mechanoreceptors   (B) Nociceptors

   (C) Thermoreceptors   (D) All of the above

Answer Key

Integumentary System, Skeletal System, Joints (Part-02)

Question	Answer	Question	Answer
01	A = Hair Papilla	26	A = Nail Body
02	A = Hair Shaft	27	A = 1mm/Week
03	C = Hair Follicle	28	B = Oil Gland
04	D = All of the Above	29	C = Sebum
05	C = Hair Bulb	30	C = Both A and B
06	D = All of the Above	31	D = All of the Above
07	B = Cuticle	32	D = All of the Above
08	A = Cortex	33	A = Holocrine Gland
09	B = Medulla	34	B = Stratum Basale
10	C = Cuticle	35	D = Pressure
11	A = Cortex	36	B = Fatty Cells
12	B = Medulla	37	D = All of the Above
13	A = Arrector Pili	38	D = All of the Above
14	A = Hairs Turns White	39	B = Adipocytes
15	C = Both A and B	40	B = 37^0C
16	B = Growth Stage	41	C = Both A and B
17	A = Resting Stage	42	A = Melanin
18	A = Hair Matrix	43	D = All of the Above
19	B = Isthmus	44	D = All of the Above
20	B = Infundibulum	45	A = 7-Dehydrocholesterol
21	A = Anagen	46	B = Dermatitis
22	B = Telogen	47	D = All of the above
23	A = 70-100 Hair Per Day	48	B = Basal Cell Carcinoma
24	B = Nails	49	A = Squamous Cell Carcinoma
25	D = All of the Above	50	D = All of the Above

Part-03

1. The skeletal system is the framework of
   (A) Bones
   (B) Cartilages
   (C) Both (A) and (B)
   (D) None of the above

2. The study of skeletal system is called
   (A) Osteology
   (B) Dermatology
   (C) Cardiology
   (D) Cytology

3. The branch of science concerned with the prevention or correction of disorders of the musculoskeletal system is called
   (A) Oncology
   (B) Orthopaedics
   (C) Gynaecology
   (D) Cardiology

4. The hardest connective tissue of body is
   (A) Blood
   (B) Bone
   (C) Cartilage
   (D) Tendons

5. Bone marrow present within certain bone that produce
   (A) Red blood cells
   (B) White blood cells
   (C) Platelets
   (D) All of the above

6. The process of formation of blood cells called
   (A) Haemopoiesis
   (B) Haemolysis
   (C) Hemozoin
   (D) Haematolysis

7. Bone tissue serves as the storage area of mineral salts which stores
   (A) Phosphorus and calcium
   (B) Potassium and sodium
   (C) Potassium and phosphorus
   (D) Chloride and magnesium

8. Function of skeleton system
   (A) Structure framework
   (B) Support
   (C) Protection
   (D) All of the above

9. The long cylindrical main portion of the bone that constitutes bone's shaft
   (A) Epiphysis
   (B) Diaphysis
   (C) Endosteum
   (D) Periosteum

10. The distal and proximal ends of the bone are called
    (A) Epiphysis   (B) Diaphysis
    (C) Endosteum   (D) Periosteum

11. The regions in mature bone where the diaphysis joins the epiphysis
    (A) Metaphysis   (B) Periosteum
    (C) Endosteum   (D) Medullary cavity

12. In a growing bone each metaphysis include a layer of hyaline cartilage called
    (A) Anaphyseal plate   (B) Epiphyseal plate
    (C) Diaphyseal plate   (D) Metaphyseal plate

13. A thin layer of hyaline cartilage that cover the part of epiphyses called
    (A) Diaphysis   (B) Metaphysis
    (C) Articular cartilage   (D) Endosteum

14. The tough sheath of dense irregular tissue that makes surrounding the surface of bone
    (A) Periosteum   (B) Articular cartilage
    (C) Metaphysis   (D) Diaphysis

15. Function of periosteum is
    (A) Protects the bone   (B) Helps nourish bone tissue
    (C) Helps in facture repairs   (D) All of the above

16. Bone forming cells are called
    (A) Osteoblasts   (B) Adipocytes
    (C) Nerve cell   (D) Oocytes

17. The inner layer of periosteum is also referred as
    (A) Cambium   (B) Cambium
    (C) Carrier   (D) Cuticle

18. Which of the following contains bone forming cells?
    (A) Diaphysis   (B) Metaphysis
    (C) Epiphysis   (D) Periosteum

19. Which of the following contains the blood vessels and nerve that provide nourishment and sensation to the bones?
    (A) Periosteum   (B) Metaphysis
    (C) Diaphysis   (D) Epiphysis

20. The space within diaphysis in adults that contain the fatty yellow bone marrow
    (A) Medullary cavity
    (B) Articular cartilage
    (C) Epiphysis
    (D) Diaphysis

21. Type of cells in bone tissue are
    (A) Osteocytes
    (B) Osteoblasts
    (C) Osteoclasts
    (D) All of the above

22. The resident cell type in articular cartilage is
    (A) Melanocytes
    (B) Chondrocytes
    (C) Adipocytes
    (D) Oocytes

23. The bone whose length exceed their width and consist of a shaft and two epiphyses called
    (A) Irregular bone
    (B) Flat bone
    (C) Short bone
    (D) Long bone

24. Diaphysis is mainly composed of
    (A) Compart bone
    (B) Cuticle bone
    (C) Crucial bone
    (D) Spongy bone

25. Functional units of compact bone created by network of bone cells and blood vessels is
    (A) Osteons
    (B) Osteocytes
    (C) Cancellous bone
    (D) Osteoblast

26. The softer less dense tissue that makes up the ends of bones and creates blood cells
    (A) Osteons
    (B) Osteocyte
    (C) Cancellous bone
    (D) Osteoblast

27. The bone found under the periosteum and in the diaphysis of long bones are
    (A) Compact bone
    (B) Crucial bone
    (C) Cuticle bone
    (D) Spongy bone

28. Compact bone is also called as
    (A) Cortical bone
    (B) Spongy bone
    (C) Crucial bone
    (D) Cuticle bone

29. The inner layer of long bone contains
    (A) Osteoblasts
    (B) Osteoclasts
    (C) Both (A) and (B)
    (D) All of the above

30. Longest bone of body is
    (A) Stapes bone
    (B) Femur bone
    (C) Carpal bone
    (D) Skull bones

31. Femur bone is located on
    (A) Thigh
    (B) Arms
    (C) Shoulder
    (D) Skull

32. Tibia and fibula bone are found in
    (A) Hands
    (B) Lower leg
    (C) Arms
    (D) Skull

33. Humours bone are found in
    (A) Leg
    (B) Upper arm
    (C) Thigh
    (D) Skull

34. Which bone have no shafts and have a nearly cubic shape and are almost equal in length and width is called
    (A) Long bone
    (B) Flat bone
    (C) Short bone
    (D) Irregular bone

35. Carpal bone is found in
    (A) Wrist
    (B) Skull
    (C) Pelvis
    (D) Leg

36. How many carpals bone are found in wrist
    (A) 8
    (B) 11
    (C) 7
    (D) 9

37. Which of the following is carpal bone?
    (A) Trapezoid
    (B) Capitate
    (C) Pisiform
    (D) All of the above

38. The bone located between phalanges and carpals are called
    (A) Tibia
    (B) Metacarpals
    (C) Tarsal
    (D) Fibula

39. How many bones are in the metacarpal?

(A) 10

(B) 11

(C) 5

(D) 7

40. Which of the following is not a carpal bone?

(A) Capitate

(B) Hamate

(C) Trapezium

(D) Talus

41. Tarsal bone is found in

(A) Shoulder

(B) Foot

(C) Skull

(D) Hand

42. The number of tarsal bones is

(A) 7

(B) 11

(C) 12

(D) 10

43. Which of the following is tarsal bone?

(A) Talus

(B) Navicular

(C) Calcaneus

(D) All of the above

44. Which of the following is the largest tarsal bone that projects posteriorly as the heel?

(A) Cuboid bone

(B) Calcaneus bone

(C) Cuneiform bone

(D) Talus bone

45. Which of the following bone is link between the foot and the leg through the ankle joint?

(A) Talus bone

(B) Navicular bone

(C) Cuboid bone

(D) Calcaneus bone

46. Which of the following is not a tarsal bone?

(A) Talus bone

(B) Calcaneus bone

(C) Cuneiform bone

(D) Hamate bone

47. Sternum are which type of bone

(A) Irregular bone

(B) Flat bone

(C) Long bone

(D) Short bone

48. Sternum bone are found in

(A) Chest

(B) Leg

(C) Hand

(D) Skull

49. Ribs bone is an example of

    (A) Irregular bone

    (B) Flat bone

    (C) Short bone

    (D) Long bone

50. The irregularly shaped bones that consist of spongy bone enclosed by relatively thin layers of compact bone

    (A) Long bone

    (B) Short bone

    (C) Flat bone

    (D) Irregular bone

Answer Key

Integumentary System, Skeletal System, Joints (Part-03)

Question	Answer	Question	Answer
01	C = Both A and B	26	C = Cancellous Bone
02	A = Osteology	27	A = Compact Bone
03	B = Orthopaedics	28	A = Cortical Bone
04	B = Bone	29	C = Both A and B
05	D = All of the Above	30	B = Femur Bone
06	A = Haemopoiesis	31	A = Thigh
07	A = Phosphorus and Calcium	32	B = Lower Leg
08	D = All of the Above	33	B = Upper Arm
09	B = Diaphysis	34	C = Short Bone
10	A = Epiphysis	35	A = Wrist
11	A = Metaphysis	36	A = 08
12	B = Epiphyseal Plate	37	D = All of the Above
13	C = Articular Cartilage	38	B = Metacarpals
14	A = Periosteum	39	C = 05
15	D = All of the Above	40	D = Talus
16	A = Osteoblast	41	B = Foot
17	A = Cambium	42	A = 07
18	D = Periosteum	43	D = All of the Above
19	A = Periosteum	44	B = Calcaneus Bone
20	A = Medullary Cavity	45	A = Talus Bone
21	D = All of the Above	46	D = Hamate Bone
22	B = Chondrocytes	47	B = Flat Bone
23	D = Long Bone	48	A = Chest
24	A = Compact Bone	49	B = Flat Bone
25	A = Osteons	50	D = Irregular Bone

Part-04

1. Integumentary system includes
    (A) Skin
    (B) Brain
    (C) Heart
    (D) Liver

2. The largest organ in the body is
    (A) Kidney
    (B) Skin
    (C) Liver
    (D) Lungs

3. The surface area of skin in adults is around
    (A) 1.5 – 2 square meters
    (B) 3 – 4 square meters
    (C) 2 – 3 square meters
    (D) 3.5 – 4 square meters

4. Integumentary system consists accessory structure which includes
    (A) Hair
    (B) Glands
    (C) Nails
    (D) All of the above

5. The Function of skin includes
    (A) Protects underlying structures from injury
    (B) Protects from microbial invasion
    (C) Regulation of body temperature
    (D) All of the above

6. Which of the following organ contains sensory nerve endings of pain, temperature and touch?
    (A) Liver
    (B) Heart
    (C) Stomach
    (D) Skin

7. The branch of medicine specialized for diagnosis and treatment of skin disorder
    (A) Urology
    (B) Dermatology
    (C) Neurology
    (D) Ophthalmology

8. Skin is thickest on
    (A) Palms of the hands
    (B) Soles of the feet
    (C) Both (A) and (B)
    (D) None of the above

9. Which of the following is the outermost layer of skin?
   - (A) Epidermis
   - (B) Hypodermis
   - (C) Dermis
   - (D) Subcutaneous layer

10. The epidermal layer of skin is composed of
   - (A) Simple cuboidal epithelium
   - (B) Simple squamous epithelium
   - (C) Stratified squamous keratinized epithelium
   - (D) Simple columnar epithelium

11. Which layer found below the epidermis
   - (A) Dermis
   - (B) Hypodermis
   - (C) Sweat glands
   - (D) Hair bulb

12. Which of the following is the deepest layer of skin?
   - (A) Epidermis
   - (B) Hypodermis
   - (C) Dermis
   - (D) Hair root

13. Which layer of skin provides a waterproof barrier and contribute to skin tone
   - (A) Sweat gland
   - (B) Hypodermis
   - (C) Dermis
   - (D) Epidermis

14. Which layer of skin found beneath the epidermis, contains connective tissue, hair follicles, blood vessels, lymphatic vessels and sweat glands
   - (A) Epidermis
   - (B) Dermis
   - (C) Hypodermis
   - (D) Subcutaneous tissue

15. Deeper subcutaneous tissue layer
   - (A) Hypodermis
   - (B) Epidermis
   - (C) Dermis
   - (D) Sebaceous gland

16. Which layer of skin made up of fat and connective tissue
   - (A) Epidermis
   - (B) Hypodermis
   - (C) Dermis
   - (D) Sebaceous gland

17. Skin is made up of
   - (A) Water
   - (B) Proteins
   - (C) Fats
   - (D) All of the above

18. Which cell is responsible for imparting colour of skin?

(A) Osteocytes

(B) Melanocytes

(C) Leukocytes

(D) Adipocytes

19. Which part of skin does not contain any blood vessels?

(A) Epidermis

(B) Dermis

(C) Hypodermis

(D) Sebaceous gland

20. The small rounded bones that assist in the functioning of muscles

(A) Sesamoid bone

(B) Flat bone

(C) Short bone

(D) Long bone

21. Patella bone is example of which type of bone

(A) Flat bone

(B) Short bone

(C) Sesamoid bone

(D) Long bone

22. Patella bone are found in

(A) Skull

(B) Arms

(C) Knee joint

(D) Shoulder

23. Bone is a strong and durable connective tissue the consists of the

(A) Extracellular matrix

(B) The bone cells

(C) Both (A) and (B)

(D) None of the above

24. The amount of water in extracellular matrix is around

(A) 25 %

(B) 60 %

(C) 5 %

(D) 11 %

25. The amount of collagen fibers in extracellular matrix is

(A) 60 %

(B) 50%

(C) 25 %

(D) 06 %

26. The amount of crystallized mineral salts in extracellular matrix is

(A) 05 %

(B) 50 %

(C) 25 %

(D) 15 %

27. Which of the following crystallized mineral salts present in extracellular matrix?

(A) Calcium phosphate

(B) Calcium hydroxide

(C) Calcium carbonate

(D) All of the above

28. A large multinuclear cell associated with the reabsorption of bone

    (A) Osteoblasts   (B) Osteoclasts
    (C) Osteocytes   (D) Osteogenic cells

29. A mature bone cell involved with the maintenance of bone

    (A) Osteocytes   (B) Osteoblasts
    (C) Osteoclasts   (D) Osteogenic cells

30. A mononucleated cell from which bone develops

    (A) Osteoclasts   (B) Osteoblasts
    (C) Osteocytes   (D) Osteogenic cells

31. Which of the following is only bone cell that divides?

    (A) Osteogenic cells   (B) Osteoblasts
    (C) Osteoclasts   (D) Osteocytes

32. Osteoblasts are present in

    (A) Deeper layers of periosteum   (B) Ends of diaphysis
    (C) At the fracture site   (D) All of the above

33. Which bone cells breakdown and release calcium and phosphate

    (A) Osteoblasts   (B) Osteoclasts
    (C) Osteogenic cells   (D) Osteocytes

34. Osteoclasts are giant cells with up to

    (A) 50 nuclei   (B) 10 nuclei
    (C) 5 nuclei   (D) 15 nuclei

35. The bone – reabsorbing cells are

    (A) Osteoblasts   (B) Osteoclasts
    (C) Osteocytes   (D) Osteogenic cells

36. Between the rings of matrix, the osteocytes are located in spaces called

    (A) Lacunae   (B) Lamina
    (C) Cisternae   (D) Cristae

37. Which cells secrete collagen and other organic components required to
    build extracellular matrix of bone tissues

    (A) Osteoclasts   (B) Osteoblasts
    (C) Osteogenic cells   (D) Osteocytes

38. Which bone cells are entrapped in matrix?
    (A) Osteocytes
    (B) Osteoblasts
    (C) Osteocytes
    (D) Osteogenic cells

39. Which of the following are types of bone tissues?
    (A) Compact or dense bone
    (B) Cancellous or spongy bone
    (C) Both (A) and (B)
    (D) None of the above

40. How much body bone mass makes up compact bone tissue?
    (A) 80 %
    (B) 20 %
    (C) 30 %
    (D) 15 %

41. Each osteon is made up of a
    (A) Cuticle canal
    (B) Central canal
    (C) Crucial canal
    (D) Critical canal

42. Which bone cells contains powerful lysosomal enzymes and acids that digest the protein and mineral components of the bone matrix
    (A) Osteoclasts
    (B) Osteoblasts
    (C) Osteocytes
    (D) Osteogenic cells

43. Osteon consists central canal which is called as
    (A) Tubular canal
    (B) Alimentary canal
    (C) Volkmann's canal
    (D) Osteonic canal

44. Osteonic canal is also known as
    (A) Harversian canal
    (B) Volkmann's canal
    (C) Tubular canal
    (D) Alimentary canal

45. Which canal run parallel to the surface of bone and contain blood vessels
    (A) Osteonic canal
    (B) Tubular canal
    (C) Volkmann's canal
    (D) Sesamoid canal

46. Which blood vessels contains in osteonic canal
    (A) Capillaries
    (B) Arterioles
    (C) Venules
    (D) All of the above

47. The blood vessels in central canal brings

     (A) Oxygen   (B) Nutrient

     (C) Waste products   (D) All of the above

48. The lacunae are connecting to each other and to larger harversian canals by small canals called

     (A) Canaliculi   (B) Calcaneus

     (C) Cuneiform   (D) Cuticle

49. Compact bone is made up of concentric rings of osteocytes called

     (A) Lamellae   (B) Osteons

     (C) Canaliculi   (D) Cuticle

50. Osteocyte receive their nutrients via

     (A) Canaliculi   (B) Cuticle

     (C) Calcaneus   (D) Cuneiform

Answer Key

Integumentary System, Skeletal System, Joints (Part-04)

Question	Answer	Question	Answer
01	A = Skin	26	B = 50%
02	B = Skin	27	D = All of the Above
03	A = 1.5 to 2 Square Meter	28	B = Osteoclasts
04	D = All of the Above	29	A = Osteocytes
05	D = All of the Above	30	B = Osteoblast
06	D = Skin	31	A = Osteogenic Cells
07	B = Dermatology	32	D = All of the Above
08	C = Both A and B	33	B = Osteoclasts
09	A = Epidermis	34	A = 50 Nuclei
10	C = Stratified Squamous Keratinized Epithelium	35	B = Osteoclast
11	A = Dermis	36	A = Lacunae
12	B = Hypodermis	37	B = Osteoblasts
13	B = Hypodermis	38	C = Osteocytes
14	B = Dermis	39	C = Both A and B
15	A = Hypodermis	40	A = 80%
16	B = Hypodermis	41	B = Central Canal
17	D = All of the Above	42	A = Osteoclast
18	B = Melanocytes	43	D = Osteonic Canal
19	A = Epidermis	44	A = Haversian Canal
20	A = Sesamoid Bone	45	A = Osteonic Canal
21	C = Sesamoid Bone	46	D = All of the Above
22	C = Knee Joint	47	D = All of the Above
23	C = Both A and B	48	A = Canaliculi
24	A = 25%	49	A = Lamellae
25	C = 25%	50	A = Canaliculi

Part-05

1. Each central canal is linked with neighbouring canals that run horizontally to the central canal
   - (A) Volkmann's canals
   - (B) Haversian canals
   - (C) Osteonic canals
   - (D) Tubular canals

2. The spaces between adjacent osteons are filled with
   - (A) Canaliculi
   - (B) Lamella
   - (C) Interstitial lamellae
   - (D) Fontanelle

3. Which of the following contain fragments of older osteons that have been partially destroyed during bone remodelling or growth?
   - (A) Canaliculi
   - (B) Interstitial lamellae
   - (C) Fontanelle
   - (D) Lacunae

4. Which of the following allows the circulation of interstitial fluid through the bone and make direct contact between the osteocytes?
   - (A) Canaliculi
   - (B) Lamella
   - (C) Osteons
   - (D) Endosteum

5. Volkmann's canals are also known as
   - (A) Perforating holes
   - (B) Haversian canal
   - (C) Osteonic canal
   - (D) Tubular canal

6. Which canal connect adjacent osteons and also connect the blood vessels of haversian canals with the periosteum
   - (A) Osteonic canal
   - (B) Haversian canal
   - (C) Volkmann's canals
   - (D) Alimentary canal

7. Volkmann's canals also contain nutritional vessels arising from the
   - (A) Periosteal bone surface
   - (B) Endosteal bone surface
   - (C) Both (A) and (B)
   - (D) None of the above

8. Volkmann's canal found in
   - (A) Spongy bone
   - (B) Trabecular bone
   - (C) Compact bone
   - (D) Cancellous bone

9. Volkmann's canal contains capillaries that bring
   - (A) Oxygen
   - (B) Nutrients
   - (C) Remove waste
   - (D) All of the above

10. Which bone located at the ends of long bones and forms the centre of all other bones
   - (A) Spongy bone
   - (B) Compact bone
   - (C) Cortical bone
   - (D) Cortex bone

11. Spongy bone is also called as
   - (A) Tubular bone
   - (B) Compact bone
   - (C) Trabecular bone
   - (D) Cortical cone

12. Spongy bone consists of a framework of interconnecting sections called
   - (A) Tubular
   - (B) Cisternae
   - (C) Trabeculae
   - (D) Cuticle

13. How much of skeletal bone mass is spongy bone
   - (A) 50%
   - (B) 20%
   - (C) 80%
   - (D) 60%

14. Spongy bone is composed of cells called
   - (A) Osteoblasts
   - (B) Osteoclasts
   - (C) Osteocytes
   - (D) Osteogenic cells

15. Which bone tissue does not contain osteons?
   - (A) Cortical bone tissue
   - (B) Compact bone tissue
   - (C) Dense bone tissue
   - (D) Spongy bone tissue

16. Function of trabecular bone
   - (A) Bone strength
   - (B) Structural stability
   - (C) Flexibility
   - (D) All of the above

17. The spaces between the trabeculae are filled with
   - (A) Yellow collagen fibres
   - (B) Red bone marrow
   - (C) White collagen fibres
   - (D) Cartilage fibrous

18. The process of formation of bone is called
   - (A) Ossification
   - (B) Haematopoiesis
   - (C) Erythropoiesis
   - (D) Thrombopoiesis

19. The skeleton of a developing foetus is completely formed by the end of the
    (A) Ninth month of pregnancy
    (B) Eight months of pregnancy
    (C) First month of pregnancy
    (D) Third month of pregnancy

20. Ossification is also called
    (A) Osteogenesis
    (B) Histogenesis
    (C) Glucogenesis
    (D) Haematopoiesis

21. Type of ossification is/are
    (A) Intramembranous ossification
    (B) Endochondral ossification
    (C) Both (A) and (B)
    (D) None of the above

22. The method of bone formation results in the formation of flat bones as in the skull and mandible
    (A) Endochondral ossification
    (B) Intramembranous ossification
    (C) Extra membranous ossification
    (D) Extra chondral ossification

23. The direct conversion of mesenchymal tissue into bone is called
    (A) Intramembranous ossification
    (B) Endochondral ossification
    (C) Extra membranous ossification
    (D) Extra chondral ossification

24. Which of the following involves the replacement of sheet like connective tissue membranes with bony tissue?
    (A) Extra membranous ossification
    (B) Endochondral ossification
    (C) Intramembranous ossification
    (D) Extra chondral ossification

25. Which bones formed via intramembranous ossification
    (A) Flat bones of the face
    (B) Most of the cranial bones
    (C) Clavicles
    (D) All of the above

26. Which spots help the fatal skull pass through the birth canal
   (A) Soft spots
   (B) Hard spots
   (C) Flat spots
   (D) Long spots

27. The mesenchymal cells cluster together at the site of bone development is called as
   (A) Ossification centre
   (B) Fontanelle
   (C) Interstitial lamellae
   (D) Canaliculi

28. At ossification centre, the mesenchymal cells differentiate into osteogenic cell and then further differentiate into
   (A) Osteoclasts
   (B) Osteoblasts
   (C) Periosteum
   (D) Metaphysis

29. During intramembranous ossification osteoblasts secretes
   (A) Extracellular matrix
   (B) Intracellular matrix
   (C) Interstitial fluids
   (D) Intracellular fluids

30. Which extracellular matrix protein secreted by osteoblasts during intramembranous ossification
   (A) Collagen
   (B) Keratin
   (C) Ferritin
   (D) Alanine

31. The osteoblasts get surrounded by the extracellular matrix and develop into
   (A) Osteogenic cells
   (B) Osteoclasts
   (C) Osteocytes
   (D) Fontanelle

32. Which organic matrix are contained in extracellular matrix?
   (A) Proteoglycans
   (B) Glycoproteins
   (C) Glycosaminoglycans
   (D) All of the above

33. The process in which bone formation occurs by the replacement of cartilage with bone is called
   (A) Endochondral ossification
   (B) Intramembranous ossification
   (C) Extra membranous ossification
   (D) Interstitial ossification

34. The chondroblasts secrete the cartilage extracellular matrix and develop into a
    (A) Tendons model
    (B) Ligament model
    (C) Cartilage model
    (D) Endosteum model

35. Cartilage model consists
    (A) Hyaline cartilage
    (B) Elastic cartilage
    (C) Thyroid cartilage
    (D) Cricoid cartilage

36. At the site of bone development, the mesenchymal cells cluster together and differentiate into
    (A) Osteoblast
    (B) Osteocyte
    (C) Chondrocytes
    (D) Osteogenic cells

37. Blood vessels penetrate the cartilage and new osteoblasts form a
    (A) Primary ossification centre
    (B) Secondary ossification centre
    (C) Tertiary ossification centre
    (D) Quaternary ossification centre

38. Blood vessels invade the epiphyses and osteoblasts form
    (A) Primary ossification centre
    (B) Secondary ossification centre
    (C) Tertiary ossification centre
    (D) Quaternary ossification centre

39. Primary ossification proceeds inward from the external surface of the forming
    (A) Fontanelle
    (B) Spongy trabeculae
    (C) Lamella
    (D) Lacunae

40. Around birth secondary centres of ossification develop in the
    (A) Epiphyses
    (B) Endosteum
    (C) Diaphysis
    (D) Metaphysis

41. The osteoblasts break down some of the newly formed spongy trabeculae in the centre and form a
    (A) Medullary canal
    (B) Tubular canal
    (C) Cuticle canal
    (D) Laminar canal

42. Most of the walls of diaphysis are replaced by

    (A) Compact bone
    (B) Trabecular bone
    (C) Cuticle bone
    (D) Crucial bone

43. Which cells are responsible for bone deposition

    (A) Osteoclasts
    (B) Osteoblasts
    (C) Osteocytes
    (D) Osteogenic cells

44. The process of addition of minerals and collagen fibres to the bone resulting in formation of the bone extracellular matrix is called

    (A) Bone resorption
    (B) Bone deposition
    (C) Bone destruction
    (D) Bone removal

45. The growing bone need small amount of minerals, which are

    (A) Fluoride
    (B) Magnesium
    (C) Iron
    (D) All of the above

46. Which vitamin is required for collagen synthesis in bone?

    (A) Vitamin A
    (B) Vitamin C
    (C) Vitamin K
    (D) Vitamin B

47. Which of the following hormone regulate the growth and remodelling of bone?

    (A) Growth hormones
    (B) Thyroxin
    (C) Tri - iodothyronine
    (D) All of the above

48. Which hormones control the level of calcium in blood

    (A) Parathyroid hormones
    (B) Calcitonin
    (C) Both (A) and (B)
    (D) None of the above

49. Parathyroid hormone maintains the blood calcium levels by

    (A) Release of calcium from the bone into blood
    (B) Decrease loss of calcium from the urine
    (C) Promote the absorption of calcium from food
    (D) All of the above

50. The increase in the blood calcium level stimulates the thyroid gland to secrete

    (A) Oxytocin
    (B) Calcitonin
    (C) Follicle stimulating hormone
    (D) Melatonin

Answer Key

Integumentary System, Skeletal System, Joints (Part-05)

Question	Answer	Question	Answer
01	A = Volkmann's canals	26	A = Soft Sports
02	C = Interstitial Lamellae	27	A = Ossification Centre
03	B = Interstitial Lamellae	28	B = Osteoblast
04	A = Canaliculi	29	A = Extracellular Matrix
05	A = Perforating Holes	30	A = Collagen
06	C = Volkmann's Canals	31	C = Osteocytes
07	C = Both A and B	32	D = All of the above
08	C = Compact Bone	33	A = Endochondral Ossification
09	D = All of the Above	34	C = Cartilage Model
10	A = Spongy Bone	35	A = Hyaline Cartilage
11	C = Trabeculae	36	C = Chondrocytes
12	C = Trabeculae	37	A = Primary Ossification Centre
13	B = 20%	38	B = Secondary Ossification Centre
14	C = Osteocytes	39	B = Spongy Trabeculae
15	D = Spongy Bone Tissue	40	A = Epiphyses
16	D = All of the Above	41	A = Medullary Canal
17	B = Red Bone Marrow	42	A = Compact Bone
18	A = Ossification	43	B = Osteoblast
19	D = Third Month of Pregnancy	44	B = Bone Deposition
20	A = Osteogenesis	45	D = All of the Above
21	C = Both A and B	46	B = Vitamin C
22	B = Intramembranous Ossification	47	D = All of the Above
23	A = Intramembranous Ossification	48	C = Both A and B
24	C = Intramembranous Ossification	49	D = All of the Above
25	D = All of the Above	50	B = Calcitonin

Part-06

1. The broken end of the bone protrudes through the skin is called
   - (A) Impacted fracture
   - (B) Open fracture
   - (C) Comminated fracture
   - (D) Closed fracture

2. Open fracture is also called as
   - (A) Compound fracture
   - (B) Impacted fracture
   - (C) Closed fracture
   - (D) Comminated fracture

3. The broken bone ends do not protrude through the skin
   - (A) Closed fracture
   - (B) Open fracture
   - (C) Simple fracture
   - (D) Impacted fracture

4. Closed fracture is also called as
   - (A) Open fracture
   - (B) Compound fracture
   - (C) Simple fracture
   - (D) Impacted fracture

5. The bone breaks into small fragments at the impact site and the smaller bone fragments lies between the two main fragments
   - (A) Simple fracture
   - (B) Comminuted fracture
   - (C) Closed fracture
   - (D) Open fracture

6. One end of the fractured bone is forcefully pushed into the interior of the other is called
   - (A) Simple fracture
   - (B) Compound fracture
   - (C) Closed fracture
   - (D) Impacted fracture

7. The break goes completely through the bone and separating it in two called
   - (A) Complete fracture
   - (B) Open fracture
   - (C) Close fracture
   - (D) Compound fracture

8. A gap forms where the bone breaks and after this injury requires surgery to fix
   - (A) Open fracture
   - (B) Closed fracture
   - (C) Displaced fracture
   - (D) Simple fracture

9. Bone segments are pulled a part as a result of twisting motion is called
    (A) Open fracture
    (B) Spiral fracture
    (C) Closed fracture
    (D) Simple fracture

10. Which fracture occurs straight across the long axis of the bone
    (A) Closed fracture
    (B) Transverse fracture
    (C) Compound fracture
    (D) Simple fracture

11. As the blood vessels break at the fracture site, the blood leaks out and forms a clot called
    (A) Fracture hyaline
    (B) Fracture haematoma
    (C) Fracture haemolysis
    (D) Fracture haematogenesis

12. Formation of fracture hematoma also called
    (A) Inflammatory phase
    (B) Intramedullary phase
    (C) Interstitial phase
    (D) Extracellular phase

13. Which of the following is first stage of healing that occurs immediately after the injury?
    (A) Reparative phase
    (B) Intramedullary phase
    (C) Inflammatory phase
    (D) Bone remodelling

14. The inflammatory phase ends approximately after what time of the fracture
    (A) 1 – 2 weeks
    (B) 4 - 6 weeks
    (C) 10 – 12 weeks
    (D) 14 – 16 weeks

15. During the formation of fracture hematoma, inflammatory reaction results in the release of
    (A) Cytokinin
    (B) Growth factors
    (C) Prostaglandins
    (D) All of the above

16. Fibroblasts and cells of periosteum invade the fracture site and begin to produce collagen fibres and fibrocartilage which lead to the development of the mass of repair tissue called
    (A) Fibrocartilaginous callus
    (B) Fibro tendonous callus
    (C) Fibroligamentenous callus
    (D) Fibro filament callus

17. Fibrocartilaginous callus mainly consists of
    (A) Collagen fibres
    (B) Cartilage fibres
    (C) Both (A) and (B)
    (D) None of the above

18. Osteoblasts convert fibrocartilage into spongy bone and the callus is the preferred as

   (A) Soft callus
   (B) Flat callus
   (C) Bony callus
   (D) Irregular callus

19. Formation of callus is also called

   (A) Inflammatory phase
   (B) Reparative phase
   (C) Remodelling phase
   (D) Intramedullary phase

20. Formation of callus stage may last up to

   (A) 2 – 16 weeks
   (B) 1 – 2 weeks
   (C) 18 – 20 weeks
   (D) 20 – 25 weeks

21. The final stage of fracture repair is

   (A) Inflammatory phase
   (B) Reparative phase
   (C) Bone remodelling
   (D) Intramedullary phase

22. In which stage the bony callus is remoded by osteoclasts and osteoblasts

   (A) Bone remodelling
   (B) Inflammatory phase
   (C) Reparative phase
   (D) Intramedullary phase

23. How many bones consists in adult human skeleton?

   (A) 200 bones
   (B) 206 bones
   (C) 210 bones
   (D) 211 bones

24. The bones of skeleton are divided into

   (A) Axial skeleton
   (B) Appendicular skeleton
   (C) Both (A) and (B)
   (D) None of the above

25. The axial skeleton consists of the

   (A) Skull
   (B) Vertebral column
   (C) Ribs and sternum
   (D) All of the above

26. How many bones consist in axial skeleton?

   (A) 80 bones
   (B) 75 bones
   (C) 85 bones
   (D) 90 bones

27. How many bones consists in appendicular skeleton?

   (A) 122 bones
   (B) 126 bones
   (C) 130 bones
   (D) 131 bones

28. The appendicular skeleton consists of
    (A) Shoulder girdle with the upper limbs
    (B) Pelvic girdle with the lower limbs
    (C) Both (A) and (B)
    (D) None of the above

29. The bone structure that forms the head in vertebrates called
    (A) Skull   (B) Pelvic
    (C) Ribs   (D) Arms

30. The bones of the skull are divided into
    (A) Cranial bones   (B) Facial bones
    (C) Both (A) and (B)   (D) None of the above

31. Total number of bones in the human skull is
    (A) 22   (B) 18
    (C) 14   (D) 20

32. How many cranial bones are there?
    (A) 10   (B) 8
    (C) 11   (D) 12

33. The main function of cranial bone is
    (A) Enclose and protect the brain
    (B) Enclose and protect the liver
    (C) Enclose and protect the kidney
    (D) Enclose and protect the lungs

34. Cranial bones are united or joined by immovable joints called
    (A) Socket   (B) Ball
    (C) Sutures   (D) Hinge

35. Which of the following is cranial bones?
    (A) Frontal bones   (B) Parietal bones
    (C) Temporal bones   (D) All of the above

36. Which bone forms the forehead
    (A) Frontal bone   (B) Sternum bone
    (C) Mandible   (D) Maxilla

37. How many frontal bones are there?
    (A) 4
    (B) 3
    (C) 5
    (D) 1

38. The bone markings on the frontal bone are
    (A) Orbital margin
    (B) Suborbital margin
    (C) Both (A) and (B)
    (D) None of the above

39. The frontal bone and parietal bone are joined by suture called
    (A) Cortical suture
    (B) Coronal suture
    (C) Squamous suture
    (D) Sagittal suture

40. Which bones form the sides and roof of the skull
    (A) Maxilla
    (B) Parietal bone
    (C) Sternum bone
    (D) Mandible

41. The parietal bone and temporal bone are joined by a suture called
    (A) Coronal suture
    (B) Squamous suture
    (C) Lambdoidal suture
    (D) Sagittal suture

42. The parietal bone and occipital bone are joined by a suture called
    (A) Squamous suture
    (B) Sagittal suture
    (C) Coronal suture
    (D) Lambdoidal suture

43. Which of the following is part of temporal bone?
    (A) Squamous
    (B) Petrous
    (C) Mastoid
    (D) All of the above

44. Largest and most superior part of temporal bone
    (A) Squamous
    (B) Petrous
    (C) Mastoid
    (D) Coronal

45. Which part of the temporal bone is thin fan – shaped area that articulates with the parietal bone?
    (A) Petrous
    (B) Mastoid
    (C) Squamous
    (D) Coronal

46. Which bone surrounds the ears and protects nerves and structures that play a role in controlling hearing and balance
    (A) Frontal bone
    (B) Nasal bone
    (C) Lacrimal bone
    (D) Temporal bone

47. Which bone articulate with the mandible at the temporomandibular joint

   (A) Temporal bone   (B) Frontal bone

   (C) Nasal bone   (D) Lacrimal bone

48. Which bone forms the back of the head and part of the base of the skull

   (A) Nasal bone   (B) Lacrimal bone

   (C) Occipital bone   (D) Mandible

49. The inferior portion of occipital bone has a large opening called

   (A) Foramen magnum   (B) Coronal

   (C) Orbital margin   (D) Suture

50. Which bone occupies the middle portion of the base of the skull

   (A) Maxilla   (B) Sphenoid bone

   (C) Nasal bone   (D) Mandible

Answer Key

Integumentary System, Skeletal System, Joints (Part-06)

Question	Answer	Question	Answer
01	B = Open Fracture	26	A = 80 Bones
02	A = Compound Fracture	27	B = 126 Bones
03	A = Closed Fracture	28	C = Both A and B
04	C = Simple Fracture	29	A = Skull
05	B = Comminuted Fracture	30	C = Both A and B
06	D = Impacted Fracture	31	A = 22
07	A = Complete Fracture	32	B = 08
08	C = Displaced Fracture	33	A = Enclose and Protect the Brain
09	B = Spiral Fracture	34	C = Suture
10	B = Transverse Fracture	35	D = All of the Above
11	B = Fractured Haematoma	36	A = Frontal Bone
12	A = Inflammatory Phase	37	D = 01
13	C = Inflammatory Phase	38	C = Both A and B
14	A = 1-2 Weeks	39	B = Coronal Suture
15	D = All of the Above	40	B = Parietal Bone
16	A = Fibrocartilaginous Callus	41	B = Squamous Suture
17	C = Both A and B	42	D = Lambdoidal Suture
18	C = Bony Callus	43	D = All of the Above
19	B = Reparative Phase	44	A = Squamous
20	A = 2-16 Weeks	45	C = Squamous
21	C = Bone Remodelling	46	D = Temporal Bone
22	A = Bone Remodelling	47	A = Temporal Bone
23	B = 206 Bones	48	C = Occipital Bone
24	C = Both A and B	49	A = Foramen Magnum
25	D = All of the Above	50	B = Sphenoid Bone

Part-07

1. Which bone acts as an anchor binding all the cranial bones together
   (A) Nasal bone
   (B) Frontal bone
   (C) Parietal bone
   (D) Sphenoid bone

2. Which of the bone shape resembles a bat with outstretched wings?
   (A) Sphenoid bone
   (B) Parietal bone
   (C) Nasal bone
   (D) Lacrimal bone

3. The body of the sphenoid bone contains
   (A) Occipital sinuses
   (B) Sphenoid sinuses
   (C) Temporal sinuses
   (D) Frontal sinuses

4. Sphenoidal sinuses open into
   (A) Nasal cavity
   (B) Parietal cavity
   (C) Coronal suture
   (D) Temporal cavity

5. The middle portion of the sphenoid bone has a little saddle – shaped depression on the superior surface called as
   (A) Hypophyseal fossa
   (B) Hypoglossal fossa
   (C) Hyperglossal fossa
   (D) Hyperphysea fossa

6. In hypophyseal fossa which gland rests
   (A) Thyroid gland
   (B) Adrenal gland
   (C) Pituitary gland
   (D) Salivary gland

7. Hypophyseal gland of sphenoid bone also contain
   (A) Optic foramen
   (B) Passage of the optic (II) nerve
   (C) Ophthalmic artery
   (D) All of the above

8. Which of the following is the lightest of the cranial bones?
   (A) Ethmoid bone
   (B) Parietal bone
   (C) Temporal bone
   (D) Occipital bone

9. Ethmoid bone helps form
   - (A) Orbital cavity
   - (B) Nasa septum
   - (C) Lateral walls of the nasal cavity
   - (D) All of the above

10. The horizontal part of ethmoid bone called
   - (A) Cribriform plate
   - (B) Crucible plate
   - (C) Crucial plate
   - (D) Cortex plate

11. On each side of the ethmoid bone have projections into nasal cavity which are
   - (A) The superior conchae
   - (B) The middle conchae
   - (C) Both (A) and (B)
   - (D) None of the above

12. How many facial bones are there?
   - (A) 14
   - (B) 20
   - (C) 21
   - (D) 22

13. Which bone is commonly called cheek bones?
   - (A) Zygomatic bones
   - (B) Parietal bones
   - (C) Frontal bone
   - (D) Temporal bone

14. Which bone form the prominences of the cheeks and part of the floor and lateral walls of orbital cavities
   - (A) Parietal bones
   - (B) Zygomatic bones
   - (C) Frontal bones
   - (D) Lacrimal bones

15. Zygomatic bones articulate with the
   - (A) Frontal bone
   - (B) Maxilla
   - (C) Sphenoid bone
   - (D) All of the above

16. Which bones forms the zygomatic arch by articulation with the temporal bone
   - (A) Zygomatic bones
   - (B) Frontal bones
   - (C) Mandible
   - (D) Lumbar bones

17. Which of the following bone is upper jaw bone?
   - (A) Maxilla
   - (B) Mandible
   - (C) Frontal bone
   - (D) Parietal bone

18. How many maxilla bone is there
    (A) 3
    (B) 2
    (C) 4
    (D) 5

19. Maxilla articulate with every bone of the face except
    (A) Nasal bone
    (B) Mandible
    (C) Lacrimal bone
    (D) Frontal bone

20. Maxilla forms the
    (A) Upper jaw
    (B) Part of the floor of orbital cavities
    (C) Part of the lateral walls
    (D) All of the above

21. Which sinus contain maxilla that opens into the nasal cavity
    (A) Maxillary sinus
    (B) Sphenoidal sinus
    (C) Parietal sinus
    (D) Occipital sinus

22. Which bones meet at the midline of the face and form the bridge of the nose
    (A) Mandible
    (B) Parietal bone
    (C) Nasal bone
    (D) Occipital bone

23. The rest of the supporting tissues of the nose consist of
    (A) Cartilage
    (B) Ligament
    (C) Tendons
    (D) Fats

24. The two smallest bones located in the face are
    (A) Parietal bone
    (B) Lacrimal bone
    (C) Mandible
    (D) Occipital bone

25. Which bones is posterior and lateral to the nasal bones and form part of the medial walls of the orbital cavities?
    (A) Frontal bone
    (B) Temporal bone
    (C) Parietal bone
    (D) Lacrimal bone

26. Which duct carries the tears from the eyes towards nasal cavity
    (A) Nasolacrimal duct
    (B) Parotid duct
    (C) Sublingual duct
    (D) Cystic duct

27. Nasolacrimal duct is also called

   (A) Saliva duct   (B) Tear duct
   (C) Bile duct   (D) Parotid duct

28. A thin flat bone on the floor of the nasal cavity that articulates superiorly with the perpendicular plate of the ethmoid bone is called

   (A) Vomer bone   (B) Parietal bone
   (C) Nasal bone   (D) Mandible

29. Which bone forms the inferior portion of the nasal septum

   (A) Parietal bone   (B) Maxilla
   (C) Vomer bone   (D) Mandible

30. Which of the following bone is a paired, L – shaped facial bone?

   (A) Nasal bone   (B) Lacrimal bone
   (C) Palatine bone   (D) Mandible

31. Palatine bones form the

   (A) Posterior portion of hard palate
   (B) Part of the floor and lateral walls of the nasal cavity
   (C) A small portion of the floor of the orbital cavities
   (D) All of the above

32. The bones are very thin and fragile and present on the lateral side of each nostril

   (A) Parietal bone   (B) Inferior conchae
   (C) Mandible   (D) Zygomatic bone

33. The superior and middle conchae are parts of the

   (A) Ethmoid bone   (B) Parietal bone
   (C) Occipital bone   (D) Temporal bone

34. Function of nasal conchae

   (A) Increase the surface are of nasal cavity
   (B) Providing rapid warming
   (C) Filtered air before it passes into lungs
   (D) All of the above

35. Which of the following is largest and strongest facial bone?

   (A) Nasal bone   (B) Mandible

   (C) Vomer bone   (D) Lacrimal bone

36. Which of the following is lower jaw bone?

   (A) Mandible   (B) Maxilla

   (C) Nasal bone   (D) Lacrimal bone

37. Which bone is only movable bone of the skull?

   (A) Nasal bone   (B) Palatine bone

   (C) Vomer bone   (D) Mandible

38. The mandible is composed of

   (A) The curved body   (B) The ramus

   (C) Both (A) and (B)   (D) None of the above

39. At the upper end the ramus divides into the condylar process the articulates
    with the temporal bone to form

   (A) Temporomandibular joint   (B) Temporoparietal joint

   (C) Nasal mandibular joint   (D) Parietal mandibular joint

40. A variety of movement occurs at the temporomandibular joint and the
    movements are

   (A) Mandibular depression   (B) Elevation

   (C) Lateral deviation   (D) All of the above

41. Which bone is vertical partition that divides the inside of the nose into the
    right and left sides?

   (A) Nasal septum   (B) Hyoid bone

   (C) Fontanelles   (D) Sinuses

42. The component of nasal septum is

   (A) Vomer

   (B) Septal cartilage

   (C) The perpendicular plate of the ethmoid bone

   (D) All of the above

43. The term "broken nose" often refers to the damage to the

   (A) Septal cartilage   (B) Meniscal cartilage

   (C) Articular cartilage   (D) Lateral cartilage

44. The single horse – shoe shaped bone located in the anterior neck between the mandible and the larynx
    (A) Nasal septum
    (B) Parietal bone
    (C) Hyoid bone
    (D) Temporal bone

45. The only bone in humans that does not articulate with any other bone are
    (A) Temporal bone
    (B) Mandible
    (C) Frontal bone
    (D) Hyoid bone

46. Which bone acts as a support for tongue and its associated muscles
    (A) Hyoid bone
    (B) Maxilla
    (C) Temporal bone
    (D) Nasal septum

47. Which bone helps elevate the larynx during swallowing and speech
    (A) Nasal septum
    (B) Hyoid bone
    (C) Frontal bone
    (D) Temporal bone

48. The major fontanelles present in the skull at birth are
    (A) Anterior fontanelle
    (B) Posterior fontanelle
    (C) Both (A) and (B)
    (D) None of the above

49. Which of the following is the largest fontanelle and is located between parietal bones and the cranial bone?
    (A) Anterior fontanelle
    (B) Posterior fontanelle
    (C) Lateral fontanelle
    (D) Inferior fontanelle

50. Which fontanelle usually closes 18 – 24 months after birth
    (A) Posterior fontanelle
    (B) Anterior fontanelle
    (C) Lateral fontanelle
    (D) Distal fontanelle

Answer Key

Integumentary System, Skeletal System, Joints (Part-07)

Question	Answer	Question	Answer
01	D = Sphenoid Bone	26	A = Nasolacrimal Duct
02	A = Sphenoid Bone	27	B = Tear Duct
03	B = Sphenoid Bone	28	A = Vomer Bone
04	A = Nasal Cavity	29	C = Vomer Bone
05	A = Hypophyseal Fossa	30	C = Palatine Bone
06	C = Pituitary Gland	31	D = All of the Above
07	D = All of the Above	32	B = Inferior Conchae
08	A = Ethmoid Bone	33	A = Ethmoid Bone
09	D = All of the Above	34	D = All of the Above
10	A = Cribriform Plate	35	B = Mandible
11	C = Both A and B	36	A = Mandible
12	A = 14	37	D = Mandible
13	A = Zygomatic Bone	38	C = Both A and B
14	B = Zygomatic Bone	39	A = Temporomandibular Joint
15	D = All of the Above	40	D = All of the Above
16	A = Zygomatic Bones	41	A = Nasal Septum
17	A = Maxilla	42	D = All of the Above
18	B = 02	43	A = Septal Cartilage
19	B = Mandible	44	C = Hyoid Bone
20	D = All of the Above	45	D = Hyoid Bone
21	A = Maxillary Sinus	46	A = Hyoid Bone
22	C = Nasal Bone	47	B = Hyoid Bone
23	A = Cartilage	48	C = Both A and B
24	B = Lacrimal Bone	49	A = Anterior Fontanelle
25	D = Lacrimal Bone	50	B = Anterior Fontanelle

Part-08

1. Which fontanelle located at the midline between the parietal bones and occipital bone
   - (A) Anterior fontanelle
   - (B) Posterior fontanelle
   - (C) Lateral fontanelle
   - (D) Distal fontanelle

2. Which of the following fontanelle generally closes 2 months after birth
   - (A) Posterior fontanelle
   - (B) Anterior fontanelle
   - (C) Lateral fontanelle
   - (D) Inferior fontanelle

3. The sinuses are air - filled cavities which are present in
   - (A) Sphenoid bone
   - (B) Ethmoid bone
   - (C) Maxillary bone
   - (D) All of the above

4. Which of the following are lined with ciliated mucous membrane and are continuous with nasal cavity?
   - (A) Suture
   - (B) Sinuses
   - (C) Ramus
   - (D) Curved body

5. The major function of sinus involves
   - (A) Providing resonance to the voice
   - (B) Reducing the weight of the skull
   - (C) Both (A) and (B)
   - (D) None of the above

6. How many sacrum consists in sacral region?
   - (A) 10
   - (B) 8
   - (C) 12
   - (D) 5

7. Vertebral column is also called
   - (A) Backbone
   - (B) Thighbone
   - (C) Arm bone
   - (D) Front bone

8. Function of vertebral column is/are
   (A) Enclosed and protect the spinal cord
   (B) Supports the head
   (C) Servers as point of attachment for the ribs, pelvic girdle and muscles of the back
   (D) All of the above

9. Which of the following is region of vertebral column?
   (A) Cervical region
   (B) Thoracic region
   (C) Lumbar region
   (D) All of the above

10. Total number of vertebrae is
    (A) 36
    (B) 33
    (C) 39
    (D) 31

11. The movable vertebrae are
    (A) Cervical vertebrae
    (B) Thoracic vertebrae
    (C) Lumbar vertebrae
    (D) All of the above

12. In each vertebrae the thick disc – shaped anterior portion that varies in size in different regions is called
    (A) The body
    (B) Vertebral neural
    (C) Vertebral arch
    (D) Processes

13. The area behind the body and forms the posterior and lateral walls of the vertebral foramen called
    (A) Vertebral coronal
    (B) Vertebral arch
    (C) Processes
    (D) Sinuses

14. In vertebral arch the lateral walls are formed from plates of bone called
    (A) Pedicles
    (B) Medulla
    (C) Sinuses
    (D) Suture

15. The large space present between the vertebral arch and the body is called
    (A) Vertebral sinus
    (B) Vertebral foramen
    (C) Vertebral suture
    (D) Vertebral septum

16. How many cervical vertebrae contain in cervical region?
    (A) 7
    (B) 12
    (C) 10
    (D) 3

17. Which of the following is the smallest vertebrae?
    (A) Thoracic vertebrae   (B) Lumbar vertebrae
    (C) Cervical vertebrae   (D) Sacrum

18. Which vertebrae present in the neck
    (A) Cervical vertebrae   (B) Coccyx
    (C) Sacrum   (D) Lumbar vertebrae

19. All cervical vertebrae have foramina which are
    (A) One vertebral foramen   (B) Two transverse foramen
    (C) Both (A) and (B)   (D) None of the above

20. Which of the following have transverse processes through which a vertebral artery passes upwards to the brain?
    (A) Transverse foramina   (B) Vertebral foramen
    (C) Lateral foramen   (D) Proximal foramen

21. The first cervical vertebrae (C_1) are called
    (A) Odontoid   (B) Prominins
    (C) Atlas   (D) Costae

22. The 7th cervical vertebrae (C7) are also known as
    (A) Vertebrae prominens   (B) Vertebrae predominant
    (C) Vertebrae capitulum   (D) Vertebrae sternal

23. How many thoracic vertebrae contain in thoracic region?
    (A) 10   (B) 12
    (C) 15   (D) 16

24. The largest and strongest vertebrae in the vertebral column is
    (A) Sacrum   (B) Coccyx
    (C) Cervical vertebrae   (D) Lumbar vertebrae

25. Which vertebrae have to support the weight of the upper body
    (A) Lumbar vertebrae   (B) Cervical vertebrae
    (C) Coccyx   (D) Sacrum

26. How many lumbar vertebrae contains in lumbar region?
    (A) 5   (B) 7
    (C) 12   (D) 10

27. Which of the following is the triangular and slightly curve bone formed by the union of five sacral vertebrae?

    (A) Sacrum

    (B) Thoracic vertebrae

    (C) Lumbar vertebrae

    (D) Cervical vertebrae

28. The upper part of sacrum articulates with the fifth lumbar vertebra to form

    (A) Sacroiliac joint

    (B) Lumbosacral joint

    (C) Pivot joint

    (D) Hinge joint

29. At the inferior tip of sacrum articulates with the

    (A) Coccyx

    (B) Cervical vertebrae

    (C) Thoracic vertebrae

    (D) Lumbar vertebrae

30. On each side sacrum articulates with ilium to form a

    (A) Pivot joint

    (B) Ellipsoidal joint

    (C) Sacroiliac joint

    (D) Hinge joint

31. Which vertebrae have series of foramina on each side of the bone for the passage of nerves and blood vessels

    (A) Sacrum

    (B) Thoracic vertebrae

    (C) Lumbar vertebrae

    (D) Cervical vertebrae

32. Which vertebrae formed by the fusion of four coccygeal vertebrae

    (A) Cervical vertebrae

    (B) Thoracic vertebrae

    (C) Sacrum

    (D) Coccyx

33. Which of the following has a broad base that articulates with the tip of the sacrum?

    (A) Cervical vertebrae

    (B) Lumbar vertebrae

    (C) Thoracic vertebrae

    (D) Coccyx

34. The bodies of adjacent vertebra are separated by

    (A) Intermediate discs

    (B) Intervertebral discs

    (C) Intervertebral foramina

    (D) Intermedullary discs

35. Intervertebral discs are composed of

    (A) Annulus fibrosus

    (B) Nucleus pulposus

    (C) Both (A) and (B)

    (D) None of the above

36. Total number of vertebral discs in vertebral column are
    - (A) 23
    - (B) 30
    - (C) 29
    - (D) 31

37. Function of intervertebral discs
    - (A) Forms strong joints
    - (B) Permit various movements of the vertebral column
    - (C) Absorb shock
    - (D) All of the above

38. The intervertebral foramina form a passage for the
    - (A) Spinal nerves
    - (B) Blood vessels
    - (C) Lymph vessels
    - (D) All of the above

39. The side view of the vertebral column shows curves, which are
    - (A) Two primary curves
    - (B) Two secondary curves
    - (C) Both (A) and (B)
    - (D) None of the above

40. The fetus in the uterus shows only a single anterior curve called
    - (A) Primary curve
    - (B) Secondary curve
    - (C) Tertiary curve
    - (D) Quaternary curve

41. The thoracic and sacral curves are called
    - (A) Secondary curve
    - (B) Primary curve
    - (C) Tertiary curve
    - (D) Quaternary curve

42. The cervical and lumbar curves are called
    - (A) Primary curve
    - (B) Tertiary curve
    - (C) Secondary curve
    - (D) Quaternary curve

43. Which curve develops when the child sits up, stands and walks
    - (A) Primary thoracic curve
    - (B) Primary sacral curve
    - (C) Secondary cervical curve
    - (D) Secondary lumbar curve

44. Secondary cervical curve develops after birth that time is about
    - (A) 3 months
    - (B) 10 months
    - (C) 15 months
    - (D) 20 months

45. Which curve develops when the infant begins to hold its head erect
    - (A) Secondary lumbar curve
    - (B) Secondary cervical curve
    - (C) Primary thoracic curve
    - (D) Primary sacral curve

46. The thoracic cage (thorax) is formed by
    - (A) Sternum
    - (B) Ribs
    - (C) Thoracic vertebrae
    - (D) All of the above

47. Which of the following bone is a long, narrow, flat vertical bone located in the middle of the front of the chest?
    - (A) Sternum
    - (B) Ribs
    - (C) Carpal
    - (D) Femur

48. The sternum consists of the part
    - (A) The manubrium
    - (B) The body
    - (C) The xiphoid
    - (D) All of the above

49. Which of the following is the uppermost part of the sternum?
    - (A) Manubrium
    - (B) Xiphoid
    - (C) Body
    - (D) Middle

50. The manubrium articulates with the clavicles at which joint
    - (A) Sacroiliac joints
    - (B) Ellipsoidal joints
    - (C) Pivot joints
    - (D) Sternoclavicular joints

Answer Key

Integumentary System, Skeletal System, Joints (Part-08)

Question	Answer	Question	Answer
01	B = Posterior Fontanelle	26	A = 05
02	A = Posterior Fontanelle	27	A = Sacrum
03	D = All of the Above	28	B = Lumbosacral Joint
04	B = Sinus	29	A = Coccyx
05	C = Both A and B	30	C = Sacroiliac Joint
06	D = 05	31	A = Sacrum
07	A = Backbone	32	D = Coccyx
08	D = All of the Above	33	D = Coccyx
09	D = All of the Above	34	B = Intervertebral Discs
10	B = 33	35	C = Both A and B
11	D = All of the Above	36	A = 23
12	A = The Body	37	D = All of the Above
13	B = Vertebral Arch	38	D = All of the Above
14	A = Pedicles	39	C = Both A and B
15	B = Vertebral Foramen	40	A = Primary Curve
16	A = 07	41	B = Primary Curve
17	C = Cervical Vertebrae	42	C = Secondary Curve
18	A = Cervical Vertebrae	43	D = Secondary Lumbar Curve
19	C = Both A and B	44	A = 03 Months
20	A = Transverse Foramina	45	B = Secondary Cervical Curve
21	C = Atlas	46	D = All of the Above
22	A = Vertebrae Prominens	47	A = Sternum
23	B = 12	48	D = All of the Above
24	D = Lumbar Vertebrae	49	A = Manubrium
25	A = Lumbar Vertebrae	50	D = Sternoclavicular Joints

Part-09

1. The junction of manubrium and the body forms
   - (A) Sternal angle
   - (B) Coronal angle
   - (C) Vertebral angle
   - (D) Cervical angle

2. The manubrium articulates with the
   - (A) Scapula
   - (B) Carpal
   - (C) Clavicle
   - (D) Metacarpal bones

3. The body or middle part of the sternum attached to the
   - (A) Ribs
   - (B) Carpal
   - (C) Phalanges
   - (D) Ulna and radius

4. The inferior tip of the sternum is
   - (A) Manubrium
   - (B) The body
   - (C) Xiphoid process
   - (D) Ribs

5. The xiphoid process gives attachment to the
   - (A) Diaphragm
   - (B) Muscles of the anterior abdominal wall
   - (C) The Linea alba
   - (D) All of the above

6. How many pairs of ribs are there?
   - (A) 9 pairs
   - (B) 12 pairs
   - (C) 10 pairs
   - (D) 6 pairs

7. The upper 7 pairs of ribs attach directly to the sternum are called
   - (A) True ribs
   - (B) False ribs
   - (C) Shock ribs
   - (D) Core ribs

8. The lower 3 pairs (8th, 9th and 10th) of ribs that indirectly articulates with sternum are called
   - (A) Shock ribs
   - (B) Core ribs
   - (C) True ribs
   - (D) False ribs

9. The lowest 2 pairs (11th and 12th) of ribs that do not articulates with sternum are called

   (A) Blotting ribs

   (B) Floating ribs

   (C) Predominant ribs

   (D) Crucial ribs

10. Typical ribs consist of

   (A) Vertebral part

   (B) Sternal part

   (C) Both (A) and (B)

   (D) None of the above

11. The vertebral part of ribs is articulating with the thoracic vertebrae by two facets are

   (A) Capitulum and tubercle

   (B) Cortex and tubular

   (C) Cuticle and carpal

   (D) Ulna and radius

12. The spaces between ribs arecalled

   (A) Intervertebral discs

   (B) Intercostal spaces

   (C) Intercarpal spaces

   (D) Intercortex spaces

13. The intercostal spacesareoccupied by

   (A) Intercostal muscles

   (B) Blood vessels

   (C) Nerves

   (D) All of the above

14. The appendicular skeleton consists of

   (A) Shoulder girdle

   (B) Pelvic girdle

   (C) Both (A) and (B)

   (D) None of the above

15. How many shoulders girdle is there?

   (A) 2

   (B) 3

   (C) 4

   (D) 5

16. Shoulder girdle attached the bones of the

   (A) Lower limbs to the axial skeleton

   (B) Carpal bone

   (C) Upper limbs to the axial skeleton

   (D) Tibia and fibula

17. Shoulder girdle is also called

   (A) Ulna girdle

   (B) Fibula girdle

   (C) Pubis girdle

   (D) Pectoral girdle

18. The shoulder girdle consists of
   - (A) Clavicle
   - (B) Scapulae
   - (C) Both (A) and (B)
   - (D) None of the above

19. The S – shaped long bone located horizontally across the anterior part of the thorax superior to the first rib is called
   - (A) Clavicle
   - (B) Carpal
   - (C) Metacarpal
   - (D) Ilium

20. How many clavicles bone are there
   - (A) 1
   - (B) 2
   - (C) 3
   - (D) 4

21. Clavicle bone is also called
   - (A) Scapula bone
   - (B) Ulna bone
   - (C) Carpal bone
   - (D) Collar bone

22. The clavicle articulates with the acromion of the scapula to form the
   - (A) Acromioclavicular joint
   - (B) Pivot joint
   - (C) Sacroiliac joint
   - (D) Ellipsoidal joint

23. Which bone is also called as beauty bone of the body?
   - (A) Ulna
   - (B) Humerus
   - (C) Clavicle
   - (D) Carpal

24. Which bone is large, flat, triangular located in the superior part of the posterior thorax?
   - (A) Scapula
   - (B) Carpal
   - (C) Ulna
   - (D) Patella

25. Scapula has lateral angle and a shallow concavity called
   - (A) Glandular cavity
   - (B) Glenoid cavity
   - (C) Giant cavity
   - (D) Cuticle cavity

26. The glenoid cavity of the scapula articulates with the head of the humerus to form the
   - (A) Acromioclavicular joint
   - (B) Sternoclavicular joint
   - (C) Glenohumeral joint
   - (D) Ellipsoidal joint

27. Scapula prominent ridge is called
    - (A) Spine
    - (B) Suture
    - (C) Curve
    - (D) Arch

28. The prominent overhang which can be easily felt as the highest point of the shoulder is called
    - (A) Coronal process
    - (B) Cambium process
    - (C) Acromion process
    - (D) Sacrum process

29. How many bones contain in each upper limb?
    - (A) 20 bones
    - (B) 30 bones
    - (C) 40 bones
    - (D) 45 bones

30. The bone of upper arm is called
    - (A) Humerus
    - (B) Femur
    - (C) Tibia
    - (D) Patella

31. The longest and largest bone of upper limb is
    - (A) Carpal
    - (B) Humerus
    - (C) Tibia
    - (D) Patella

32. The proximal end of the humerus has a rounded head that articulates with the glenoid cavity of the scapula to form
    - (A) Shoulder joint
    - (B) Carpal joint
    - (C) Ulna joint
    - (D) Fibula joint

33. Scapula is also called as
    - (A) Carpal blade
    - (B) Shoulder blade
    - (C) Tibia blade
    - (D) Phalanges blade

34. Ulna and radius articulate with the humerus at which of the following joint
    - (A) Shoulder joint
    - (B) Elbow joint
    - (C) Carpal joint
    - (D) Patella joint

35. Ulna and radius articulate with carpal bone at this joint
    - (A) Wrist joint
    - (B) Shoulder joint
    - (C) Patella joint
    - (D) Ulna joint

36. How many carpal bones are there?
    - (A) 10
    - (B) 12
    - (C) 8
    - (D) 4

37. The bone of the wrist is called
  (A) Patella
  (B) Femur
  (C) Tibia
  (D) Carpals

38. The carpals joined to one another by ligaments to form
  (A) Carpometacarpal joint
  (B) Interphalangeal joint
  (C) Intercarpal joints
  (D) Sternoclavicular joint

39. Carpals are arranged in rows of
  (A) Proximal row
  (B) Distal row
  (C) Both (A) and (B)
  (D) None of the above

40. The bones of proximal row of carpals are
  (A) Scaphoid
  (B) Lunate
  (C) Triquetrum
  (D) All of the above

41. Which of the following bone is not a bone of distal row of carpals?
  (A) Trapezium
  (B) Capitate
  (C) Lunate
  (D) Hamate

42. The bone of proximal row of carpal are associated with
  (A) Wrist joint
  (B) Elbow joint
  (C) Shoulder joint
  (D) Knees joint

43. The bones of distal row of carpal are articulate with
  (A) Elbow joint
  (B) Shoulder bones
  (C) Metacarpal bone
  (D) Tibia bone

44. The bone of distal row is
  (A) Trapezium
  (B) Trapezoid
  (C) Capitate
  (D) All of the above

45. How many bones found in metacarpal of the palm of the hand
  (A) Seven
  (B) Five
  (C) Eight
  (D) Nine

46. The proximal ends of metacarpal bones articulate with the carpal bones to form
  (A) Carpometacarpal joints
  (B) Intercarpal joints
  (C) Sternoclavicular joint
  (D) Ellipsoidal joint

47. The distal end of metacarpal bone articulates with the proximal phalanges to form
   (A) Sternoclavicular joint
   (B) Metacarpophalangeal joint
   (C) Intercarpal joint
   (D) Sternal

48. How many phalanges found in the fingers?
   (A) 10
   (B) 8
   (C) 14
   (D) 18

49. The phalanges are joined to each other by
   (A) Sternoclavicular joint
   (B) Sternal joint
   (C) Glenohumeral joint
   (D) Interphalangeal joint

50. Each hip bone consists of fused bone which is
   (A) Ilium
   (B) Ischium
   (C) Pubis
   (D) All of the above

Answer Key

Integumentary System, Skeletal System, Joints (Part-09)

Question	Answer	Question	Answer
01	A = Sternum Angle	26	C = Glenohumeral Joint
02	C = Clavicle	27	A = Spine
03	A = Ribs	28	C = Acromion Process
04	C = Xiphoid Process	29	B = 30 Bones
05	D = All of the Above	30	A = Humerus
06	B = 12 Pairs	31	B = Humerus
07	A = True Ribs	32	A = Shoulder Bone
08	D = False Ribs	33	B = Shoulder Bone
09	B = Floating Ribs	34	B = Elbow Bone
10	C = Both A and B	35	A = Wrist Bone
11	A = Capitulum and Tubercle	36	C = 08
12	B = Intercostal Spaces	37	D = Carpals
13	D = All of the Above	38	C = Intercarpal Joints
14	C = Both A and B	39	C = Both A and B
15	A = 02	40	D = All of the Above
16	C = Upper Limbs & Axial Skeleton	41	C = Lunate
17	D = Pectoral Girdle	42	A = Wrist Joint
18	C = Both A and B	43	C = Metacarpal Bone
19	A = Clavicle	44	D = All of the Above
20	B = 02	45	B = Five
21	D = Collar Bone	46	A = Carpometacarpal Joints
22	A = Acromioclavicular Joint	47	B = Metacarpophalangeal Joints
23	C = Clavicle	48	C = 14
24	A = Scapula	49	D = Interphalangeal Joint
25	B = Glenoid Cavity	50	D = All of the Above

Part-10

1. Pelvic girdle attached the bones of the
   - (A) Lower limbs to the axial skeleton
   - (B) Carpal bone
   - (C) Upper limbs to the axial skeleton
   - (D) Scapula

2. The pelvic girdle is formed by
   - (A) Elbow bone
   - (B) Shoulder bone
   - (C) Hip bone
   - (D) Carpal bone

3. The basin – shaped structure formed by pelvic girdle is called
   - (A) Pelvis
   - (B) Clavicle
   - (C) Ulna
   - (D) Radius

4. The hip bones are joined anteriorly to one another at the
   - (A) Metacarpophalangeal joint
   - (B) Pubic symphysis
   - (C) Carpometacarpal joint
   - (D) Pivot joint

5. The hip bones are joined posteriorly with the sacrum at the
   - (A) Sacroiliac joints
   - (B) Shoulder joint
   - (C) Carpometacarpal joint
   - (D) Intercarpal joint

6. The uppermost and largest portion of the hip bone is
   - (A) Ischium
   - (B) Ilium
   - (C) Pubic
   - (D) Carpal

7. The curved upper margin of the ilium is called
   - (A) Iliac crest
   - (B) Iliac fossa
   - (C) Posterior inferior spine
   - (D) Posterior superior spine

8. A bony projection making limit of the iliac crest in the front of
   - (A) Anterior superior spine
   - (B) Iliac fossa
   - (C) Iliac crest
   - (D) Posterior inferior spine

9. The ilium forms a synovial joint with the sacrum this is the
   - (A) Intercarpal joint
   - (B) Carpometacarpal joint
   - (C) Sacroiliac joint
   - (D) Shoulder joint

10. The inferior and posterior portion of hip bone is called
    (A) Ilium
    (B) Ischium
    (C) Pubis
    (D) Carpal

11. The bony inferior projection of the body of ischium and its ramus is called
    (A) Ischial ilium
    (B) Ilium crest
    (C) Ilium fossa
    (D) Ischial tuberosity

12. Which of the following bear the body weight in sitting position?
    (A) Ischial tuberosity
    (B) Carpal
    (C) Scapula
    (D) Ilium

13. Which of the following is present between the pubis and ischium?
    (A) Carpometacarpal joint
    (B) Intercarpal joint
    (C) Glenoid cavity
    (D) Obturator foramen

14. The largest foramen in the human skeleton is
    (A) Obturator foramen
    (B) Rotundum foramen
    (C) Spinosum foramen
    (D) Jugular foramen

15. Obturator foramen serves as the passage for
    (A) Nerves
    (B) Blood vessels
    (C) Tendons
    (D) All of the above

16. On the lateral surface of the hip bone just above the obturator foramen is a deep depression called
    (A) Acetabulum
    (B) Spine
    (C) Manubrium
    (D) Sternal

17. Which of the following is formed by the fusion of ilium, ischium and pubis
    (A) Manubrium
    (B) Neural arch
    (C) Fontanelles
    (D) Acetabulum

18. The pelvis is divided into upper and lower parts by the
    (A) Lunate
    (B) Intertubercular sulcus
    (C) Pelvic brim
    (D) Capitulum

19. The portion of the pelvis superior to pelvic brim which does not contain pelvis organ is referred
    (A) False pelvis
    (B) Core pelvis
    (C) True pelvis
    (D) Broad pelvis

20. The portion of inferior to the pelvic brim that surrounds the pelvic cavity is referred as
    - (A) Core pelvis
    - (B) True pelvis
    - (C) False pelvis
    - (D) Trunk pelvis

21. How many bones consists in each lower limb?
    - (A) 20
    - (B) 25
    - (C) 30
    - (D) 40

22. The proximal end of the femur consists of a rounded head that articulates with the acetabulum of the hip bone to form
    - (A) Hip joint
    - (B) Ribs joint
    - (C) Elbow joint
    - (D) Shoulder joint

23. The distal end of the femur is widened into a
    - (A) Medial condyle
    - (B) Lateral condyle
    - (C) Both (A) and (B)
    - (D) None of the above

24. Which of the following is the longest and heaviest bone of the body?
    - (A) Femur
    - (B) Patella
    - (C) Carpal
    - (D) Tibia

25. The femur is which type of bone
    - (A) Long bone
    - (B) Short bone
    - (C) Irregular bone
    - (D) Sesamoid bone

26. Function of femur bone is/are
    - (A) Holds body weight
    - (B) Stabilizing movement
    - (C) Connecting muscles, tendons and ligament of hips
    - (D) All of the above

27. The long portion of the femur that supports weight and forms structure of thigh called
    - (A) Femur shaft
    - (B) Femur sternal
    - (C) Femur sulcus
    - (D) Femur tubular

28. A small, triangular bone located anterior to the knee joint is called
    - (A) Tibia
    - (B) Ulna
    - (C) Patella
    - (D) Carpal

29. The posterior surface of patella articulates with the femur in the
    (A) Knee joint   (B) Carpal joint
    (C) Elbow joint   (D) Tarsal joint

30. The posterior surface of the patella articulates with the femur and is
    marked by
    (A) Medial facet   (B) Lateral facet
    (C) Both (A) and (B)   (D) None of the above

31. Which of the following articulates with the medial condyle of the femur?
    (A) Medial facet   (B) Distal facet
    (C) Superior facet   (D) Lateral facet

32. Which of the following articulates with the lateral condyle of the femur?
    (A) Distal facet   (B) Superior facet
    (C) Proximal facet   (D) Lateral facet

33. Function of patella is/are
    (A) Leg extension   (B) Protection of knee
    (C) Allows smooth movement   (D) All of the above

34. Patella is a which type of bone
    (A) Sesamoid bone   (B) Irregular bone
    (C) Short bone   (D) Long bone

35. The larger medial bone of lower leg is
    (A) Carpal   (B) Metacarpal
    (C) Humerus   (D) Tibia

36. The tibia and femur articulate to form
    (A) Tibiofemoral joint   (B) Intercarpal joint
    (C) Sternoclavicular joint   (D) Ellipsoidal joint

37. The distal end of tibia articulates with the talus to form
    (A) Intercarpal joint   (B) Talocrural joint
    (C) Ellipsoidal joint   (D) Elbow joint

38. Tibia is which type of bone
    (A) Long bone   (B) Irregular bone
    (C) Short bone   (D) Sesamoid bone

39. Which bone is lateral to the tibia?
    - (A) Clavicle
    - (B) Sternum
    - (C) Fibula
    - (D) Carpal

40. The head of the fibula articulates with the lateral condyle of the tibia to form
    - (A) Intercarpal joint
    - (B) Ellipsoidal joint
    - (C) Sacroiliac joint
    - (D) Tibiofibular joint

41. The distal end of fibula articulates with the
    - (A) Talus
    - (B) Carpal
    - (C) Sternal
    - (D) Clavicle

42. The bone of ankle is also known as
    - (A) Tibia bone
    - (B) Femur bone
    - (C) Tarsal bone
    - (D) Patella bone

43. How many tarsal bones present in the ankle?
    - (A) 10
    - (B) 7
    - (C) 3
    - (D) 9

44. Which of the following is tarsal bone?
    - (A) Calcaneus
    - (B) Cuboid
    - (C) Talus
    - (D) All of the above

45. The strongest and the largest tarsal bone is
    - (A) Cuneiforms
    - (B) Talus
    - (C) Navicular
    - (D) Calcaneus

46. The talus is the only bone of the foot that articulates with the fibula and tibia to form
    - (A) Ankle joint
    - (B) Elbow joint
    - (C) Shoulder joint
    - (D) Carpal joint

47. Which type of bone is tarsal bone
    - (A) Long bone
    - (B) Short bone
    - (C) Irregular bone
    - (D) Flat bone

48. How many metatarsal bones are there?
    - (A) 10
    - (B) 8
    - (C) 5
    - (D) 9

49. The proximal end of metatarsal bone articulates with

    (A) Tarsal bone   (B) Elbow bone

    (C) Patella bone   (D) Femur bone

50. The distal end of metatarsal bone articulates with

    (A) Elbow bone   (B) Patella bone

    (C) Phalanges   (D) Tibia bone

Answer Key

Integumentary System, Skeletal System, Joints (Part-10)

Question	Answer	Question	Answer
01	A = Lower Limbs to the Axial Skeleton	26	D = All of the Above
02	C = Hip Bone	27	A = Femur Shaft
03	A = Pelvis	28	C = Patella
04	B = Pubic Symphysis	29	A = Knee Joints
05	A = Sacroiliac Joints	30	C = Both A and B
06	B = Ilium	31	A = Medial Facet
07	A = Iliac Crest	32	D = Lateral Facet
08	A = Anterior Superior Spine	33	D = All of the Above
09	C = Sacroiliac Joints	34	A = Sesamoid Bone
10	B = Ischium	35	D = Tibia
11	D = Ischial Tuberosity	36	A = Tibiofemoral Joint
12	A = Ischial Tuberosity	37	B = Talocrural Joint
13	D = Obturator Foramen	38	A = Long Bone
14	A = Obturator Foramen	39	C = Fibula
15	D = All of the Above	40	D = Tibiofibular Joint
16	A = Acetabulum	41	A = Talus
17	D = Acetabulum	42	C = Tarsal Bone
18	C = Pelvic Brim	43	B = 07
19	A = False Pelvis	44	D = All of the Above
20	B = True Pelvis	45	D = Calcaneus
21	C = 30	46	A = Ankle Joint
22	A = Hip Joint	47	B = Short Bone
23	C = Both A and B	48	C = 05
24	A = Femur	49	A = Tarsal Bone
25	A = Long Bone	50	C = Phalanges

Part-11

1. The scientific study of muscle is called
   - (A) Myology
   - (B) Cytology
   - (C) Histology
   - (D) Osteology

2. The muscular system comprises the specialized contractile tissue called
   - (A) Nerve tissue
   - (B) Bone tissue
   - (C) Muscle tissue
   - (D) Cardiac tissue

3. How much of the total body weight is of muscle tissue?
   - (A) 5 – 6 %
   - (B) 30 – 40 %
   - (C) 70 – 80 %
   - (D) 80 – 90 %

4. Functions of muscle tissue is/are
   - (A) Body movement
   - (B) Body posture
   - (C) Heat generation
   - (D) All of the above

5. The muscle cells are specialized contractile cells also called
   - (A) Fibres
   - (B) Joint
   - (C) Bone
   - (D) Organ

6. Properties of muscle tissue are
   - (A) Excitability
   - (B) Contractibility
   - (C) Elasticity
   - (D) All of the above

7. Types of muscle tissue are
   - (A) Skeletal muscle tissue
   - (B) Smooth muscle tissue
   - (C) Cardiac muscle tissue
   - (D) All of the above

8. Which muscles are attached to the bone and are used to move the bones of the skeleton?
   - (A) Smooth muscle tissue
   - (B) Skeletal muscle tissue
   - (C) Visceral muscle tissue
   - (D) Cardiac muscle tissue

9. Skeletal muscle tissue is also called as
   - (A) Striated muscle tissue
   - (B) Smooth muscle tissue
   - (C) Cardiac muscle tissue
   - (D) Visceral muscle tissue

10. Which of the following muscle is voluntary muscle in nature?
    (A) Skeletal muscle tissue
    (B) Smooth muscle tissue
    (C) Visceral muscle tissue
    (D) Cardiac muscle tissue

11. Which muscle tissue show striations when it is examined under microscope
    (A) Smooth muscle tissue
    (B) Visceral muscle tissue
    (C) Skeletal muscle tissue
    (D) Cardiac muscle tissue

12. Which muscle tissue is also called visceral muscle?
    (A) Striated muscle tissue
    (B) Cardiac muscle tissue
    (C) Skeletal muscle tissue
    (D) Smooth muscle tissue

13. The smooth muscle is found in
    (A) Digestive tract
    (B) Respiratory tract
    (C) Excretory system
    (D) All of the above

14. Which muscle tissue found only in the wall of heart
    (A) Cardiac muscle tissue
    (B) Smooth muscle tissue
    (C) Skeletal muscle tissue
    (D) Striated muscle tissue

15. Skeletal muscle tissue found in
    (A) Digestive tract
    (B) Respiratory tract
    (C) Reproductive system
    (D) Shoulder muscle

16. A thick layer of fibrous connective tissue that surrounds the whole muscle trunk is called
    (A) Pivot
    (B) Suture
    (C) Fascia
    (D) Hinge

17. Fascia provides the pathway for
    (A) Nerves
    (B) Blood vessels
    (C) Lymphatic vessels
    (D) All of the above

18. The layers of connective tissue extend from the fascia to support and strengthen skeletal muscles
    (A) Epimysium
    (B) Perimysium
    (C) Endomysium
    (D) All of the above

19. The outermost layer of connective tissue presents beneath the fascia and it encircles the entire muscle
    (A) Epimysium
    (B) Endomysium
    (C) Perimysium
    (D) Exomysium

20. Within the muscle the cells are collected into separate bundles which are called as

    (A) Follicle
    (B) Fascicles
    (C) Capitulum
    (D) Cuticle

21. Each fascicle is covered in a connective tissue sheath called as

    (A) Endomysium
    (B) Exomysium
    (C) Perimysium
    (D) Epimysium

22. The individual muscle cells lie within the fascicles each wrapped in a fine areolar connective tissue layer called

    (A) Perimysium
    (B) Endomysium
    (C) Epimysium
    (D) Exomysium

23. Each skeletal muscle cell is multinucleated and is surrounded by

    (A) Sarcolemma
    (B) Carcinoma
    (C) Stratum
    (D) Cuticle

24. Thousands of tiny invaginations of sarcolemma are called

    (A) Renal tubules
    (B) Transverse tubules
    (C) Transit tubules
    (D) Vertical tubules

25. Which of the following helps in rapid transmission of the nerve impulse along the muscle fibre?

    (A) Proximal tubules
    (B) Vertical tubules
    (C) Transverse tubules
    (D) Distal tubules

26. The sarcolemma contains

    (A) Glycogen
    (B) Mitochondria
    (C) Myoglobulin
    (D) All of the above

27. A red – coloured protein that is found in striated muscle is called

    (A) Myoglobulin
    (B) Collagen
    (C) Alanine
    (D) Tubulin

28. At high magnification the sarcoplasm appears to be stuffed with thousands of smaller units which are called

    (A) Myofibrils
    (B) Myoclonic
    (C) Myometrium
    (D) Myocyte

29. Each myofibril is made up of
    (A) Thick (dark) filaments
    (B) Thin (light) filaments
    (C) Both (A) and (B)
    (D) None of the above

30. The dark bands are made up of thick filaments made up of the protein is
    (A) Actin
    (B) Tubulin
    (C) Alanine
    (D) Myosin

31. The light bands are made up of thin filaments made up of protein is
    (A) Tubulin
    (B) Actin
    (C) Keratin
    (D) Elastin

32. The region of a striated muscle sarcomere that contains myosin thick filament is called
    (A) A bands
    (B) C bands
    (C) F bands
    (D) P bands

33. The region of a striated muscle sarcomere that contains actin thin filaments is called
    (A) C bands
    (B) I band
    (C) L bands
    (D) T bands

34. The dark A band has a middle light zone called
    (A) H line
    (B) P line
    (C) D line
    (D) T line

35. Electron microscopy has revealed that muscle fibrils are surrounded by a fluid – filled system of membranous sacs which is called
    (A) Golgi body
    (B) Sarcoplasmic reticulum
    (C) Nuclear membrane
    (D) Ribosomes

36. Sarcoplasmic reticulum is specialized for storage of
    (A) Chloride
    (B) Potassium
    (C) Calcium
    (D) Iron

37. A group of muscle fibres innovated by one motor neuron is called
    (A) Motor core
    (B) Motor unit
    (C) Motor discs
    (D) Motor sacs

38. How many muscle fibres are there in eyeball muscle?
    - (A) 10 muscle fibres
    - (B) 30 muscle fibres
    - (C) 40 muscle fibres
    - (D) 35 muscle fibres

39. The contractile protein is
    - (A) Myosin
    - (B) Actin
    - (C) Both (A) and (B)
    - (D) None of the above

40. The actin molecule contains a site on which a myosin head can attach and the site is called
    - (A) Tubulin – binding site
    - (B) Alanine – binding site
    - (C) Elastin – binding site
    - (D) Myosin – binding site

41. The theory about the contraction of skeletal muscle is called
    - (A) Sliding filament theory
    - (B) Fluid – mosaic theory
    - (C) Endosymbiotic theory
    - (D) Watson and crick model

42. The muscle contraction results from the sliding of thin actin filaments over the thick
    - (A) Tubulin filaments
    - (B) Keratin filaments
    - (C) Alanine filaments
    - (D) Myosin filaments

43. During muscle contraction the thin filaments pulled towards the
    - (A) I band
    - (B) A band
    - (C) M line
    - (D) H zone

44. The thin filaments mainly composed of
    - (A) Actin
    - (B) Tropomyosin
    - (C) Troponin
    - (D) All of the above

45. In resting potential which ion present predominantly outside the sarcolemma
    - (A) Na^+
    - (B) Cl^-
    - (C) K^+
    - (D) Fe^{2+}

46. In resting potential which ion present predominantly inside the sarcolemma
    - (A) Cl^-
    - (B) Na^+
    - (C) Fe^{2-}
    - (D) K^+

47. When a muscle fibre stimulate which ions moves inside the muscle cells

    (A) Sodium   (B) Potassium

    (C) Iron   (D) Magnesium

48. When a muscle fibre stimulate which ions moves outside the muscle's cells

    (A) Magnesium   (B) Chloride

    (C) Potassium   (D) Iron

49. The calcium ions released from sarcoplasmic reticulum and binds to

    (A) Keratin   (B) Tubulin

    (C) Alanine   (D) Troponin

50. In relaxed muscle the myosin – binding site on the actin is occupied by inhibitors proteins are

    (A) Tropomyosin   (B) Troponin

    (C) Both (A) and (B)   (D) None of the above

Answer Key

Integumentary System, Skeletal System, Joints (Part-11)

Question	Answer	Question	Answer
01	A = Myology	26	D = All of the Above
02	C = Muscle Tissue	27	A = Myoglobulin
03	B = 30-40%	28	A = Myofibrils
04	D = All of the Above	29	C = Both A and B
05	A = Fibres	30	D = Myosin
06	D = All of the Above	31	B = Actin
07	D = All of the Above	32	A = A Bands
08	B = Skeletal Muscle Tissue	33	B = I Bands
09	A = Straited Muscle Tissue	34	A = H Line
10	A = Skeletal Muscle Tissue	35	B = Sarcoplasmic Reticulum
11	C = Skeletal Muscle Tissue	36	C = Calcium
12	D = Smooth Muscle Tissue	37	B = Motor Disc
13	D = All of the Above	38	A = 10 Muscle Fibres
14	A = Cardiac Muscle Tissue	39	C = Both A and B
15	D = Shoulder Muscle	40	D = Myosin- Binding Site
16	C = Fascia	41	A = Sliding Filament Theory
17	D = All of the Above	42	D = Myosin Filaments
18	D = All of the Above	43	C = M Line
19	A = Epimysium	44	D = All of the Above
20	B = Fascicles	45	A = NA$^+$
21	C = Perimysium	46	D = K$^+$
22	B = Endomysium	47	A = Sodium
23	A = Sarcolemma	48	C = Potassium
24	B = Transverse Tubules	49	D = Troponin
25	C = Transverse Tubules	50	C = Both A and B

Part-12

1. Which enzyme contain in myosin head
   (A) ATPase
   (B) Lipase Amylase
   (C) Maltase

2. Which contractile protein of skeletal muscle involving ATPase activity
   (A) Actin
   (B) Myosin
   (C) Tubulin
   (D) Alanine

3. In the presence of ATPase enzyme in myosin then the ATP is hydrolysed into
   (A) ADP
   (B) Phosphate group
   (C) Both (A) and (B)
   (D) None of the above

4. The energized myosin head attaches to the
   (A) Tubulin
   (B) Actin
   (C) Keratin
   (D) Alanine

5. Which of the following formed when the myosin heads attach to actin
   (A) Cross bridges
   (B) Junction
   (C) Synapses
   (D) Interstitial space

6. The thin filament slides over the thick filament towards
   (A) T – line
   (B) P – line
   (C) S – line
   (D) M – line

7. The region where the nerve and muscle come into the closest proximity and the transmission of the action potential take place is called
   (A) Interstitial space
   (B) Gap junction
   (C) Neuromuscular junction
   (D) Extracellular space

8. Where stimulation of muscle fibres by a motor neuron take place
   (A) Neuromuscular junction
   (B) Gap junction
   (C) Intracellular space
   (D) Interstitial space

9. The synaptic end bulb that contains hundreds of membranes – enclosed sacs is called

   (A) Fluids vesicles
   (B) Tubular canal
   (C) Synaptic vesicles
   (D) Cuticle vesicles

10. Each synaptic vesicle contains thousands of neurotransmitters that is

    (A) Acetylcholine
    (B) Melatonin
    (C) Thyroxine
    (D) Melanin

11. The neuromuscular junction includes

    (A) Synaptic end bulbs
    (B) Motor end plate
    (C) Both (A) and (B)
    (D) None of the above

12. The gap between two neuron is called

    (A) Synaptic vesicles
    (B) Synaptic cleft
    (C) Interstitial space
    (D) Intracellular space

13. Which of the following receptor is present in motor end plate

    (A) Adrenaline receptor
    (B) Oxytocin receptor
    (C) Melatonin receptor
    (D) Acetylcholine receptor

14. The arrival of the nerve impulse at the neuromuscular junction causes many synaptic vesicles to release

    (A) Adrenaline
    (B) Acetylcholine
    (C) Glutamate
    (D) Serotonin

15. Acetylcholine is rapidly broken down by which of the following enzyme

    (A) Maltase
    (B) Amylase
    (C) Acetyl cholinesterase
    (D) Trypsin

16. The muscle cells convert chemical energy into

    (A) Heat energy
    (B) Mechanical energy
    (C) Kinetic energy
    (D) Potential energy

17. The muscle fibres produce ATP by which of the following process

    (A) Glycolysis
    (B) Krebs citric acid cycle and electron transport
    (C) From phosphocreatine
    (D) All of the above

18. The glycolysis process converts glucose into

    (A) Acetic acid   (B) Hydrochloric acid

    (C) Pyruvic acid   (D) Malic acid

19. How many ATP release in glycolysis process

    (A) 10 ATP   (B) 2 ATP

    (C) 5 ATP   (D) 9 ATP

20. In Krebs citric acid cycle and electron transportcycle, pyruvic acid is further breakdown into

    (A) CO_2 (B) H_2O

    (C) Both (A) and (B)   (D) None of the above

21. The inability of a muscle to maintain force of contraction after prolonged activity is called

    (A) Muscle fatigue   (B) Muscle tone

    (C) Muscle discharge   (D) Muscle twitch

22. The facts that contribute to muscle fatigue include

    (A) Insufficient oxygen   (B) Depletion of glucose

    (C) Deposition of lactic acid   (D) All of the above

23. The strength of contraction of muscle fibres depends up on

    (A) Strength of stimulus   (B) Duration of stimulus

    (C) Speed of stimulus   (D) All of the above

24. The type of skeletal muscle fibres is

    (A) Tonic muscle fibres   (B) Twitch muscle fibres

    (C) Both (A) and (B)   (D) None of the above

25. Which muscle fibres are thin, dark red and slow – contracting muscle fibres?

    (A) Tonic muscle fibres   (B) Twitch muscle fibres

    (C) White muscle fibres   (D) Fast muscle fibres

26. Which muscle fibres contain a high amount of myoglobulin, abundant mitochondria and poorly formed sarcoplasmic reticulum

    (A) Twitch muscle fibres   (B) Fast muscle fibres

    (C) Tonic muscle fibres   (D) White muscle fibres

27. Tonic muscle fibres is also called

    (A) Red muscle fibres
    (B) White muscle fibres
    (C) Twitch muscle fibres
    (D) Fast muscle fibres

28. Which muscle fibres are much thicker, lighter in colour and fast constricting in nature?

    (A) Tonic muscle fibres
    (B) Red muscle fibres
    (C) Twitch muscle fibres
    (D) Slow muscle fibres

29. Which muscle fibres have low myoglobulin content, few mitochondria and well – formed sarcoplasmic reticulum

    (A) Red muscle fibres
    (B) Tonic muscle fibres
    (C) Slow muscle fibres
    (D) Twitch muscle fibres

30. Which muscle fibres also called white / fast muscle fibres

    (A) Twitch muscle fibres
    (B) Tonic muscle fibres
    (C) Red muscle fibres
    (D) Slow muscle fibres

31. Which muscle fibres carry on slow and sustained contraction for long time periods without fatigue

    (A) White muscle fibres
    (B) Fast muscle fibres
    (C) Twitch muscle fibres
    (D) Tonic muscle fibres

32. The example of tonic muscle fibres is

    (A) Extensor muscles in the back
    (B) To maintain erect posture against gravity
    (C) Long – distance running
    (D) All of the above

33. The body muscles meant for fast and strenuous work for short durations are composed mostly of

    (A) Twitch muscle fibres
    (B) Slow muscle fibres
    (C) Red muscle fibres
    (D) Tonic muscle fibres

34. The example of twitch muscle fibres

    (A) Weightlifting
    (B) Throwing a ball
    (C) Both (A) and (B)
    (D) None of the above

35. The intercalated disc found in

    (A) Smooth muscle tissue
    (B) Skeletal muscle tissue
    (C) Striated muscle tissue
    (D) Cardiac muscle tissue

36. Which of the following connect the end of cardiac muscle fibres to one another?

   (A) Intercalated disc   (B) Intervertebral disc

   (C) Sternal disc   (D) Intertubercular sulcus

37. Which of the following is type of smooth muscle tissue?

   (A) Single – unit smooth muscle tissue

   (B) Multiunit smooth muscle tissue

   (C) Both (A) and (B)

   (D) None of the above

38. Single – unit smooth muscle tissue is found in

   (A) Walls of arteries   (B) Stomach

   (C) Uterus   (D) All of the above

39. Multiunit smooth muscle tissue is found in

   (A) Ciliary body   (B) Iris muscle

   (C) Arrector pill   (D) All of the above

40. How long a single relaxed smooth muscle fibre is

   (A) $30 - 200$ μm long   (B) $250 - 300$ μm long

   (C) $2 - 6$ μm long   (D) $500 - 600$ μm long

41. Smooth muscle fibres contain thin filament called

   (A) Core bodies   (B) Dense bodies

   (C) Cuticle   (D) Cortex

42. The smooth muscle tissue contains a protein called

   (A) Calmodulin   (B) Tubulin

   (C) Alanine   (D) Keratin

43. Calmodulin protein of smooth muscle binds to Ca^{2+} and activates the enzyme are

   (A) Lipoxygenases   (B) Myosin light chain kinase

   (C) Oxidoreductases   (D) Carboxylase

44. Myosin light chain kinase enzyme bind ATP to the myosin in the interaction between

   (A) Myosin   (B) Actin

   (C) Both (A) and (B)   (D) None of the above

45. The attachment of a muscle's tendon to the stationary bone is called

(A) Origin

(B) Insertion

(C) Ulna

(D) Margin

46. The attachment of the muscle's other tendon to the movable bone is called

(A) Margin

(B) Ulna

(C) Insertion

(D) Origin

47. The fleshy portion of the muscle between the tendons is called

(A) Fontanelle

(B) Lacunae

(C) Osteon

(D) Belly

48. The muscle that performing actual movement

(A) Prime mover

(B) Flexors

(C) Extensors

(D) Abductors

49. The muscles that assist the prime mover

(A) Trapezium

(B) Lunate

(C) Capitate

(D) Synergists

50. Which of the following is bend one part of a limb on another at a joint?

(A) Supinator's

(B) Pronators

(C) Flexors

(D) Rotators

Answer Key

Integumentary System, Skeletal System, Joints (Part-12)

Question	Answer	Question	Answer
01	A = ATPase	26	C = Tonic Muscle Fibres
02	B = Myosin	27	A = Red Muscle Fibres
03	C = Both A and B	28	C = Twitch Muscle Fibres
04	B = Actin	29	D = Twitch Muscle Fibres
05	A = Cross Bridge	30	A = Twitch Muscle Fibres
06	D = M Line	31	D = Tonic Muscle Fibres
07	C = Neuromuscular Junction	32	D = All of the Above
08	A = Neuromuscular Junction	33	A = Twitch Muscle Fibres
09	C = Synaptic Vesicles	34	C = Both A and B
10	A = Acetylcholine	35	D = Cardiac Muscle Tissue
11	C = Both A and B	36	A = Intercalated Disc
12	B = Synaptic Cleft	37	C = Both A and B
13	D = Acetylcholine Receptor	38	D = All of the Above
14	B = Acetylcholine	39	D = All of the Above
15	C = Acetylcholine Cholinesterase	40	A = 30 to 200 μm long
16	B = Mechanical Energy	41	B = Dense Bodies
17	D = All of the Above	42	A = Calmodulin
18	C = Pyruvic Acid	43	B = Myosin Light Chain Kinase
19	B = 2 ATP	44	C = Both A and B
20	C = Both A and B	45	A = Origin
21	A = Muscle fatigue	46	C = Insertion
22	D = All of the Above	47	D = Belly
23	D = All of the Above	48	A = prime Mover
24	C = Both A and B	49	D = Synergists
25	A = Tonic Muscle Fibres	50	C = Flexors

Part-13

1. Which muscles is present over occipital bone?
   - (A) Occipitalis
   - (B) Buccinator
   - (C) Rhomboid
   - (D) Deltoid

2. Which of the following muscles is found in cheeks?
   - (A) Rhomboid
   - (B) Buccinator
   - (C) Serratus anterior
   - (D) Pectoralis minor

3. Which muscle surrounds the opening of mouth
   - (A) Brachialis
   - (B) Anconaeus
   - (C) Orbicularis orris
   - (D) Palmarus logus

4. Which muscle found in zygomatic bone
   - (A) Soleus
   - (B) Zygomaticus
   - (C) Gastrocnemius
   - (D) Peroneus longus

5. Which muscle is responsible to closes the eye?
   - (A) Orbicularis oculi
   - (B) Plantaris
   - (C) Popliteus
   - (D) Sartorius

6. Which muscle is located in maxilla?
   - (A) Sartorius
   - (B) Levator labii superioris
   - (C) Semitendinosus
   - (D) Plantaris

7. Which muscle is present over frontal bone?
   - (A) Frontalis
   - (B) Soleus
   - (C) Plantaris
   - (D) Pectineus

8. Which muscle is involved in smiling and laughing?
   - (A) Zygomaticus
   - (B) Pectineus
   - (C) Soleus
   - (D) Sartorius

9. Which muscle closes the jaw and exerts considerable pressure on the food
   - (A) Levator scapulae
   - (B) Pectoralis minor
   - (C) Masseter
   - (D) Superior rectus

10. Whichmuscle is found in temporal bone?

(A) Trapezius
(B) Rhomboid
(C) Temporalis
(D) Sartorius

11. Which muscle extends from sphenoid bone to mandible

(A) Pterygoid
(B) Masseter
(C) Rhomboid
(D) Plantaris

12. Which muscle found in superior and central part of eyeball

(A) Soleus
(B) Plantaris
(C) Supinator
(D) Superior rectus

13. Which muscle moves eyeball downwards

(A) Inferior rectus
(B) Soleus
(C) Deltoid
(D) Plantaris

14. Which muscle found in lateral side of eyeball

(A) Scalene
(B) Lateral rectus
(C) Sartorius
(D) Soleus

15. Which of the following is the origin of trapezius muscle?

(A) Ribs
(B) Humerus
(C) Scapula
(D) Occipital bone

16. Which of the following is insertion of trapezius muscle?

(A) Clavicle
(B) Ulna
(C) Radius
(D) Humerus

17. Which of the following muscle pulls head backwards and rotates scapula?

(A) Rectus abdominis
(B) Pollicis
(C) Supinator
(D) Trapezius

18. Which muscle originates from lower eight ribs

(A) External oblique
(B) Adductor magnus
(C) Abductor brevis
(D) Adductor longus

19. The insertion of triceps brachii are

(A) Patella
(B) Femur
(C) Ulna
(D) Metacarpal

20. The origin of serratus anterior muscle is
    (A) Occipital bone   (B) Temporal bone
    (C) Humerus   (D) Ribs

21. The insertion of rhomboid muscle is
    (A) Ulna   (B) Scapula
    (C) Radius   (D) Thumb

22. Which muscle abducts and rotates the arm
    (A) Scalene   (B) Diaphragm
    (C) Rectus abdominis   (D) Deltoid

23. Which muscle flexes the shoulder joint
    (A) Coracobrachialis   (B) Scalene
    (C) Pterygoid   (D) Triceps brachii

24. The origin of coracobrachialis muscle is
    (A) Scapula   (B) Ulna
    (C) Radius   (D) Clavicle

25. Which muscle flexes the elbow joint
    (A) Anconeus   (B) Brachioradialis
    (C) Deltoid   (D) Pectoralis major

26. The insertion of biceps brachii muscle are
    (A) Patella   (B) Ulna
    (C) Humerus   (D) Femur

27. Which muscle flexes the wrist joint
    (A) Palmarus longus   (B) Occipitalis
    (C) Zygomaticus   (D) Orbicularis oculi

28. The insertion of flexor carpi radialis muscle are
    (A) Humerus   (B) Metacarpal bones
    (C) Femur   (D) Patella

29. The insertion of supinator muscle is
    (A) Radius   (B) Thumb
    (C) Clavicle   (D) Femur

30. Which muscle pronates the forearm
    (A) Adductor pollicis   (B) Pronator teres
    (C) Palmarus longus   (D) Occipitalis

31. The origin of pronator quadratus muscle is
   (A) Patella
   (B) Femur
   (C) Ulna
   (D) Clavicle

32. The origin of opponens pollicis are
   (A) Radius
   (B) Ulna
   (C) Both (A) and (B)
   (D) None of the above

33. The insertion of extensor indicis muscle are
   (A) Index finger
   (B) Occipital bone
   (C) Clavicle
   (D) Femur

34. Which muscle abducts and extends the fingers
   (A) Dorsal interossei
   (B) Supinator
   (C) Occipitalis
   (D) Zygomaticus

35. The insertion of splenius capitis muscle is
   (A) Occipital bone
   (B) Temporal bone
   (C) Both (A) and (B)
   (D) None of the above

36. The origin of splenius capitis muscle is
   (A) Cervical vertebrae
   (B) Thoracic vertebrae
   (C) Both (A) and (B)
   (D) None of the above

37. The origin of scalene muscle is
   (A) Cervical vertebrae
   (B) Femur
   (C) Patella
   (D) Carpal

38. Which muscle flexes and rotates the head
   (A) Diaphragm
   (B) Scalene
   (C) Internal oblique
   (D) Gluteus minimus

39. The Pectineus muscle originate from
   (A) Pubis
   (B) Tibia
   (C) Humerus
   (D) Clavicle

40. The origin of soleus muscle is
   (A) Tibia
   (B) Fibula
   (C) Both (A) and (B)
   (D) None of the above

41. The insertion of peroneus brevis muscle is
    (A) Carpal
    (B) Metatarsals
    (C) Clavicle
    (D) Elbow

42. Which muscle flexes, rotates the hip joint
    (A) Iliacus
    (B) Scalene
    (C) Buccinator
    (D) Occipitalis

43. Which disease is characterized by massive muscle necrosis due to sustained pressure on the trunk or limbs?
    (A) Myasthenia gravis
    (B) Crush syndrome
    (C) Arthritis
    (D) Osteoporosis

44. The abnormal contractions of skeletal muscles include
    (A) Spasm
    (B) Cramp
    (C) Tremor
    (D) All of the above

45. Which of the following is an autoimmune disorder that cause chronic, progressive damage to the neuromuscular junction?
    (A) Myasthenia gravis
    (B) Glaucoma
    (C) Crush syndrome
    (D) Myositis

46. The symptoms of myasthenia gravis is
    (A) Muscle weakness
    (B) Diplopia
    (C) Difficulty in chewing
    (D) All of the above

47. The drug's use in myasthenia gravis are
    (A) Pyridostigmine
    (B) Neostigmine
    (C) Both (A) and (B)
    (D) None of the above

48. The inflammation of muscular tissue is called
    (A) Arthritis
    (B) Myositis
    (C) Osteoporosis
    (D) Glaucoma

49. The process of increase in size of muscle is called
    (A) Muscle atrophy
    (B) Muscle hypertrophy
    (C) Muscle hyperplasia
    (D) Apoptosis

50. The process of decrease in size of muscle is called
    (A) Muscle atrophy
    (B) Muscle hyperplasia
    (C) Muscle hypertrophy
    (D) Apoptosis

Answer Key

Integumentary System, Skeletal System, Joints (Part-13)

Question	Answer	Question	Answer
01	A = Occipitalis	26	C = Humerus
02	B = Buccinator	27	A = Palmarus Longus
03	C = Orbicularis Orris	28	B = Metacarpal Bone
04	B = Zygomaticus	29	A = Radius
05	A = Orbicularis Oculi	30	B = Pronator Teres
06	B = Levator Labii Superioris	31	C = Ulna
07	A = Frontalis	32	C = Both A and B
08	A = Zygomaticus	33	A = Index Finger
09	C = Masseter	34	A = Dorsal Interossei
10	C = Temporalis	35	C = Both A and B
11	A = Pterygoid	36	C = Both A and B
12	D = Superior Rectus	37	A = Cervical Vertebrae
13	A = Inferior Rectus	38	B = Scalene
14	B = Lateral Rectus	39	A = Pubis
15	D = Occipital Bone	40	C = Both A and B
16	A = Clavicle	41	B = Metatarsals
17	D = Trapezius	42	A = Iliacus
18	A = External Oblique	43	B = Crush Syndrome
19	C = Ulna	44	D = All of the Above
20	D = Ribs	45	A = Myasthenia Gravis
21	B = Scapula	46	D = All of the Above
22	D = Deltoid	47	C = Both A and B
23	A = Coracobrachialis	48	B = Myositis
24	A = Scapula	49	B = Muscle Hypertrophy
25	B = Brachioradialis	50	A = Muscle Atrophy

Part-14

1. The place of union or junction between two or more bones called
   (A) Joints
   (B) Sternal
   (C) Pubis
   (D) Synapse

2. Joint is also called
   (A) Articulation
   (B) Condyle
   (C) Capitulum
   (D) Glenoid cavity

3. Joints allow the
   (A) Flexibility of the skeleton
   (B) Movement of the skeleton
   (C) Attachment between bones
   (D) All of the above

4. The scientific study of joints is called
   (A) Ophthalmology
   (B) Arthrology
   (C) Neurology
   (D) Cardiology

5. The main type of joints is
   (A) Immovable joints
   (B) Slightly movable joints
   (C) Freely movable joints
   (D) All of the above

6. The type of tissue that covers the surface of a bone at a joint is called
   (A) Ligaments
   (B) Bursas
   (C) Cartilage
   (D) Tendons

7. A tissue lines the joint and seals it into a joint capsule is called
   (A) Synovial membrane
   (B) Ligament
   (C) Tendons
   (D) Cartilage

8. The synovial membrane secretes a clear, sticky fluid around the joint to lubricate is called
   (A) Saliva
   (B) Hormones
   (C) Bile
   (D) Synovial fluid

9. The tough, elastic bands of connective tissue that surrounds the joint to give support and limit the joint's movement is called
   (A) Ligaments
   (B) Synovial membrane
   (C) Bursas
   (D) Meniscus

10. The fluid – filled sacs between bones, ligament or other nearby structures and the help cushion the friction in a joint is called
    (A) Tendons
    (B) Ligaments
    (C) Cartilage
    (D) Bursas

11. The bones forming the joints that are held together by fibrous connective tissue is called
    (A) Cartilaginous joint
    (B) Fibrous joint
    (C) Saddle joint
    (D) Hinge joint

12. Fibrous joint is also called
    (A) Immovable joint
    (B) Slightly movable joint
    (C) Partially movable joint
    (D) Freely movable joint

13. The joint between the tibia and fibula formed by a sheet of fibrous tissue is called
    (A) Periodontal ligament
    (B) Intervertebral discs
    (C) Intraosseous membrane
    (D) Intervertebral foramina

14. The joint between the tooth and the mandible formed by dense connective tissues called
    (A) Periodontal ligament
    (B) Intervertebral discs
    (C) Intraosseous membrane
    (D) Capitulum

15. The example of immovable joint is
    (A) Sutures
    (B) Gomphoses
    (C) Syndesmosis
    (D) All of the above

16. Suture joint are found in
    (A) Elbow
    (B) Femur
    (C) Skull
    (D) Carpal

17. The bones forming the joints that are held together by fibrocartilage or hyaline cartilage is called
    (A) Cartilaginous joint
    (B) Fibrous joint
    (C) Synovial joint
    (D) Pivot joint

18. The example of cartilaginous joint is
    (A) Pubis symphysis
    (B) Joint between the vertebra
    (C) Both (A) and (B)
    (D) None of the above

19. Synovial joints are characterized by the presence of space called
    (A) Synovial cavity   (B) Dorsal cavity
    (C) Cranial cavity   (D) Spinal cavity

20. The end of the bone at the joints are covered by a layer of hyaline cartilage called
    (A) Articular capsule   (B) Articular cartilage
    (C) Cortex cartilage   (D) Fibrous cartilage

21. The function of articular cartilage in synovial joint is/are
    (A) Absorb shock   (B) Provide elastic surface
    (C) Reduces friction   (D) All of the above

22. The synovial joint is surrounded and enclosed by a sleeve – like capsule called
    (A) Articular capsule   (B) Articular cartilage
    (C) Synovial membrane   (D) Accessory ligaments

23. The articular capsule composed of the layers of
    (A) Outer fibrous capsule   (B) Inner synovial membrane
    (C) Both (A) and (B)   (D) None of the above

24. Which of the following consists of dense, fibrous tissue that attaches to the periosteum of the articulating bone?
    (A) Outer fibrous capsule   (B) Outer cartilage capsule
    (C) Inner tendons capsule   (D) Inner ligament capsule

25. Which of the following composed of areolar connective tissue and elastic fibres
    (A) Outer fibrous capsule   (B) Inner synovial membrane
    (C) Inner tendons capsule   (D) Outer cartilage capsule

26. Function of synovial fluid is/are
    (A) Lubrication   (B) Nutrient distribution
    (C) Shock absorption   (D) All of the above

27. The synovial fluid is secreted by the synovial membrane into the
    (A) Synovial cavity   (B) Cranial cavity
    (C) Spinal cavity   (D) Dorsal cavity

28. Synovial joints are also called
   (A) Freely movable joint
   (B) Slightly movable joint
   (C) Immovable joint
   (D) Partially movable joint

29. Synovial joint is found in
   (A) Shoulder
   (B) Skull
   (C) Ribs
   (D) Suture

30. Many synovial joints also contain accessory ligaments called
   (A) Extracapsular ligaments
   (B) Intracapsular ligaments
   (C) Both (A) and (B)
   (D) None of the above

31. Which ligaments lies outside the articular capsule and provide additional stability in synovial joint
   (A) Intracapsular ligaments
   (B) Extracapsular ligaments
   (C) Intracellular ligaments
   (D) Interstitial ligaments

32. Which ligaments occur within the articular capsule but outside the synovial membrane
   (A) Intracellular ligament
   (B) Interstitial ligament
   (C) Intracapsular ligament
   (D) Extracapsular ligament

33. Which of the following joint consists of a ball – like head of one bone fitted into socket or cuplike depression of another bone?
   (A) Ball and socket joint
   (B) Hinge joint
   (C) Pivot join
   (D) Saddle joint

34. Ball and socket allow wide range of movement including
   (A) Flexion
   (B) Extension
   (C) Rotation
   (D) All of the above

35. Ball and socket joint are found in
   (A) Ankle joint
   (B) Wrist joint
   (C) Shoulder joint
   (D) Carpometacarpal joint

36. In which joint the convex surface of one bone fits into the concave surface of another bone
   (A) Hinge joint
   (B) Ball and socket joint
   (C) Saddle joint
   (D) Pivot joint

37. Hinge joint are found in
    (A) Knee joint
    (B) Elbow joint
    (C) Ankle joint
    (D) All of the above

38. The ball and socket joint are also called as
    (A) Ellipsoidal joint
    (B) Spheroidal joint
    (C) Hinge joint
    (D) Pivot joint

39. In which joint the convex oval – shaped projection of one bone fits into the cup – shaped depression of another bone
    (A) Ball and socket joint
    (B) Saddle joint
    (C) Condyloid joint
    (D) Pivot joint

40. Which joint are found in wrist joint?
    (A) Condyloid joint
    (B) Saddle joint
    (C) Ball and socket joint
    (D) Pivot joint

41. Condyloid joint is also called
    (A) Ginglymoid joint
    (B) Ellipsoid joint
    (C) Spheroidal joint
    (D) Pivot joint

42. The joints permit sliding movement of two bones over each other and the articular surfaces are usually flat and slightly curved called
    (A) Ball and socket joint
    (B) Hinge joint
    (C) Condyloid joint
    (D) Gliding joint

43. Which joints found between carpals in wrist, tarsals in foot and between the sternum and clavicle bone
    (A) Gliding joint
    (B) Hinge joint
    (C) Ball and socket joint
    (D) Spheroidal joint

44. In which joint the rounded end of one bone fits into a shallow pit of another and allow only rotatory movement one bone on the other
    (A) Hinge joint
    (B) Ball and socket joint
    (C) Pivot joint
    (D) Gliding joint

45. Which joint found between the atlas and the axis
    (A) Pivot joint
    (B) Ball and socket joint
    (C) Hinge joint
    (D) Condyloid joint

46. In which joint the articular surface of one bone is saddle shaped and the articular surface of another bone fits into the saddle

    (A) Pivot joint
    (B) Ball and socket joint
    (C) Saddle joint
    (D) Gliding joint

47. Which joint found in metacarpal joint of the   thumb

    (A) Ball and socket joint
    (B) Pivot joint
    (C) Hinge joint
    (D) Saddle joint

48. The inflammation of joint is called

    (A) Gout
    (B) Arthritis
    (C) Osteoporosis
    (D) Rickets

49. The accumulation of uric acid crystal in the joint is feature of which disorder

    (A) Rickets
    (B) Gout
    (C) Osteomyelitis
    (D) Osteomalacia

50. The condition in which bone density decreases or bone tissue mass reduces, resulting in weakening of skeletal strength and increased susceptibility to bone fractures

    (A) Gout
    (B) Arthritis
    (C) Bursitis
    (D) Osteoporosis

Answer Key

Integumentary System, Skeletal System, Joints (Part-14)

Question	Answer	Question	Answer
01	A = Joints	26	D = All of the Above
02	A = Articulation	27	A = Synovial Cavity
03	D = All of the Above	28	A = Freely Movable Joints
04	B = Arthrology	29	A = Shoulder
05	D = All of the Above	30	C = Both A and B
06	C = Cartilage	31	B = Extracapsular Ligaments
07	A = Synovial Membrane	32	C = Intracapsular Ligaments
08	D = Synovial Fluid	33	A = Ball and Socket Joints
09	A = Ligaments	34	D = All of the Above
10	D = Bursas	35	C = Shoulder Joints
11	B = Fibrous Joint	36	A = Hinge Joint
12	A = Immovable Joint	37	D = All of the Above
13	C = Intraosseous Membrane	38	B = Spheroidal Joint
14	A = Periodontal Ligament	39	C = Condyloid Joint
15	D = All of the Above	40	A = Condyloid Joint
16	C = Skull	41	B = Ellipsoidal Joint
17	A = Cartilaginous Joint	42	D = Gliding Joints
18	C = Both A and B	43	A = Gliding Joints
19	A = Synovial Cavity	44	C = Pivot Joints
20	B = Articular Cartilage	45	A = Pivot Joints
21	D = All of the Above	46	C = Saddle Joints
22	A = Articular Capsule	47	D = Saddle Joints
23	C = Both A and B	48	B = Arthritis
24	A = Outer Fibrous Capsule	49	B = Gout
25	B = Inner Synovial membrane	50	D = Osteoporosis

Notes

Nervous System, Central Nervous System

Part-01

1. The nervous system consists of
   - (A) Brain
   - (B) Spinal cord
   - (C) Peripheral nerves
   - (D) All of the above

2. For descriptive purpose the parts of the nervous system are grouped into
   - (A) Central nervous system
   - (B) Peripheral nervous system
   - (C) Both (A) and (B)
   - (D) None of the above

3. The central nervous system consists of
   - (A) Brain
   - (B) Spinal cord
   - (C) Both (A) and (B)
   - (D) None of the above

4. Which nervous system consisting all the nerves outside the brain and spinal cord
   - (A) Peripheral nervous system
   - (B) Central nervous system
   - (C) Both (A) and (B)
   - (D) None of the above

5. Which nerve participate in transmitting impulses to the central nervous system
   - (A) Sensory nerve
   - (B) Motor nerve
   - (C) Efferent nerve
   - (D) Effective nerve

6. Which nerve transmit impulses from the central nervous system
   - (A) Afferent nerve
   - (B) Motor nerve
   - (C) Sensory nerve
   - (D) Effective nerve

7. Which nerve relay messages between neurons in the CNS
   - (A) Interneurons
   - (B) External neurons
   - (C) Exoneurons
   - (D) Endoneurons

8. Peripheral nervous system comprises of

    (A) Cranial nerve

    (B) Sacral nerve

    (C) Both (A) and (B)

    (D) None of the above

9. The spinal nerves and cranial nerves are collectively termed as

    (A) Cerebrospinal nerves

    (B) Vertebrospinal nerve

    (C) Sternospinal nerve

    (D) Spinovertebral nerve

10. Functions of the nervous system is/are

    (A) Neural signalling

    (B) Integrative function

    (C) Perception

    (D) All of the above

11. The fastest nerve signal travels at a speed of

    (A) 10 m/sec

    (B) 20 m/sec

    (C) 100 m/sec

    (D) 15 m/sec

12. Each neuron consists of

    (A) Cell body

    (B) Axon

    (C) Dendrites

    (D) All of the above

13. The longest axon, a cluster of nerve cell bodies that carries information from the skin to the brain

    (A) Dorsal root ganglion

    (B) Lateral ganglion

    (C) Proximal ganglion

    (D) Inferior root ganglion

14. Bundles of axon are bound together are called

    (A) Nerves

    (B) Vessels

    (C) Bone

    (D) Cartilage

15. Neurones are commonly referred are

    (A) Bone cells

    (B) Blood cells

    (C) Nerve cells

    (D) Stem cells

16. Which of the following is type of nervous tissue is

    (A) Neurones

    (B) Neuroglia

    (C) Both (A) and (B)

    (D) None of the above

17. Neurones are supported by connective tissue and are collectively known as

    (A) Neuroglia

    (B) Cartilage

    (C) Tendons

    (D) Ligaments

18. Which of the following cells are not able to divide?
    - (A) White blood cells
    - (B) Red blood cells
    - (C) Platelets
    - (D) Nerve cells

19. Function of neurones are
    - (A) Transmit information
    - (B) Regulating glandular secretions
    - (C) Thinking and remembering
    - (D) All of the above

20. How much percent constitute the neuroglia or glial cells of all brain cells
    - (A) 10 %
    - (B) 20 %
    - (C) 60 %
    - (D) 5 %

21. The neurons need continuous supply of
    - (A) Oxygen
    - (B) Glucose
    - (C) Both (A) and (B)
    - (D) None of the above

22. The ability to initiate nerve impulses in response to stimuli is called
    - (A) Electrical excitability
    - (B) Conductivity
    - (C) Potential conductance
    - (D) Kinetic movement

23. The ability to transmit the impulse from one part of the body to another is called
    - (A) Electrical excitability
    - (B) Conductivity
    - (C) Potential conductance
    - (D) Kinetic movement

24. Which of the following is the kind of nerve fibres are
    - (A) Dendrites
    - (B) Axons
    - (C) Both (A) and (B)
    - (D) None of the above

25. An axon is a single long extension that begins as a slight enlargement of the cell body called
    - (A) Axonal hillock
    - (B) Axoplasm
    - (C) Axolemma
    - (D) Axial

26. The cytoplasm in axon is called
    - (A) Axolemma
    - (B) Axoplasm
    - (C) Endoplasm
    - (D) Axonal hillock

27. The axoplasm of axon is surrounded by a plasma membrane called

    (A) Axoplasm

    (B) Axonal hillock

    (C) Axolemma

    (D) Endolemma

28. An axon consists of

    (A) Mitochondria

    (B) Neurofibrils

    (C) Both (A) and (B)

    (D) None of the above

29. The axon begins singly but may branch and it has many fine extensions at its end called

    (A) Axon terminals

    (B) Axon tension

    (C) Axial tension

    (D) Axonal hillock

30. The site of transmission of nerve impulse between two neurons is called

    (A) Synapse

    (B) Junction

    (C) Filament

    (D) Interstitial space

31. What type of transmission of nerve signals are?

    (A) Electrical

    (B) Chemical

    (C) Both (A) and (B)

    (D) None of the above

32. The large peripheral neurons are surrounded by myelin sheath produced by the

    (A) Bone cells

    (B) Blood cells

    (C) Schwann cells

    (D) Stem cells

33. The myelin sheath consists of Schwann cells arranged along the length of the axon that produce fatty sheets lipoprotein called

    (A) Actin

    (B) Myelin

    (C) Myosin

    (D) Alanine

34. The outermost layer of Schwann cell plasma membrane is called

    (A) Neurilemma

    (B) Axolemma

    (C) Axoplasm

    (D) Axonal hillock

35. There are some narrow gaps in the myelin sheaths is called

    (A) Cell body

    (B) Dendrites

    (C) Nucleus

    (D) Nodes of Ranvier

36. Which neurons having single process

(A) Bipolar
(B) Unipolar
(C) Multipolar
(D) Tripolar

37. Which neuron found in the nervous system of embryos

(A) Tripolar
(B) Bipolar
(C) Unipolar
(D) Multipolar

38. Which neurons having one dendron and one axon

(A) Bipolar
(B) Multipolar
(C) Tripolar
(D) Unipolar

39. Which neuron found in the retina of eye

(A) Unipolar
(B) Bipolar
(C) Tripolar
(D) Multipolar

40. Which neuron having many dendron and one axon

(A) Multipolar
(B) Unipolar
(C) Tripolar
(D) Bipolar

41. The single extension of unipolar neuron divides into branches, which are

(A) Central branch
(B) Peripheral branch
(C) Both (A) and (B)
(D) None of the above

42. Which branch of unipolar neuron enters the brain or spinal cord

(A) Central branch
(B) Peripheral branch
(C) Medial branch
(D) Lateral branch

43. Which branch of unipolar neuron connects to the peripheral part of the body

(A) Central branch
(B) Peripheral branch
(C) Medial branch
(D) Lateral branch

44. The bipolar neurons are found in

(A) Retina of eye
(B) Inner ear
(C) Olfactory area of nose
(D) All of the above

45. The nature of sensory or afferent neurons are

(A) Multipolar
(B) Unipolar
(C) Tripolar
(D) Bipolar

46. Which nerve involved in skeletal muscle contraction
    (A) Sensory nerve
    (B) Autonomic nerve
    (C) Somatic nerve
    (D) Mixed nerve

47. Which nerve involved in cardiac and smooth muscle contraction and glandular secretion
    (A) Autonomic nerve
    (B) Somatic nerve
    (C) Mixed nerve
    (D) Sensory nerve

48. The sensory receptors respond to different types of stimuli such as
    (A) Cutaneous
    (B) Proprioceptor
    (C) Special senses
    (D) All of the above

49. Which sensory receptor originate in the skin due to pain, touch, heat and cold
    (A) Proprioceptor
    (B) Cutaneous
    (C) Special senses
    (D) Surface receptor

50. Which receptor originate in the muscles and joints and is responsible for the maintenance of balance and posture
    (A) Proprioceptor
    (B) Cutaneous
    (C) Surface receptor
    (D) Special senses

Answer Key

Nervous System, Central Nervous System (Part-01)

Question	Answer	Question	Answer
01	D = All of the Above	26	B = Axoplasm
02	C = Both A and B	27	C = Axolemma
03	C = Both A and B	28	C = Both A and B
04	A = Peripheral Nervous System	29	A = Axon Terminals
05	A = Sensory Nerve	30	A = Synapse
06	B = Motor Nerve	31	C = Both A and B
07	A = Interneurons	32	C = Schwann Cells
08	C = Both A and B	33	B = Myelin
09	A = Cerebrospinal Nerve	34	A = Neurilemma
10	D = All of the Above	35	D = Nodes of Ranvier
11	C = 100m/Sec	36	B = Unipolar
12	D = All of the Above	37	C = Unipolar
13	A = Dorsal Root Ganglion	38	A = Bipolar
14	A = Nerves	39	B = Bipolar
15	C = Nerve Cells	40	A = Multipolar
16	C = Both A and B	41	C = Both A and B
17	A = Neuroglia	42	A = Central Branch
18	D = Nerve Cells	43	B = Peripheral Branch
19	D = All of the Above	44	D = All of the Above
20	C = 60%	45	B = Unipolar
21	C = Both A and B	46	C = Somatic Nerve
22	A = Electrical Excitability	47	A = Autonomic Nerve
23	B = Conductivity	48	D = All of the Above
24	C = Both A and B	49	B = Cutaneous
25	A = Axonal Hillock	50	A = Proprioceptor

Part-02

1. Each nerve bundles have protective covering of connective tissue which are
   - (A) Endoneurium
   - (B) Perineurium
   - (C) Epineurium
   - (D) All of the above

2. The innermost layer of nerve is
   - (A) Endoneurium
   - (B) Perineurium
   - (C) Epineurium
   - (D) Endometrium

3. The nerve is arranged in bundles called
   - (A) Fascicles
   - (B) Follicle
   - (C) Cisternae
   - (D) Cuticles

4. Each bundle of nerve fibres is wrapped in
   - (A) Endoneurium
   - (B) Perineurium
   - (C) Endometrium
   - (D) Epineurium

5. The outermost covering over the entire nerve is
   - (A) Endometrium
   - (B) Endoneurium
   - (C) Epineurium
   - (D) Perineurium

6. The axons of the most mammalian neurons are surrounded by a multi-layered lipid and protein covering called
   - (A) Myelin sheath
   - (B) Actin sheath
   - (C) Myosin sheath
   - (D) Alanine sheath

7. Axons with myelin sheath covering are said to be
   - (A) Myofilament
   - (B) Myoligament
   - (C) Myelinated
   - (D) Myolined

8. Type of neuroglia produce myelin sheath are
   - (A) Schwann cells
   - (B) Oligodendrocytes
   - (C) Both (A) and (B)
   - (D) None of the above

9. Which of the following produce myelin sheath around nerves in the PNS?

   (A) Melanocytes

   (B) Schwann cells

   (C) Oligodendrocytes

   (D) Osteocytes

10. Which of the following produce and maintain myelin sheath around nerves in the CNS?

    (A) Oligodendrocytes

    (B) Osteocytes

    (C) Osteoblast

    (D) Melanocytes

11. An impulse on a myelinated nerve fibres can travel about

    (A) 5 m/sec

    (B) 8 m/sec

    (C) 120 m/sec

    (D) 10 m/sec

12. An impulse on anunmyelinated nerve fibre can travel about

    (A) 20 m/sec

    (B) 0.5 m/sec

    (C) 30 m/sec

    (D) 35 m/sec

13. Neuroglia is also called as

    (A) Fragile cells

    (B) Glial cells

    (C) Mast cells

    (D) Synapse

14. Types of neuroglia are

    (A) Astrocytes

    (B) Oligodendrocytes

    (C) Microglia

    (D) All of the above

15. Which neuroglia are star – shaped cells that wrap around the nerve cells?

    (A) Schwann cells

    (B) Astrocytes

    (C) Microglia

    (D) Ependymal cells

16. Which neuroglia help in the formation of blood brain barrier

    (A) Schwann cells

    (B) Oligodendrocytes

    (C) Microglia

    (D) Astrocytes

17. Which neuroglia are small cells derived from monocytes that migrate from the blood into the nervous system before birth?

    (A) Astrocytes

    (B) Microglia

    (C) Oligodendrocytes

    (D) Schwann cells

18. Which neuroglia protect CNS cells from disease by engulfing the invading microbes and clear away the debris of dead cells

    (A) Astrocytes

    (B) Oligodendrocytes

    (C) Microglia

    (D) Ependymal cells

19. Which neuroglia form the epithelial lining of the ventricles of the brain
    - (A) Microglia
    - (B) Ependymal cells
    - (C) Astrocytes
    - (D) Schwann cells

20. Which neuroglia produce cerebrospinal fluid and help in its circulation
    - (A) Astrocytes
    - (B) Ependymal cells
    - (C) Microglia
    - (D) Schwann cells

21. Which matter is the collection of the myelinated neurons and it appears whitish?
    - (A) Yellow matter
    - (B) White matter
    - (C) Grey matter
    - (D) Brown matter

22. The grey matter of nervous system contains
    - (A) Cell bodies of neurons
    - (B) Dendrites
    - (C) Unmyelinated axons
    - (D) All of the above

23. The phases of membrane action potential in the nerve are
    - (A) Resting potential
    - (B) Depolarization
    - (C) Repolarization
    - (D) All of the above

24. The main extracellular cation in nervous system is
    - (A) Sodium
    - (B) Potassium
    - (C) Chloride
    - (D) Calcium

25. The main intracellular cation in nervous system is
    - (A) Chloride
    - (B) Calcium
    - (C) Potassium
    - (D) Sodium

26. The difference in electrical potential across the plasma membrane when the cell is not stimulated or when the cell is in a state of relaxation is called
    - (A) Depolarization
    - (B) Resting potential
    - (C) Repolarization
    - (D) Hyperpolarization

27. The value of resting potential is
    - (A) -10 mV
    - (B) -70 mV
    - (C) +5 mV
    - (D) -5 mV

28. In response to the arrival of an action potential, Sodium channels in the membrane open and sodium floods into the neuron from the extracellular fluid is called
    - (A) Depolarization
    - (B) Resting potential
    - (C) Repolarization
    - (D) Hyperpolarization

29. The depolarization cause by opening of
    - (A) Potassium ion channels
    - (B) Sodium ion channels
    - (C) Chloride ion channels
    - (D) Calcium ion channels

30. In which phase both voltage – gated sodium and voltage – gated potassium ions channels are closed
    - (A) Depolarization
    - (B) Repolarization
    - (C) Hyperpolarization
    - (D) Resting potential

31. In which phase potassium channel open and potassium ions flows out the membrane
    - (A) Depolarization
    - (B) Resting potential
    - (C) Repolarization
    - (D) Hypo polarization

32. Which of the following cause by closing of sodium channels and opening of potassium channels?
    - (A) Depolarization
    - (B) Repolarization
    - (C) Hypo polarization
    - (D) Resting potential

33. In which phase the neuron cell body has positive charge
    - (A) Depolarization
    - (B) Resting potential
    - (C) Repolarization
    - (D) Hyperpolarization

34. In which phase neuron cell body has negative charge
    - (A) Resting potential
    - (B) Depolarization
    - (C) Repolarization
    - (D) Hypo polarization

35. Hyperpolarization occurs due to excessive efflux of
    - (A) Sodium
    - (B) Potassium
    - (C) Chloride
    - (D) Calcium

36. The point where the nerve impulse passes from one nerve to another is called
    - (A) Synapse
    - (B) Gap junction
    - (C) Interstitial space
    - (D) Extracellular space

37. The neuron that sends the impulse is called
    (A) Postsynaptic neuron
    (B) Presynaptic neuron
    (C) Juxtaposition
    (D) Relay synaptic neuron

38. The neuron that receives the impulse is called
    (A) Juxtaposition
    (B) Presynaptic neuron
    (C) Postsynaptic neuron
    (D) Delay synaptic neuron

39. The axon terminal of the presynaptic neuron breaks into minute branches that end in small endings called
    (A) Synaptic knobs
    (B) Synaptic gap
    (C) Node of Ranvier
    (D) Synapses

40. The synaptic knobs are close to the dendrites of the postsynaptic neuron and the space between these synaptic knobs and dendrites is called
    (A) Synaptic gap
    (B) Synaptic cleft
    (C) Synapses
    (D) Node of Ranvier

41. The chemical messenger that allows nerve cells to communicate with each other
    (A) Neurotransmitters
    (B) Receptors
    (C) Coenzymes
    (D) Synapses

42. The neurotransmitter which is synthesized by nerve cells and stores in the
    (A) Cell body
    (B) Dendrites
    (C) Synaptic vesicles
    (D) Synapses

43. The synaptic vesicles release neurotransmitter into
    (A) Synaptic cleft
    (B) Dendrites
    (C) Axon
    (D) Nucleus

44. Which of the following is a type of classification of neurotransmitter
    (A) Excitatory neurotransmitter
    (B) Inhibitory neurotransmitter
    (C) Modulatory neurotransmitter
    (D) All of the above

45. The neurotransmitter in the brain and spinal cord includes
    (A) Noradrenaline
    (B) Dopamine
    (C) Acetylcholine
    (D) All of the above

46. The Examples of neuromodulator is/are
    (A) Enkephalins
    (B) Endorphins
    (C) Dynorphins
    (D) All of the above

47. Noradrenaline is also called
    (A) Histamine
    (B) Serotonin
    (C) Norepinephrine
    (D) Dopamine

48. Epinephrine is also called
    (A) Adrenaline
    (B) Dopamine
    (C) Serotonin
    (D) Acetylcholine

49. Which of the following is excitatory neurotransmitter?
    (A) GABA
    (B) Serotonin
    (C) Glycine
    (D) Adrenaline

50. Which of the following is inhibitory neurotransmitter?
    (A) Glutamate
    (B) Adrenaline
    (C) GABA
    (D) Noradrenaline

Answer Key

Nervous System, Central Nervous System (Part-02)

Question	Answer	Question	Answer
01	D = All of the Above	26	B = Resting Potential
02	A = Endoneurium	27	B = -70mV
03	A = Fascicles	28	A = Depolarization
04	B = Perineurium	29	B = Sodium Ion Channel
05	C = Epineurium	30	D = Resting Potential
06	A = Myelin Sheath	31	C = Repolarization
07	C = Myelinated	32	B = Repolarization
08	C = Both A and B	33	A = Depolarization
09	B = Schwann Cells	34	A = Resting Potential
10	A = Oligodendrocytes	35	B = Potassium
11	C = 120 m/Sec	36	A = Synapse
12	B = 0.5 m/Sec	37	B = Presynaptic Neuron
13	B = Glial Cells	38	C = Post Synaptic Neuron
14	D = All of the Above	39	A = Synaptic Knobs
15	B = Astrocytes	40	B = Synaptic Cleft
16	D = Astrocytes	41	A = Neurotransmitters
17	B = Microglia	42	C = Synaptic Vesicles
18	C = Microglia	43	A = Synaptic Cleft
19	B = Ependymal Cells	44	D = All of the Above
20	B = Ependymal Cells	45	D = All of the Above
21	B = White Matter	46	D = All of the Above
22	D = All of the Above	47	C = Norepinephrine
23	D = All of the Above	48	A = Adrenaline
24	A = Sodium	49	D = Adrenaline
25	C = Potassium	50	C = GABA

Part-03

1. The human brain weighs are about
   - (A) 1.4 kg
   - (B) 5 kg
   - (C) 3 kg
   - (D) 3.5 kg

2. The brain is the centre for
   - (A) Intellect
   - (B) Emotions
   - (C) Memory
   - (D) All of the above

3. The 97% of the total body's neuronal tissues present in
   - (A) Liver
   - (B) Brain
   - (C) Kidney
   - (D) Lungs

4. The major part of brain is
   - (A) Fore brain
   - (B) Mid brain
   - (C) Hind brain
   - (D) All of the above

5. The fore brain includes
   - (A) Cerebrum
   - (B) Diencephalon
   - (C) Both (A) and (B)
   - (D) None of the above

6. The hind brain includes
   - (A) Pons
   - (B) Medulla oblongata
   - (C) Cerebellum
   - (D) All of the above

7. Mid brain, pons and medulla oblongata are collectively termed as
   - (A) Brain stem
   - (B) Brain fissure
   - (C) Brain matter
   - (D) Brain plexus

8. Which of the following present in superior to the brain stem?
   - (A) Meninges
   - (B) Cerebellum
   - (C) Spinal cord
   - (D) Diencephalon

9. Diencephalon consists of
   - (A) Thalamus
   - (B) Hypothalamus
   - (C) Both (A) and (B)
   - (D) None of the above

10. The brain is protected by the
    - (A) Cranial bones
    - (B) Cranial meninges
    - (C) Both (A) and (B)
    - (D) None of the above

11. The meninges that protect the brain are termed as
    - (A) Cuticle meninges
    - (B) Cranial meninges
    - (C) Cortex meninges
    - (D) Crucial meninges

12. Which of the following present between the skull and brain?
    - (A) Diencephalon
    - (B) Cerebrum
    - (C) Cranial meninges
    - (D) Hypothalamus

13. The cranial meninges and spinal meninges have basic structure of
    - (A) Dura mater
    - (B) Pia mater
    - (C) Arachnoid mater
    - (D) All of the above

14. The outer layer of meninges is
    - (A) Dura mater
    - (B) Arachnoid mater
    - (C) Pia mater
    - (D) Fissure

15. The middle layer of meninges is
    - (A) Dura mater
    - (B) Pia mater
    - (C) Arachnoid mater
    - (D) Thalamus

16. The inner layer of meninges is
    - (A) Sulcus
    - (B) Pia mater
    - (C) Dura mater
    - (D) Arachnoid mater

17. The dura mater and arachnoid mater are separated by
    - (A) Subarachnoid space
    - (B) Subpial space
    - (C) Subdural space
    - (D) Sub carpal space

18. The arachnoid mater and pia mater are separated by
    - (A) subarachnoid space
    - (B) subdural space
    - (C) subpial space
    - (D) fissure space

19. The part of dura mater enclosing the brain is called
    - (A) Cerebral dura mater
    - (B) Spinal dura mater
    - (C) Sternal dura mater
    - (D) Fissure dura mater

20. The part of dura mater covers the spinal cord is called
    (A) Sternal duramater
    (B) Fissure dura mater
    (C) Spinal dura mater
    (D) Cerebral dura mater

21. The outer layer of cerebral dura mater attached to
    (A) Suture of the skull
    (B) Lateral ventricle
    (C) Choroid plexus
    (D) Fourth ventricle

22. The various part of the brain is separated by the extensions of cerebral dura mater are
    (A) Falx cerebri
    (B) Falx cerebelli
    (C) Tentorium cerebelli
    (D) All of the above

23. The falx cerebri separates the two hemispheres of
    (A) Cerebellum
    (B) Cerebrum
    (C) Medulla oblongata
    (D) Spinal cord

24. The cerebelli separates the two hemispheres of the
    (A) Cerebellum
    (B) Cerebrum
    (C) Spinal cord
    (D) Medulla oblongata

25. The layer of fibrous tissue that lies between the pia mater and dura mater is
    (A) Thalamus
    (B) Hypothalamus
    (C) Arachnoid mater
    (D) Choroid plexus

26. Arachnoid is a delicate membrane that passes over the
    (A) Convolutions of the cerebrum
    (B) Cerebellum
    (C) Hypothalamus
    (D) Thalamus

27. The certain protrusions of arachnoid mater accompany the inner layer of dura matter in the formation of
    (A) Pia villi
    (B) Arachnoid villi
    (C) Dura villi
    (D) Fissures villi

28. The delicate layer of connective tissue containing many minute blood vessels are called
    (A) Dura mater
    (B) Pia mater
    (C) Arachnoid mater
    (D) Fissure

29. How many ventricles are in brain?
    (A) 7   (B) 8
    (C) 4   (D) 10

30. The cavities lie within the cerebral hemispheres just below the corpus callosum
    (A) Four ventricles   (B) Lateral ventricle
    (C) Third ventricle   (D) Fifth ventricle

31. The right and left ventricles are separated from each other by a thin membrane are
    (A) Septum pellucidum   (B) Intercoastal space
    (C) Pericardium   (D) Pleura

32. Each lateral ventricle connects with third ventricle by a narrow opening called
    (A) Intervertebral foramen   (B) Intercoastal foramen
    (C) Interventricular foramen   (D) Supraorbital foramen

33. Which cavity situated below the lateral ventricle between the right left halves of the thalamus
    (A) Fifth ventricle   (B) Fourth ventricle
    (C) Sixth ventricle   (D) Third ventricle

34. The third ventricle connects with the fourth ventricle by a canal known as
    (A) Cerebral aqueduct   (B) Circle of Wallis
    (C) Canaliculi   (D) Cerebellum cortex

35. The diamond shaped cavity situated below and behind the third ventricle between the cerebellum and pons called
    (A) Lateral ventricle   (B) Fifth ventricle
    (C) Fourth ventricle   (D) Sixth ventricle

36. How many foramina present in roof of the fourth ventricle?
    (A) One   (B) Two
    (C) Three   (D) Four

37. The clear, colourless liquid that protects the brain and spinal cord against injuries is called
    - (A) Cerebrospinal fluid
    - (B) Synovial fluid
    - (C) Interstitial fluid
    - (D) Extracellular fluid

38. The site of cerebrospinal fluid production is
    - (A) Dural sinus
    - (B) Choroid plexus
    - (C) Arachnoid granulation
    - (D) Subdural space

39. The main cell type that produces cerebrospinal fluid is
    - (A) Ependymal cell
    - (B) Schwann cell
    - (C) Astrocytes
    - (D) Basket cell

40. Cerebrospinal fluid carries
    - (A) Oxygen
    - (B) Glucose
    - (C) Nutrients
    - (D) All of the above

41. The movement of cerebrospinal fluid occurs due to
    - (A) Pulsation of blood vessels
    - (B) Respiration
    - (C) Positive charge
    - (D) All of the above

42. Cerebrospinal fluid is continuously secreted at a rate of about
    - (A) 100 mL / day
    - (B) 720 mL / day
    - (C) 200 mL / day
    - (D) 210 mL / day

43. The function of cerebrospinal fluid is
    - (A) It supports and protects the brain and spinal cord
    - (B) It acts as a fluid buffer
    - (C) It is the medium for interchange of substances
    - (D) All of the above

44. How many cardiac outputs receives by brain?
    - (A) 15 %
    - (B) 50 %
    - (C) 60 %
    - (D) 70 %

45. The major part of the brain is supplied with arterial blood by an arrangement of arteries called
    - (A) Auricular arteries
    - (B) Circulus arteriosus
    - (C) Carotid arteries
    - (D) Radial arteries

46. The largest volume of cerebrospinal fluid is contained within the
    (A) Lateral ventricles
    (B) Third ventricles
    (C) Fourth ventricles
    (D) Subarachnoid space

47. Cerebrospinal fluid is reabsorbed by
    (A) Arachnoid granulations
    (B) Pia granulations
    (C) Dura granulations
    (D) Fissure granulations

48. The circle of Willis comprises large arteries are
    (A) Two internal carotid arteries
    (B) Two vertebral arteries
    (C) Both (A) and (B)
    (D) None of the above

49. The circulus arteriosus also called
    (A) Circle of Willis
    (B) Circle of villi
    (C) Circle of fissure
    (D) Circle of pons

50. Circle of Willis and its contributing arteries which maintain a constant supply of
    (A) Oxygen
    (B) Glucose
    (C) Both (A) and (B)
    (D) None of the above

Answer Key

Nervous System, Central Nervous System (Part-03)

Question	Answer	Question	Answer
01	A = 1.4 kg	26	A = Convolution of the Cerebrum
02	D = All of the Above	27	B = Arachnoid Villi
03	B = Brain	28	B = Pia Mater
04	D = All of the Above	29	C = 04
05	C = Both A and B	30	B = Lateral Ventricle
06	D = All of the Above	31	A = Septum Pellucidum
07	A = Brain Stem	32	C = Interventricular Foramen
08	D = Diencephalon	33	D = Third Ventricles
09	C = Both A and B	34	A = Cerebral Aqueduct
10	C = Both A and B	35	C = Fourth Ventricles
11	B = Cranial Meninges	36	C = Three
12	C = Cranial Meninges	37	A = Cerebrospinal Fluid
13	D = All of the Above	38	B = Choroid Plexus
14	A = Dura Matter	39	A = Ependymal Cell
15	C = Arachnoid Mater	40	D = All of the Above
16	B = Pia Mater	41	D = All of the Above
17	C = Subdural Space	42	B = 720 mL/Day
18	A = Subarachnoid Space	43	D = All of the Above
19	A = Cerebral Dura Mater	44	A = 15 %
20	C = Spinal Dura Mater	45	B = Circulus Arteriosus
21	A = Suture of the Skull	46	D = Subarachnoid Space
22	D = All of the Above	47	A = Arachnoid Granulation
23	B = Cerebrum	48	C = Both A and B
24	A = Cerebellum	49	A = Circle of Willis
25	C = Arachnoid Mater	50	C = Both A and B

Part-04

1. The selective barrier between the capillary and neurons that protects the brain is
   - (A) Blood brain barrier
   - (B) Blood placental barrier
   - (C) Blood testis barrier
   - (D) Blood skin barrier

2. The blood brain barrier exists in all part of brain except in some area of the
   - (A) Cerebrum
   - (B) Hypothalamus
   - (C) Cerebellum
   - (D) Medulla oblongata

3. The substance that can cross the blood brain barrier and enter the brain tissues are
   - (A) Oxygen
   - (B) Water
   - (C) Amino acids
   - (D) All of the above

4. The blood brain barrier protects the brain from
   - (A) Toxic substance
   - (B) Chemical variation in blood
   - (C) Both (A) and (B)
   - (D) None of the above

5. The blood brain barrier is composed of
   - (A) Capillary endothelium
   - (B) Basement membrane of the endothelium
   - (C) Numerous processes of astrocytes
   - (D) All of the above

6. The drugs that cross the blood brain barrier is/are
   - (A) Reboxetine
   - (B) Viloxazine
   - (C) Melphalan
   - (D) All of the above

7. The drugs that cross the blood brain barrier must be
   - (A) Highly lipid soluble drug
   - (B) Highly aqueous soluble drug
   - (C) Hydrophilic drug
   - (D) Lipophobic drug

8. The blood brain barrier prevents the adverse CNS effects of some aqueous soluble drug which is/are

(A) Penicillin
(B) Streptomycin
(C) Thiopentone
(D) All of the above

9. The blood brain barrier is developed from which cell

(A) Schwann cells
(B) Ependymal cells
(C) Astrocytes
(D) Oligodendrocytes

10. Function of blood brain barrier

(A) Maintain constant neuronal environment
(B) Inactivates toxic metabolite
(C) Entry of hormones also restricted
(D) All of the above

11. The large part of the brain is

(A) Cerebrum
(B) Cerebellum
(C) Hypothalamus
(D) Thalamus

12. Which part is termed as 'seat of intelligence'

(A) Hypothalamus
(B) Thalamus
(C) Cerebrum
(D) Medulla oblongata

13. Cerebrum are responsible for the abilities of

(A) Reading
(B) Writing
(C) Speaking
(D) All of the above

14. The superficial part of the cerebrum is composed of nerve cell bodies or grey matter that is referred as

(A) Cerebral cortex
(B) Cerebral compact
(C) Cerebral cuticle
(D) Cerebral sponge

15. The deeper layer of cerebrum consists of

(A) Pia mater
(B) White matter
(C) Arachnoid mater
(D) Dura mater

16. Cerebral cortex is also known as

(A) Cerebral cortex
(B) Cerebral cuticle
(C) Cerebral mantle
(D) Cerebral pons

17. The surface of the cerebral cortex shows many folds, which are called
    (A) gyri
    (B) Pons
    (C) Sheaths
    (D) Fascicles

18. The gyri folds are separated by grooves which called as
    (A) Fascicles
    (B) Pons
    (C) Sheaths
    (D) Sulci

19. The cerebral hemisphere is connected internally by a mass of white matter called
    (A) Corpus callosum
    (B) Corpus colon
    (C) Corpus compact
    (D) Corpus cuticle

20. Each cerebral hemisphere is divided into lobes, these are
    (A) Frontal lobe
    (B) Parietal lobe
    (C) Temporal lobe
    (D) All of the above

21. Which of the following separates the frontal lobe from the parietal lobe of cerebrum?
    (A) Central sulci
    (B) Lateral sulci
    (C) Parietooccipital sulci
    (D) Distal sulci

22. Which of the following separates the frontal lobe from the temporal lobe of cerebrum?
    (A) Central sulci
    (B) Lateral sulci
    (C) Distal sulci
    (D) Parietooccipital sulci

23. Which of the following separates the parietal lobe from the occipital lobe of cerebrum?
    (A) Distal sulci
    (B) Lateral sulci
    (C) Central sulci
    (D) Parietooccipital sulci

24. The nerve fibres of cerebrum are organised into tracts which are
    (A) Association tract
    (B) Commissural tract
    (C) Projection tract
    (D) All of the above

25. Which tracts connect different parts of a cerebral hemisphere and transmit nerve impulses between gyri in the same hemisphere
    (A) Association tract
    (B) Projection tract
    (C) Commissural tract
    (D) Dilation tract

26. Which of the following connects the corresponding areas of two hemispheres by transmitting impulses from gyri in one hemisphere to the corresponding gyri in another hemisphere?

    (A) Projection tract

    (B) Commissural tract

    (C) Association tract

    (D) Dilation tract

27. Which of the following connects the cerebral cortex with the brain stem and the spinal cord?

    (A) Dilation tract

    (B) Commissural tract

    (C) Projection tract

    (D) Association tract

28. Which of the following may transmit impulses either from the cerebrum to the spinal cord or from the spinal cord to the brain?

    (A) Association tract

    (B) Projection tract

    (C) Commissural tract

    (D) Dilation tract

29. Functions of cerebral cortex is/are

    (A) Mental activities

    (B) Sensory perception

    (C) Skeletal muscle movement

    (D) All of the above

30. The association area of the cerebral cortex deals with complex mental functions such as

    (A) Intelligence

    (B) Memory

    (C) Reasoning

    (D) All of the above

31. The motor areas of the cerebral cortex

    (A) The primary motor area

    (B) Broca's speech area

    (C) Both (A) and (B)

    (D) None of the above

32. The primary motor area located in which lobe of the cerebral cortex

    (A) Frontal lobe

    (B) Parietal lobe

    (C) Temporal lobe

    (D) Distal lobe

33. In which area the Betz cell initiate the contraction of skeletal muscle and a nerve fibre

    (A) The primary motor area

    (B) Broca's speech area

    (C) The somatosensory are

    (D) The visual area

34. The nerve impulse in the primary motor area results in
    (A) Contraction of specific muscle fibres
    (B) Control temperature
    (C) Visual information
    (D) Smell perception

35. Which of the following located in the frontal lobe immediately anterior to the central sulcus and control the voluntary contraction of specific muscle?
    (A) The somatosensory area
    (B) The visual area
    (C) The auditory area
    (D) The primary motor area

36. Which of the following located in the frontal lobe just above the lateral sulcus and controls the muscle movements necessary for speech?
    (A) The auditory area
    (B) The Broca's speech area
    (C) The olfactory area
    (D) The visual area

37. Which of the area of the cerebral cortex dominant in the left hemisphere in the right – handed people
    (A) The olfactory area
    (B) The visual area
    (C) The Broca's speech area
    (D) The auditory area

38. Which area are coordinated contractions of the speech and breathing muscles help us speak out our thoughts?
    (A) The Broca's speech area
    (B) The auditory area
    (C) The olfactory area
    (D) The gustatory area

39. Which area is also known as primary sensory area?
    (A) The auditory area
    (B) The olfactory area
    (C) The somatosensory area
    (D) The visual area

40. The somatosensory area receives information about
    (A) Touch
    (B) Pain
    (C) Temperature
    (D) All of the above

41. Which area located at the posterior tip of the occipital lobe, behind the parietooccipital sulcus
    (A) The visual area
    (B) The olfactory area
    (C) The gustatory area
    (D) The somatosensory area

42. Which area receives the impulses of the visual information
    (A) The olfactory area
    (B) The gustatory area
    (C) The visual area
    (D) The somatosensory area

43. Which area located within the temporal lobe, immediately below the lateral sulcus
    (A) The olfactory area
    (B) The auditory area
    (C) The gustatory area
    (D) The somatosensory area

44. Which area receives impulses for sound and interprets them for auditory perception
    (A) The gustatory area
    (B) The somatosensory area
    (C) The auditory area
    (D) The olfactory area

45. The olfactory area located in
    (A) Temporal lobe
    (B) Occipital lobe
    (C) Distal lobe
    (D) Frontal lobe

46. The area receives impulses for smell and interprets them for olfactory perception
    (A) The auditory area
    (B) The olfactory area
    (C) The somatosensory area
    (D) The gustatory area

47. Which area located deep within the somatosensory area, just above the lateral sulcus in the parietal lobe
    (A) The somatosensory area
    (B) The gustatory area
    (C) The olfactory area
    (D) The auditory area

48. Which area receives impulses from taste buds' receptors and interprets them for taste
    (A) The gustatory area
    (B) The olfactory area
    (C) The visual area
    (D) The auditory area

49. The various association areas of the cerebral cortex are
    (A) Premotor area
    (B) Prefrontal area
    (C) Visual association area
    (D) All of the above

50. Wernicke's (sensory speech) area located in
    (A) Temporal lobe
    (B) Occipital lobe
    (C) Frontal lobe
    (D) Distal lobe

Answer Key

Nervous System, Central Nervous System (Part-04)

Question	Answer	Question	Answer
01	A = Blood Brain Barrier	26	B = Commissural Tract
02	B = Hypothalamus	27	C = Projection Tract
03	D = All of the Above	28	B = Projection Tract
04	C = Both A and B	29	D = All of the Above
05	D = All of the Above	30	D = All of the Above
06	D = All of the Above	31	C = Both A and B
07	A = Highly Lipid Soluble Drugs	32	A = Frontal Lobe
08	D = All of the Above	33	A = The Primary Motor Area
09	C = Astrocytes	34	A = Contraction of Specific Muscle Fibres
10	D = All of the Above	35	D = The Primary Motor Area
11	A = Cerebrum	36	B = The Broca's Speech Area
12	C = Cerebrum	37	C = The Broca's Speech Area
13	D = All of the Above	38	A = The Broca's Speech Area
14	A = Cerebral Cortex	39	C = The Somatosensory Area
15	B = White Mater	40	D = All of the Above
16	C = Cerebral Mantle	41	A = The Visual Area
17	A = Gyri	42	C = The Visual Area
18	D = Sulci	43	B = The Auditory Area
19	A = Corpus Callosum	44	C = The Auditory Area
20	D = All of the Above	45	A = Temporal Lobe
21	A = Central Sulci	46	B = The Olfactory Area
22	B = Lateral Sulci	47	B = The Gustatory Area
23	D = Parietooccipital Sulci	48	A = The Gustatory Area
24	D = All of the Above	49	D = All of the Above
25	A = Association Tract	50	A = Temporal Lobe

Part-05

1. Which areas of the cerebral cortex regulate the higher cognitive abilities by coordinating the nerve impulses from the sensory and motor areas
   (A) Association area
   (B) Olfactory area
   (C) Primary motor area
   (D) Auditory area

2. The different association areas of the cerebral cortex are connected to each other by
   (A) Association routes
   (B) Association gap
   (C) Association tracts
   (D) Association path

3. Which association area of cerebral cortex located in the frontal area immediately anterior to the primary motor area
   (A) Olfactory area
   (B) Premotor area
   (C) Auditory area
   (D) Gustatory area

4. Which area is concerned with learned motor skills that require a sequence of movements?
   (A) Premotor area
   (B) Olfactory area
   (C) Gustatory area
   (D) Auditory area

5. Which area located anterior to the premotor area just behind the eyes
   (A) Premotor area
   (B) Olfactory area
   (C) Auditory area
   (D) Prefrontal area

6. Wernicke's (sensory speech) area located in the
   (A) Occipital area
   (B) Temporal area
   (C) Distal area
   (D) Frontal area

7. Which area concerned with the interpretation of the meaning of speech by perceiving spoken words and various sound
   (A) Wernicke's (sensory speech area)
   (B) Auditory area
   (C) Gustatory area
   (D) Olfactory area

8. The main component of basal ganglia is
   (A) Striatum pallidum
   (B) Substantia nigra
   (C) Subthalamic nucleus
   (D) All of the above

9. The most common disorder of the basal ganglia is

   (A) Meningitis
   (B) Parkinson's disease
   (C) Epilepsy
   (D) Alzheimer's disease

10. The group of cortical and subcortical structure that form ring on the inner border of the cerebrum called

    (A) Limbic system
    (B) Medulla oblongata
    (C) cerebellum
    (D) Spinal cord

11. Limbic system includes

    (A) Hypothalamus
    (B) Hippocampus
    (C) Amygdala
    (D) All of the above

12. Limbic system plays a primary role in maintaining emotional state including

    (A) Pain
    (B) Pleasure
    (C) Affection
    (D) All of the above

13. Which of the following is present between the two cerebral hemispheres, superior to the mid brain

    (A) Diencephalon
    (B) Meninges
    (C) Spinal cord
    (D) Medulla oblongata

14. The diencephalon includes

    (A) Optic tracts and optic chiasma
    (B) Infundibulum
    (C) Pineal gland
    (D) All of the above

15. The diencephalon is divided into

    (A) Thalamus
    (B) Hypothalamus
    (C) Both (A) and (B)
    (D) None of the above

16. The superior part of the diencephalon is

    (A) Thalamus
    (B) Medulla oblongata
    (C) Cerebellum
    (D) Spinal cord

17. Thalamus plays an important role as an interpretation centre for conscious awareness of

    (A) Pain
    (B) Temperature
    (C) Touch
    (D) All of the above

18. The small part of the diencephalon and is composed of number of groups of nerve cells are
    (A) Hypothalamus
    (B) Pons
    (C) Meninges
    (D) Spinal cord

19. Which of the following situated below and in front of the thalamus immediately above the pituitary gland
    (A) Spinal cord
    (B) Medulla oblongata
    (C) Hypothalamus
    (D) Pons

20. The chief function of the hypothalamus is
    (A) Control of the pituitary
    (B) Regulation of body temperature
    (C) Regulation of food intake and water balance
    (D) All of the above

21. The supraoptic and paraventricular nuclei of the hypothalamus secrete
    (A) Antidiuretic hormones
    (B) Oxytocin
    (C) Both (A) and (B)
    (D) None of the above

22. Example of anterior pituitary hormones are
    (A) Growth hormones releasing hormones
    (B) Prolactin-inhibitory hormone
    (C) Corticotropin- releasing hormone
    (D) All of the above

23. The hypothalamus regulates food intake through the centres
    (A) Feeding centre
    (B) Satiety centre
    (C) Both (A) and (B)
    (D) None of the above

24. The hypothalamus regulates water balance through
    (A) Thirst mechanism
    (B) ADH mechanism
    (C) Both (A) and (B)
    (D) None of the above

25. The hypothalamus along with the limbic system regulates the feelings of
    (A) Rage
    (B) Aggression
    (C) Pleasure
    (D) All of the above

26. Which of the following present between the diencephalon and the spinal cord

    (A) Brain stem
    (B) Cerebrum
    (C) Convolution
    (D) Skull

27. The brain stem consists of

    (A) Midbrain
    (B) Pons
    (C) Medulla oblongata
    (D) All of the above

28. The brain stem serves function are

    (A) Regulates heart rate
    (B) Regulates breathing
    (C) Regulates balance
    (D) All of the above

29. Which of the following situated below the cerebrum and above the pons

    (A) Meninges
    (B) Spinal cord
    (C) Mid brain
    (D) Sulcus

30. The mid brain contains

    (A) Cerebral peduncles
    (B) Tectum
    (C) Substantia nigra
    (D) All of the above

31. Which of the following conduct nerve impulses from the cerebral cortex to the pons and spinal cord?

    (A) Tectum
    (B) Cerebral peduncles
    (C) Substantia nigra
    (D) Fissures

32. Tectum serves as a reflex centre that controls the

    (A) Movement of eye balls and head
    (B) Movement of head and trunk
    (C) Both (A) and (B)
    (D) None of the above

33. Which of the following release dopamine and control subconscious muscle activities

    (A) Substantia nigra
    (B) Cerebral peduncles
    (C) Tectum
    (D) Fissures

34. Which of the following situated in front of the cerebellum, below the midbrain and above the medulla oblongata

    (A) Tectum
    (B) Midbrain
    (C) Pons
    (D) Medulla oblongata

35. Which areas consist in pons that help to regulate breathing
    (A) Pneumotaxic areas   (B) Apneustic areas
    (C) Both (A) and (B)   (D) None of the above

36. Which of the following extends from the pons above and is continuous
    with the spinal cord below?
    (A) Medulla oblongata   (B) Cerebrum
    (C) Hypothalamus   (D) Thalamus

37. The medulla oblongata forms the main pathway for the
    (A) Ascending (sensory) tracts   (B) Descending (motor) tracts
    (C) Both (A) and (B)   (D) None of the above

38. The special features of medulla are
    (A) Reflex centre   (B) Vasomotor centre
    (C) Respiratory centre   (D) All of the above

39. Which centre regulates the force of cardiac contraction and heart rate
    (A) Respiratory centre   (B) Cardiovascular centre
    (C) Vasomotor centre   (D) Reflex centre

40. Reflex centre controls
    (A) Sneezing   (B) Coughing
    (C) Swallowing   (D) All of the above

41. Which centre controls the rate and depth of respiration
    (A) Vasomotor centre   (B) Cardiovascular centre
    (C) Respiratory centre   (D) Reflex centre

42. Which centre regulates the diameter of the blood vessels
    (A) Vasomotor centre   (B) Reflex centre
    (C) Respiratory centre   (D) Digestion centre

43. The collection of neurons extending throughout the brainstem and into
    the spinal cord is called
    (A) Reticular formation   (B) Sensory decussation
    (C) Reflex centre   (D) Respiratory centre

44. Reticular formation maintains
    - (A) Consciousness and arousal
    - (B) Helps regulate the muscle tone
    - (C) Both (A) and (B)
    - (D) None of the above

45. The second largest portion of the brain and is situated below the posterior portion of the cerebrum and behind the pons and medulla of the brainstem
    - (A) Cerebrum
    - (B) Cerebellum
    - (C) Medulla oblongata
    - (D) Hypothalamus

46. The cerebellum consists of two partially separated hemispheres connected by a narrow strip called
    - (A) Vermis
    - (B) Cisternae
    - (C) Pons
    - (D) Fissures

47. The surface of cerebellum composed of
    - (A) Dura mater
    - (B) Pia mater
    - (C) Arachnoid mater
    - (D) Grey matter

48. The deeper layer of cerebellum consists of
    - (A) Pia mater
    - (B) Arachnoid mater
    - (C) White matter
    - (D) Dura mater

49. Functions of cerebellum is
    - (A) Maintenance pf posture
    - (B) Balance and equilibrium
    - (C) Learning and language processing
    - (D) All of the above

50. The damage of the cerebellum results in
    - (A) Clumsy
    - (B) Uncoordinated muscular movement
    - (C) Tremors
    - (D) All of the above

Answer Key

Nervous System, Central Nervous System (Part-05)

Question	Answer	Question	Answer
01	A = Association Area	26	A = Brain Stem
02	C = Association Tract	27	D = All of the Above
03	B = Premotor Area	28	D = All of the Above
04	A = Premotor Area	29	C = Mid Brain
05	D = Prefrontal Area	30	D = All of the Above
06	B = Temporal Area	31	B = Cerebral Peduncles
07	A = Wernicke's (Sensory Speech Area)	32	C = Both A and B
08	D = All of the Above	33	A = Substantia Nigra
09	B = Parkinson's Disease	34	C = Pons
10	A = Limbic System	35	C = Both A and B
11	D = All of the Above	36	A = Medulla Oblongata
12	D = All of the Above	37	C = Both A and B
13	A = Diencephalon	38	D = All of the Above
14	D = All of the Above	39	B = Cardiovascular System
15	C = Both A and B	40	D = All of the Above
16	A = Thalamus	41	C = Respiratory Centre
17	D = All of the Above	42	A = Vasomotor Centre
18	A = Hypothalamus	43	A = Reticular Formation
19	C = Hypothalamus	44	C = Both A and B
20	D = All of the Above	45	B = Cerebellum
21	C = Both A and B	46	A = Vermis
22	D = All of the Above	47	D = Grey Matter
23	C = Both A and B	48	C = White Matter
24	C = Both A and B	49	D = All of the Above
25	D = All of the Above	50	D = All of the Above

Part-06

1. The elongated almost cylindrical part of the CNS is
   - (A) Spinal cord
   - (B) cerebrum
   - (C) Cerebellum
   - (D) Hypothalamus

2. Spinal cord is closed with in the
   - (A) Haversian canal
   - (B) Vertebral canal
   - (C) Reticular canal
   - (D) Medullar canal

3. Spinal cord is surrounding by
   - (A) Meninges
   - (B) Cerebrospinal fluid
   - (C) Both (A) and (B)
   - (D) None of the above

4. The length of the spinal cord is
   - (A) 42-45 cm
   - (B) 60-65 cm
   - (C) 5-10 cm
   - (D) 12-15 cm

5. Which serves as the link between the brain and rest of the body
   - (A) Spinal cord
   - (B) Cerebrum
   - (C) Thalamus
   - (D) Hypothalamus

6. Which contains neuron connection between sensory and motor neuron that facilitation rapid reaction to certain stimuli
   - (A) Spinal cord
   - (B) Hypothalamus
   - (C) Meninges
   - (D) Thalamus

7. External anatomy of spinal cord is
   - (A) Cervical enlargement
   - (B) Lumber enlargement
   - (C) Both (A) and (B)
   - (D) None of the above

8. Which extends from the fourth cervical vertebra to the first thoracic vertebra
   - (A) Cervical enlargement
   - (B) Lumber enlargement
   - (C) Coccygeal enlargement
   - (D) Sternal enlargement

9. Which extends from the 9th to 12th thoracic vertebrae
   - (A) Cervical enlargement
   - (B) Coccygeal enlargement
   - (C) Lumber enlargement
   - (D) Sternal enlargement

10. The spinal cord terminates as a tapering conical structure called
   - (A) Conus medullaris
   - (B) Corpus luteum
   - (C) Cortex medullaris
   - (D) Conus sternal

11. The fibrous band that extends from the conus medullaris to the periosteum of the coccyx called
   - (A) Cauda equina
   - (B) Filum terminale
   - (C) Reticular terminal
   - (D) Medulla terminal

12. The spinal cord terminates between the first and second lumbar vertebrae but the vertebral column extends longer till the coccyx called
   - (A) Filum terminal
   - (B) Reflex centre
   - (C) Cauda equina
   - (D) Corpus terminal

13. The arrangement of grey and white matter in the spinal cord are
   - (A) Posterior column
   - (B) Anterior column
   - (C) Lateral column
   - (D) All of the above

14. Which is composed of sensory nerve cell bodies and nerve fibres
   - (A) Anterior column
   - (B) Posterior column
   - (C) Lateral column
   - (D) Distal column

15. Which is composed of motor nerve cell bodies and nerve fibres
   - (A) Posterior column
   - (B) Distal column
   - (C) Lateral column
   - (D) Anterior column

16. Which of the following composed of connects nerves that link sensory and motor neurons to form reflux arcs
   - (A) Lateral column
   - (B) Distal column
   - (C) Posterior column
   - (D) Anterior column

17. Posterior column is called
   - (A) Dorsal root
   - (B) Ventral root
   - (C) Lateral root
   - (D) Distal root

18. Anterior column is also called
 (A) Dorsal root
 (B) Lateral root
 (C) Ventral root
 (D) Distal root

19. The stimuli of sensory impulse may be as
 (A) Cutaneous receptor
 (B) Proprioceptor
 (C) Both (A) and (B)
 (D) None of the above

20. Cutaneous receptor stimulated by
 (A) Pain
 (B) Heat
 (C) Cold
 (D) All of the above

21. Proprioceptor present in
 (A) Muscle
 (B) Tendon
 (C) Joint
 (D) All of the above

22. Proprioceptor associated with
 (A) Maintenance of body balance
 (B) Maintenance of posture
 (C) Both (A) and (B)
 (D) None of the above

23. Which nerve transmit impulses from the brain to the periphery
 (A) Motor nerve
 (B) Ascending nerve
 (C) Afferent nerve
 (D) Sensory nerve

24. The stimulation of motor neurones is responsible for contraction of
 (A) Skeleton muscle
 (B) Smooth muscle
 (C) Cardiac muscle
 (D) All of the above

25. The motor tracts from the brain to the periphery follow
 (A) Pyramidal pathway
 (B) Extrapyramidal pathway
 (C) Both (A) and (B)
 (D) None of the above

26. The pathway through which motor fibres pass through the internal capsule are
 (A) Pyramidal pathway
 (B) Extrapyramidal pathway
 (C) Bipyramidal pathway
 (D) Tripyramidal pathway

27. The pathway through which motor fibres does not pass-through internal capsule are
 (A) Bipyramidal pathway
 (B) Tripyramidal pathway
 (C) Extrapyramidal pathway
 (D) Pyramidal pathway

28. The principal mechanisms of spinal cord that regulates homeostasis
    - (A) Propagation of nerve impulse
    - (B) Integration of information
    - (C) Both (A) and (B)
    - (D) None of the above

29. The pathway followed by the nerve impulse that results in the reflex is called
    - (A) Reflex route
    - (B) Reflux arc
    - (C) Reflux tract
    - (D) Reflux path

30. Which detects the change (stimulus) in internal or external environment and generates impulse
    - (A) Sensory receptor in the skin
    - (B) Motor neuron
    - (C) Effector organs
    - (D) Integrating centre

31. What transmits the impulse from receptor to the spinal cord?
    - (A) Sensory neuron
    - (B) Motor neuron
    - (C) Efferent neuron
    - (D) Descending neuron

32. Type of spinal cord reflexes are
    - (A) Stretch reflex
    - (B) Flexor reflex
    - (C) Autonomic reflex
    - (D) All of the above

33. Autonomic reflexes maintain
    - (A) Heart beat rate
    - (B) Digestion
    - (C) Breathing rate
    - (D) All of the above

34. The touching a hot plate is an example of
    - (A) Flexor reflex
    - (B) Autonomic reflex
    - (C) Stretch reflex
    - (D) Automatic reflex

35. Flexor reflex is also called
    - (A) Autonomic reflex
    - (B) Withdrawal reflex
    - (C) Automatic reflex
    - (D) Stretch reflex

36. The patella (or knees jerk) reflex is an example of
    - (A) Flexor reflex
    - (B) Autonomic reflex
    - (C) Stretch reflex
    - (D) Withdrawal reflex

37. How many pairs of spinal nerve that emerge from spinal nerve?
    - (A) 31 pairs
    - (B) 40 pairs
    - (C) 45 pairs
    - (D) 10 pairs

38. Which of the following is spinal nerve?
   (A) Cervical nerves
   (B) Thoracic nerves
   (C) Lumbar nerves
   (D) All of the above

39. How many pair of cervical nerves are there?
   (A) 8 pairs
   (B) 5 pairs
   (C) 10 pairs
   (D) 12 pairs

40. How many pairs of sacral nerves are there?
   (A) 8 pairs
   (B) 5 pairs
   (C) 12 pairs
   (D) 14 pairs

41. Each spinal nerve has connections with the spinal cord are
   (A) Posterior nerve root
   (B) Anterior nerve root
   (C) Both (A) and (B)
   (D) None of the above

42. Which nerve root consists sensory nerve fibres
   (A) Posterior nerve root
   (B) Anterior nerve root
   (C) Proximal nerve root
   (D) Distal nerve root

43. Which nerve root contains motor nerve fibres
   (A) Posterior nerve root
   (B) Anterior nerve root
   (C) Distal nerve root
   (D) Proximal nerve root

44. The area of the skin that provides sensory input to CNS through nerves is called
   (A) Dermatome
   (B) Dermatology
   (C) Dermatitis
   (D) Dermal

45. Immediately after emerging from the intervertebral foramen, the spinal nerves divide into several branches or rami are
   (A) Posterior ramus
   (B) Anterior ramus
   (C) Ramus communicans
   (D) All of the above

46. Which ramus supplies the deep muscles and skin of the posterior trunk
   (A) Ramus communicans
   (B) Anterior ramus
   (C) Posterior ramus
   (D) Distal ramus

47. Which supplies the anterior lateral (sides) portions of the trunk and the upper and lower limbs
   (A) Anterior ramus
   (B) Distal ramus
   (C) Posterior ramus
   (D) Distal ramus

48. Which ramus forms part of the ANS
    - (A) Ramus communicans
    - (B) Distal ramus
    - (C) Posterior ramus
    - (D) Anterior ramus

49. Cervical plexus supplies the
    - (A) Neck
    - (B) Head
    - (C) Superior part of shoulder
    - (D) All of the above

50. Brachial plexus arises from
    - (A) Axillary nerve
    - (B) Radial nerve
    - (C) Medial nerve
    - (D) All of the above

Answer Key

Nervous System, Central Nervous System (Part-06)

Question	Answer	Question	Answer
01	A = Spinal Cord	26	A = Pyramidal Pathway
02	B = Vertebral Canal	27	C = Extrapyramidal Pathway
03	C = Both A and B	28	C = Both A and B
04	A = 42 to 45 cm	29	B = Reflux Arc
05	A = Spinal Cord	30	A = Sensory Receptor in Skin
06	A = Spinal Cord	31	A = Sensory Neuron
07	C = Both A and B	32	D = All of the Above
08	A = Cervical Enlargement	33	D = All of the Above
09	C = Lumber Enlargement	34	A = Flexor Reflux
10	A = Conus Medullaris	35	B = Withdrawal Reflux
11	B = Filum Terminal	36	C = Stretch Reflex
12	C = Cauda Equina	37	A = 31 Pairs
13	D = All of the Above	38	D = All of the Above
14	B = Posterior Column	39	A = 08 Pairs
15	D = Anterior Column	40	B = 05 Pairs
16	A = Lateral Column	41	C = Both A and B
17	A = Dorsal Root	42	A = Posterior Nerve Root
18	C = Ventral Root	43	B = Anterior Nerve Root
19	C = Both A and B	44	A = Dermatome
20	D = All of the Above	45	D = All of the Above
21	D = All of the Above	46	C = Posterior Ramus
22	C = Both A and B	47	A = Anterior Ramus
23	A = Motor Nerve	48	A = Ramus Communicans
24	D = All of the Above	49	D = All of the Above
25	C = Both A and B	50	D = All of the Above

Unit - IV

Peripheral Nervous System, Special Senses

Part-01

1. Peripheral nervous system is divided into
   - (A) Somatic nervous system
   - (B) Autonomic nervous system
   - (C) Both (A) and (B)
   - (D) None of the above

2. Autonomic nervous system is divided into
   - (A) Sympathetic nervous system
   - (B) Parasympathetic nervous system
   - (C) Both (A) and (B)
   - (D) None of the above

3. Autonomic nervous system regulates involuntary bodies process including
   - (A) Heart rate
   - (B) Respiration
   - (C) Digestion
   - (D) All of the above

4. Which nervous system control involuntary responses
   - (A) Somatic nervous system
   - (B) Autonomic nervous system
   - (C) Automatic nervous system
   - (D) Central nervous system

5. Which nervous system control voluntary movement
   - (A) Autonomic nervous system
   - (B) Sympathetic nervous system
   - (C) Parasympathetic nervous system
   - (D) Somatic nervous system

6. Which nervous system governs the "Fight or Flight" response
   (A) Sympathetic nervous system
   (B) Parasympathetic nervous system
   (C) Central nervous system
   (D) Somatic nervous system

7. Which nerve system the "rest and digest" response
   (A) Sympathetic nervous system
   (B) Parasympathetic nervous system
   (C) Somatic nervous system
   (D) Central nervous system

8. The autonomic activity produces rapid effects and major effector organs include
   (A) Smooth muscles
   (B) Cardiac muscles
   (C) Glands
   (D) All of the above

9. Which nervous system to predominate in stressful situation and helps deal with emergence situations
   (A) Sympathetic nervous system
   (B) Parasympathetic nervous system
   (C) Somatic nervous system
   (D) Central nervous system

10. Which nervous system trends to predominates during rest
    (A) Sympathetic nervous system
    (B) Parasympathetic nervous system
    (C) Central nervous system
    (D) Somatic nervous system

11. The first neurons from the central nervous system to the ganglion is called
    (A) Post ganglionic neurons
    (B) Preganglionic neurons
    (C) Distal ganglionic neurons
    (D) Inferior ganglionic neurons

12. The second neuron from the ganglionic to the effector organs is called
    (A) Distal ganglionic neurons
    (B) Inferior ganglionic neurons
    (C) Postganglionic neurons
    (D) Preganglionic neurons

13. Sympathetic division is also named as
    (A) Thoracolumbar division
    (B) Craniosacral division
    (C) Cerebrospinal division
    (D) Intervertebral division

14. The neurotransmitter at the sympathetic ganglia is
    (A) Serotonin
    (B) Histamine
    (C) Acetylcholine
    (D) Melanin

15. The neurotransmitter at the effector organ in postganglionic nerve fibre is
    (A) Serotonin
    (B) Noradrenaline
    (C) Melatonin
    (D) Histamine

16. The sympathetic division is dominate in stressful situation which include
    (A) Anger
    (B) Fear
    (C) Anxiety
    (D) All of the above

17. The effects caused by sympathetic stimulation is stressed condition include
    (A) Increased heath rate
    (B) Dilation in bronchioles to taken more air
    (C) Glycogenolysis to provide energy
    (D) All of the above

18. The autonomic nerve pathways have synapses
    (A) One between preganglionic and postganglionic
    (B) Other between postganglionic neurons and neurons
    (C) Both (A) and (B)
    (D) None of the above

19. The major exception is the lack of parasympathetic supply to the
    (A) Sweat gland
    (B) Skin
    (C) Blood vessels of skeletal muscles
    (D) All of the above

20. Prevertebral ganglia situated in the abdominal cavity close to the origin of arteries of

    (A) Coeliac ganglion
    (B) Superior mesenteric ganglion
    (C) Inferior mesenteric ganglion
    (D) All of the above

21. Which of the which of the following is not a part of peripheral nervous system

    (A) Cranial nerve
    (B) Ganglion
    (C) Spinal nerve
    (D) Spinal cord

22. Which cells found in PNS

    (A) Microglia
    (B) Oligodendrocytes
    (C) Schwann cells
    (D) Astrocytes

23. Parasympathetic division is also named as

    (A) Craniosacral division
    (B) Cerebrospinal division
    (C) Intercoastal division
    (D) Thoracolumbar division

24. The preganglionic neurons of PNS originate in the

    (A) Brain stem
    (B) Sacral segments of the spinal cord
    (C) Both (A) and (B)
    (D) None of the above

25. The effects caused by parasympathetic stimulation include

    (A) Increased peristalsis movement
    (B) Normal heart rate
    (C) Contraction of smooth muscles
    (D) All of the above

26. In response to sympathetic stimulation adrenal gland secretes

    (A) Noradrenaline
    (B) Thyroxine
    (C) Melatonin
    (D) Calcitonin

27. The sympathetic accelerates firing of the sinoatrial node in the heart results in
    - (A) Increase heart rate
    - (B) Increase force of heart beat
    - (C) Both (A) and (B)
    - (D) None of the above

28. The sympathetic stimulation dilates the coronary arteries results
    - (A) Increase blood supply to heart
    - (B) Increase oxygen supply to heart
    - (C) Removal of metabolic waste product
    - (D) All of the above

29. Which of the following division is not a part of the peripheral nervous system
    - (A) Sensory
    - (B) Parasympathetic
    - (C) Brainstem
    - (D) Sympathetic

30. Which of the following is not a neurotransmitter?
    - (A) Acetylcholine
    - (B) Glucose
    - (C) Dopamine
    - (D) Serotonin

31. The step of neurohumoral transmission is
    - (A) Impulse conduction
    - (B) Release of neurotransmitter
    - (C) Neurotransmitter action
    - (D) All of the above

32. Nerve stimulation cause a sudden increase in
    - (A) Sodium
    - (B) Calcium
    - (C) Chloride
    - (D) Iron

33. An unpleasant sensation and emotional experience associated with or without actual tissue damage is called
    - (A) Anger
    - (B) Pain
    - (C) Stress
    - (D) Hunger

34. Pain may be classified into
    - (A) Cutaneous pain
    - (B) Deep somatic pain
    - (C) Visceral pain
    - (D) All of the above

35. Which of the following is cutaneous pain?

    (A) Tendons
    (B) Muscle
    (C) Burning
    (D) Joints

36. An individual feels pain but the cause is emotional rather than physical called

    (A) Psychogenic pain
    (B) Cutaneous pain
    (C) Visceral pain
    (D) Deep somatic pain

37. Which of the following is deep somatic pain?

    (A) Tendons
    (B) Muscles
    (C) Joints
    (D) All of the above

38. Which pain originates from the internal organs

    (A) Deep somatic pain
    (B) Visceral pain
    (C) Psychogenic pain
    (D) Cutaneous pain

39. Which of the following is visceral pain

    (A) Appendicitis
    (B) Burning
    (C) Emotional pain
    (D) Joint

40. Which of the following is plexus?

    (A) Cervical plexus
    (B) Lumbar plexus
    (C) Brachial plexus
    (D) All of the above

41. The anterior rami of spinal nerves do not form plexus are known as

    (A) Thoracic nerve
    (B) Brachial nerve
    (C) Lumbar nerve
    (D) Cervical nerve

42. The phrenic nerve supplies the

    (A) Hand
    (B) Forearm
    (C) Diaphragm
    (D) Foot

43. Which nerve supplies the deltoid muscle and shoulder joint

    (A) Ulnar nerve
    (B) Median nerve
    (C) Radial nerve
    (D) Axillary nerve

44. Radial nerve supplies the

    (A) Posterior arm
    (B) Forearm
    (C) Hand
    (D) All of the above

45. Musculocutaneous nerve supplies the
    - (A) Muscles of forearm
    - (B) Anal area
    - (C) Foot
    - (D) Leg

46. Medial nerve supplies the
    - (A) Anterior arm
    - (B) Forearm
    - (C) Hand
    - (D) All of the above

47. Ulnar nerve supplies the
    - (A) Medial arm
    - (B) Ring finger
    - (C) Little finger
    - (D) All of the above

48. Which nerve supplies the intercostals muscles, abdominal muscle and skin of the trunk
    - (A) Intercostal nerve
    - (B) Axillary nerve
    - (C) Median nerve
    - (D) Radial nerve

49. Lumber plexus supplies the
    - (A) Abdominal wall
    - (B) External genitals
    - (C) Lower limbs
    - (D) All of the above

50. The main branches and nerve root of lumber plexus
    - (A) Iliohypogastric nerve
    - (B) ilioinguinal nerve
    - (C) femoral nerve
    - (D) All of the above

Answer Key

Peripheral Nervous System, Special Senses (Part-01)

Question	Answer	Question	Answer
01	C = Both A and B	26	A = Noradrenaline
02	C = Both A and B	27	C = Both A and B
03	D = All of the Above	28	D = All of the Above
04	B = Autonomic Nervous System	29	C = Brainstem
05	D = Somatic Nervous System	30	B = Glucose
06	A = Sympathetic Nervous System	31	D = All of the Above
07	B = Parasympathetic Nervous System	32	A = Sodium
08	D = All of the Above	33	B = Pain
09	A = Sympathetic Nervous System	34	D = All of the Above
10	B = Parasympathetic Nervous System	35	C = Burning
11	B = Preganglionic Neurons	36	A = Psychogenic Pain
12	C = Postganglionic Neurons	37	D = All of the Above
13	A = Thoracolumbar Division	38	B = Visceral Pain
14	C = Acetylcholine	39	A = Appendicitis
15	B = Noradrenaline	40	D = All of the Above
16	D = All of the Above	41	A = Thoracic Nerve
17	D = All of the Above	42	C = Diaphragm
18	C = Both A and B	43	D = Axillary Nerve
19	D = All of the Above	44	D = All of the Above
20	D = All of the Above	45	A = Muscle of Forearm
21	D = Spinal Cord	46	D = All of the Above
22	C = Schwann Cells	47	D = All of the Above
23	A = Craniosacral Division	48	A = Intercostal Nerve
24	C = Both A and B	49	D = All of the Above
25	D = All of the Above	50	D = All of the Above

Part-02

1. Which lies deep within the neck opposite the cervical vertebrae under the protection of the sternocleidomastoid muscle
   - (A) Cervical plexus
   - (B) Lumbar plexus
   - (C) Sacral plexus
   - (D) Coccygeal plexus

2. How many cervical plexuses are there?
   - (A) 9
   - (B) 10
   - (C) 4
   - (D) 15

3. The phrenic nerve originates from
   - (A) Cervical nerve roots
   - (B) Lumbar nerve roots
   - (C) Sacral nerve roots
   - (D) Coccygeal nerve roots

4. The largest branch of the brachial plexus
   - (A) Axillary nerve
   - (B) Radial nerve
   - (C) Median nerve
   - (D) Distal nerve

5. The axillary nerve divides into minute branches to supply the
   - (A) Deltoid muscle
   - (B) Shoulder muscle
   - (C) Overlying skin
   - (D) All of the above

6. The musculocutaneous nerve branches supply the
   - (A) Muscle of upper arm
   - (B) Cutaneous nerve
   - (C) Skin of the forearm
   - (D) All of the above

7. How many lumbar plexuses are there?
   - (A) 4
   - (B) 8
   - (C) 9
   - (D) 12

8. The major nerve originates via the lumbar plexus
   - (A) Femoral nerve
   - (B) Obturator nerve
   - (C) Both (A) and (B)
   - (D) None of the above

9. Which nerve come from the sacral plexus
   - (A) Sciatic nerve
   - (B) Static nerve
   - (C) Femoral nerve
   - (D) Optic nerve

10. The nerve from the coccygeal plexus supplies the skin around
    (A) The coccyx
    (B) Anal area
    (C) Both (A) and (B)
    (D) None of the above

11. The autonomic plexuses include
    (A) Celiac plexus
    (B) Auerbach's plexus
    (C) Cardiac plexus
    (D) All of the above

12. The celiac plexus is also called as
    (A) Meissner's plexus
    (B) Solar plexus
    (C) Cardiac plexus
    (D) Pharyngeal plexus

13. The celiac plexus situated in
    (A) Behind the stomach
    (B) Innervates organs of abdomen
    (C) Both (A) and (B)
    (D) None of the above

14. Which plexus provides innervation to heart muscle
    (A) Celiac plexus
    (B) Solar plexus
    (C) Auerbach's plexus
    (D) Cardiac plexus

15. Which of the following is not a plexus?
    (A) Optic nerve
    (B) Sacral plexus
    (C) Cervical plexus
    (D) Lumbar plexus

16. Which nerve arise directly from the brain
    (A) Cranial nerve
    (B) Sacral nerve
    (C) Cervical nerve
    (D) Spinal nerve

17. How many pairs of the cranial nerve are there?
    (A) 16 pairs
    (B) 12 pairs
    (C) 10 pairs
    (D) 20 pairs

18. Cranial nerve may be
    (A) Sensory nerve
    (B) Motor nerve
    (C) Mixed nerve
    (D) All of the above

19. Which of the following is not a cranial nerve?
    (A) Olfactory nerve
    (B) Vagus nerve
    (C) Cervical plexus
    (D) Optic nerve

20. The cranial nerve with both sensory and motor function are called
    - (A) Mixed nerve
    - (B) Fixed nerve
    - (C) Tough nerve
    - (D) Narrowed nerve

21. Which type of nerve are olfactory nerve
    - (A) Motor nerve
    - (B) Mixed nerve
    - (C) Sensory nerve
    - (D) Efferent nerve

22. Which of the following in motor nerve?
    - (A) Hypoglossal nerve
    - (B) Olfactory nerve
    - (C) Optic nerve
    - (D) Auditory nerve

23. Which type of nerve are vagus nerve
    - (A) Sensory nerve
    - (B) Mixed nerve
    - (C) Motor nerve
    - (D) Efferent nerve

24. Which of the following is mixed nerve?
    - (A) Trigeminal nerve
    - (B) Optic nerve
    - (C) Abducent nerve
    - (D) Auditory nerve

25. Which type of nerve are oculomotor nerve
    - (A) Mixed nerve
    - (B) Motor nerve
    - (C) Afferent nerve
    - (D) Sensory nerve

26. Which of the following is mixed nerve?
    - (A) Facial nerve
    - (B) Vagus nerve
    - (C) Trigeminal nerve
    - (D) All of the above

27. Auditory nerve is also called
    - (A) Vestibulocochlear nerve
    - (B) Hypoglossal nerve
    - (C) Vagus nerve
    - (D) Olfactory nerve

28. Which type of nerve is facial nerve
    - (A) Motor nerve
    - (B) Efferent nerve
    - (C) Mixed nerve
    - (D) Sensory nerve

29. Which of the following is motor nerve?
    - (A) Accessory nerve
    - (B) Hypoglossal nerve
    - (C) Trochlear nerve
    - (D) All of the above

30. Which of the following nerve sense the smell?
    (A) Olfactory nerve
    (B) Optic nerve
    (C) Vagus nerve
    (D) Auditory nerve

31. Olfactory bulb presents in
    (A) Optic nerve
    (B) Vagus nerve
    (C) Olfactory nerve
    (D) Accessory nerve

32. Which of the following is nerve of sight?
    (A) Optic nerve
    (B) Olfactory nerve
    (C) Oculomotor nerve
    (D) Accessory nerve

33. The nerve fibres of optic nerve originate from
    (A) Pharynx
    (B) Trachea
    (C) Bronchi
    (D) Retina of eye

34. Which nerve controls the movement of eyeball and eyelids
    (A) Vagus nerve
    (B) Oculomotor nerve
    (C) Facial nerve
    (D) Olfactory nerve

35. The trigeminal nerve originates from
    (A) Pons (motor)
    (B) Face, head and teeth (sensory)
    (C) Both (A) and (B)
    (D) None of the above

36. The trochlear nerve originates from
    (A) Midbrain
    (B) Pons
    (C) Tongue
    (D) Retina

37. The function of auditory nerve is
    (A) Posture
    (B) Balance
    (C) Hearing
    (D) All of the above

38. Accessory nerve originates from
    (A) Brain stem
    (B) Spinal cord
    (C) Both (A) and (B)
    (D) None of the above

39. Hypoglossal nerve originates from
    (A) Medulla oblongata
    (B) Inner ear
    (C) Retina of eye
    (D) Olfactory lobe

40. The branch of auditory nerve
    (A) Cochlear nerve
    (B) Vestibular nerve
    (C) Both (A) and (B)
    (D) None of the above

41. Which nerve controls movement of tongue during speaking and swallowing
    (A) Auditory nerve
    (B) Olfactory nerve
    (C) Hypoglossal nerve
    (D) Optic nerve

42. The largest cranial nerve is
    (A) Trigeminal nerves
    (B) Optic nerve
    (C) Olfactory nerve
    (D) Auditory nerve

43. The ophthalmic nerve is sensory nerve only and supply the
    (A) Lacrimal gland
    (B) Conjunctiva of the eyes
    (C) Eyelids
    (D) All of the above

44. The branches of trigeminal nerves are
    (A) Ophthalmic nerves
    (B) Maxillary nerves
    (C) Mandibular nerve
    (D) All of the above

45. The mandibular nerve supplies the
    (A) Lower gums
    (B) Retina
    (C) Ear
    (D) Stomach

46. The maxillary nerves are sensory only and supply the
    (A) Cheeks
    (B) Upper jaws
    (C) Upper teeth
    (D) All of the above

47. The smallest cranial nerve is
    (A) Trigeminal nerve
    (B) Vagus nerve
    (C) Trochlear nerve
    (D) Accessory nerve

48. Which nerve associated with the maintenance of posture and balance
    (A) Vestibular nerve
    (B) Vagus nerve
    (C) Olfactory nerve
    (D) Optic nerve

49. The fibres of accessory nerve supply the
    (A) Sternocleidomastoid
    (B) Trapezius muscles
    (C) Both (A) and (B)
    (D) None of the above

50. Abducens nerve originate from
    (A) Pons
    (B) Midbrain
    (C) Retina
    (D) Nose

Answer Key

Peripheral Nervous System, Special Senses (Part-02)

Question	Answer	Question	Answer
01	A = Cervical Plexus	26	D = All of the Above
02	C = 04	27	A = Vestibulocochlear Nerve
03	A = Cervical Nerve Roots	28	C = Mixed Nerve
04	B = Radial Nerve	29	D = All of the Above
05	D = All of the Above	30	A = Olfactory Nerve
06	D = All of the Above	31	C = Olfactory Nerve
07	A = 04	32	A = Optic Nerve
08	C = Both A and B	33	D = Retina of Eye
09	A = Sciatic Nerve	34	B = Oculomotor Nerve
10	C = Both A and B	35	C = Both A and B
11	D = All of the Above	36	A = Midbrain
12	B = Solar Plexus	37	D = All of the Above
13	C = Both A and B	38	C = Both A and B
14	D = Cardiac Plexus	39	A = Medulla Oblongata
15	A = Optic Nerve	40	C = Both A and B
16	A = Cranial Nerve	41	C = Hypoglossal Nerve
17	B = 12 Pair	42	A = Trigeminal Nerve
18	D = All of the Above	43	D = All of the Above
19	C = Cervical Plexus	44	D = All of the Above
20	A = Mixed Nerve	45	A = Lower Gums
21	C = Sensory Nerve	46	D = All of the Above
22	A = Hypoglossal Nerve	47	C = Trochlear Nerve
23	B = Mixed Nerve	48	A = Vestibular Nerve
24	A = Trigeminal Nerve	49	C = Both A and B
25	B = Motor Nerve	50	A = Pons

Part-03

1. The organ is sight is
   - (A) Nose
   - (B) Eye
   - (C) Ear
   - (D) Tongue

2. Which of the following is situated in the orbital cavity, a bony socket built into the bone of face?
   - (A) Eye
   - (B) Nose
   - (C) Tongue
   - (D) Teeth

3. Eye is supplied by
   - (A) Auditory nerve
   - (B) Optic nerve
   - (C) Accessory nerve
   - (D) Olfactory nerve

4. Which number of cranial nerves are optic nerve
   - (A) 4th
   - (B) 6th
   - (C) 2nd
   - (D) 9th

5. The diameter of eye is about
   - (A) 5 cm
   - (B) 2.5 cm
   - (C) 7 cm
   - (D) 6 cm

6. The space between eye and orbital cavity is occupied by
   - (A) Cardiac tissue
   - (B) Adipose tissue
   - (C) Epithelial tissue
   - (D) Nervous tissue

7. Eye is divided into chamber are
   - (A) Anterior chamber
   - (B) Posterior chamber
   - (C) Both (A) and (B)
   - (D) None of the above

8. The anterior chamber is filled with a clear, watery fluid called
   - (A) Aqueous humour
   - (B) Cerebrospinal fluid
   - (C) Vitreous humour
   - (D) Mucous

9. The posterior chamber is filled with a jelly – like substance called
   - (A) Aqueous humour
   - (B) Vitreous humour
   - (C) Cerebrospinal fluid
   - (D) Sebum

10. The layer of tissue in the walls of the eye
    (A) The outer fibrous layer
    (B) The middle vascular layer
    (C) The inner nervous tissue layer
    (D) All of the above

11. The outer fibrous layer consists
    (A) Sclera
    (B) Cornea
    (C) Both (A) and (B)
    (D) None of the above

12. The transparent, avascular, watch glass – like structure with smooth shining surface called
    (A) Cornea
    (B) Retina
    (C) Iris
    (D) Sclera

13. The average diameter of the cornea is
    (A) 11 – 12 cm
    (B) 19 – 20 cm
    (C) 23 – 24 cm
    (D) 30 – 31 cm

14. Which of the following is responsible for focusing most of the light that enters the eye
    (A) Optic nerve
    (B) Retina
    (C) Optic disc
    (D) Cornea

15. Which of the following does not contain blood vessels?
    (A) Cornea
    (B) Lobule
    (C) Sclera
    (D) Retina

16. The cornea is comprised of layer are
    (A) Epithelium
    (B) Endothelium
    (C) Stroma
    (D) All of the above

17. The strong, opaque, white fibrous outermost layer of eye
    (A) Cornea
    (B) Sclera
    (C) Iris
    (D) Retina

18. Which part of eye is commonly known as "white"
    (A) Sclera
    (B) Iris
    (C) Retina
    (D) Cornea

19. The sclera is made up of divisions are
    (A) Episclera
    (B) Sclera proper
    (C) Lamina fusca
    (D) All of the above

20. The middle vascular coat is also known as
    - (A) Uveal tract
    - (B) Oval tract
    - (C) Round tract
    - (D) Ovual tract

21. The middle vascular layer consists of
    - (A) Choroid
    - (B) Ciliary body
    - (C) Iris
    - (D) All of the above

22. The dark brown highly vascular layer situated between sclera and retina
    - (A) Sclera
    - (B) Cornea
    - (C) Choroid
    - (D) Retina

23. Which of the following supplies nutrition to the outer layer of the retina?
    - (A) Choroid
    - (B) Cornea
    - (C) Optic nerve
    - (D) Optic disc

24. The visible coloured ring at the front of eye and extend anteriorly from the ciliary body
    - (A) Retina
    - (B) Optic nerve
    - (C) Iris
    - (D) Optic disc

25. The opening at the centre of the iris called
    - (A) Pupil
    - (B) Retina
    - (C) Cornea
    - (D) Choroid

26. The iris composed of the
    - (A) Pigment cells
    - (B) Smooth muscle fibres
    - (C) Both (A) and (B)
    - (D) None of the above

27. Which allow the light to enter the eye so it can be focused on the retina
    - (A) Choroid
    - (B) Sclera
    - (C) Pupil
    - (D) Optic disc

28. The muscle of pupil is
    - (A) Sphincter pupillae
    - (B) Dilator pupillae
    - (C) Both (A) and (B)
    - (D) None of the above

29. The anterior continuation of the choroid consisting ciliary muscle
    - (A) Ciliary body
    - (B) Circular body
    - (C) Semi-circular canal
    - (D) Semilunar canal

30. How many finger-like projections from the ciliary body are there?
    (A) 10 – 20
    (B) 70 – 80
    (C) 5 – 10
    (D) 15 – 20

31. The ciliary body is supplied by parasympathetic branches of the
    (A) Accessory nerve
    (B) Olfactory neve
    (C) Oculomotor nerve
    (D) Vagus nerve

32. The highly elastic circular biconvex body, lying immediately behind the pupil
    (A) Choroid
    (B) Retina
    (C) Lens
    (D) Sclera

33. The structure makeup the lens is
    (A) Capsule
    (B) Cortex
    (C) Epithelium
    (D) All of the above

34. The eye lens is mostly made up of
    (A) Lipid
    (B) Proteins
    (C) Fats
    (D) Vitamins

35. The inner most layer of eye
    (A) Retina
    (B) Sclera
    (C) Lens
    (D) Iris

36. Which of the following receive light and convert the light into neural signals?
    (A) Iris
    (B) Sclera
    (C) Retina
    (D) Cornea

37. The part of retina is
    (A) Peripheral retina
    (B) Photoreceptors
    (C) Rods
    (D) All of the above

38. The retina is the back part of the eye that contains the specialised cells that respond to light called
    (A) Photoreceptors
    (B) Cutaneous receptor
    (C) Thermoreceptor
    (D) Mechanoreceptor

39. Type of photoreceptor reside in the retina
    (A) Cones
    (B) Rods
    (C) Both (A) and (B)
    (D) None of the above

40. Which nerve cells are more sensitive to the bright light?
    - (A) Cones
    - (B) Rods
    - (C) Bands
    - (D) Rim

41. Which nerve cells are more sensitive to the dim light?
    - (A) Cones
    - (B) Rim
    - (C) Rods
    - (D) Bands

42. How many rods present in human retina?
    - (A) 120 million
    - (B) 300 million
    - (C) 290 million
    - (D) 400 million

43. The accessory organ of the eye includes
    - (A) Eyebrows
    - (B) Eyelids
    - (C) Conjunctiva
    - (D) All of the above

44. The eyebrows protect the eyeball from
    - (A) Sweat
    - (B) Dust
    - (C) Foreign bodies
    - (D) All of the above

45. The mobile tissue curtains placed in front of the eyeballs called
    - (A) Eyelids
    - (B) Conjunctiva
    - (C) Retina
    - (D) Choroid

46. From anterior to posterior the eyelids consist of
    - (A) Skin
    - (B) Subcutaneous loose areolar tissue
    - (C) Layer of striated muscles
    - (D) All of the above

47. The transparent mucous membrane that covers the inner surface of the eyelids and the surface of the aye are called
    - (A) Conjunctiva
    - (B) Retina
    - (C) Choroid
    - (D) Optic nerve

48. The parts of conjunctiva are
    - (A) Palpebral conjunctiva
    - (B) Bulbar conjunctiva
    - (C) Plica semilunaris
    - (D) All of the above

49. The lacrimal gland produces

    (A) Saliva

    (B) Mucous

    (C) Tear

    (D) Sebum

50. The layer of tissue that lies between the conjunctiva and the surface of the eye

    (A) Tendon's capsule

    (B) Tenon's capsule

    (C) Renal capsule

    (D) Tubule capsule

Answer Key

Peripheral Nervous System, Special Senses (Part-03)

Question	Answer	Question	Answer
01	B = Eye	26	C = Both A and B
02	A = Eye	27	C = Pupil
03	B = Optic Nerve	28	C = Both A and B
04	C = 2nd	29	A = Ciliary Body
05	B = 2.5 cm	30	B = 70 to 80
06	B = Adipose Tissue	31	C = Oculomotor Nerve
07	C = Both A and B	32	C = Lens
08	A = Aqueous Humour	33	D = All of the Above
09	B = Vitreous Humour	34	B = Proteins
10	D = All of the Above	35	A = Retina
11	C = Both A and B	36	C = Retina
12	A = Cornea	37	D = All of the Above
13	A = 11-12 cm	38	A = Photoreceptors
14	D = Cornea	39	C = Both A and B
15	A = Cornea	40	A = Cones
16	D = All of the Above	41	C = Rods
17	B = Sclera	42	A = 120 Million
18	A = Sclera	43	D = All of the Above
19	D = All of the Above	44	D = All of the Above
20	A = Uveal Tract	45	A = Eyelids
21	D = All of the Above	46	D = All of the Above
22	C = Choroid	47	A = Conjunctiva
23	A = Choroid	48	D = All of the Above
24	C = Iris	49	C = Tear
25	A = Pupil	50	B = Tenon's Capsule

Part-04

1. The lacrimal apparatus consists of the structures
   - (A) Lacrimal canaliculi
   - (B) Lacrimal sacs
   - (C) Nasolacrimal duct
   - (D) All of the above

2. Which type of gland is lacrimal gland
   - (A) Exocrine gland
   - (B) Endocrine gland
   - (C) Ductless gland
   - (D) External gland

3. The lacrimal gland secretes tear composed of
   - (A) Water
   - (B) Mineral salts
   - (C) Antibodies
   - (D) All of the above

4. Retina can be divided into
   - (A) Optic nerve
   - (B) Macula lutea
   - (C) Peripheral retina
   - (D) All of the above

5. The comparatively dark area situated at the posterior pole temporal to the optic disc
   - (A) Macula lutea
   - (B) Optic nerve
   - (C) Sclera
   - (D) Choroid

6. The well -defined circular, pink coloured disc of 1.5 mm diameter
   - (A) Rectangle disc
   - (B) Spherical disc
   - (C) Optic disc
   - (D) Olfactory disc

7. Vitreous humour consists of
   - (A) Water
   - (B) Salts
   - (C) Mucoproteins
   - (D) All of the above

8. Visual pathway comprises
   - (A) Optic nerve
   - (B) Optic chiasma
   - (C) Optic tract
   - (D) All of the above

9. The length of optic nerve is about
   - (A) $47 - 50$ mm
   - (B) $100 - 200$ mm
   - (C) $5 - 6$ mm
   - (D) $200 - 230$

10. Which is situated immediately in front of and above the pituitary gland, which lies hypoglossal fossa of the sphenoid bone

    (A) Sclera   (B) Cornea
    (C) Optic chiasma   (D) Retina

11. The cylindrical bundles of the nerve fibres which originate from posterolateral angle of the chiasma

    (A) Optic tracts   (B) Optic way
    (C) Optic path   (D) Optic route

12. The eyeballs are able to perform their function with the help of physiological activities are

    (A) Maintenance of clear media of the eye
    (B) Maintenance of normal intraocular pressure
    (C) Neurophysiology of vision
    (D) All of the above

13. Maintenance of the clear media of the eye include

    (A) Tear film   (B) Cornea
    (C) Aqueous humour   (D) All of the above

14. The photosensitive visual pigment present in the disc of the rods outer segment

    (A) Rhodopsin   (B) Band pigment
    (C) Rod pigment   (D) Cone pigment

15. The absorption spectrum of rhodopsin lies within the narrow limits of

    (A) 300 – 312 nm   (B) 493 – 505 nm
    (C) 102 – 107 nm   (D) 310 – 312 nm

16. The special senses are

    (A) Hearing   (B) Sight
    (C) Smell   (D) All of the above

17. Which of the following is organ of hearing?

    (A) Ear   (B) Eye
    (C) Nose   (D) Tongue

18. Ear is supplied by the cochlear branch of

    (A) Vestibulocochlear nerve   (B) Olfactory nerve
    (C) Optic nerve   (D) Accessory nerve

19. Vestibulocochlear nerve responds to the vibrations generated by
    - (A) Radio waves
    - (B) Microwaves
    - (C) Sound waves
    - (D) Ultraviolet waves

20. The ear is divided into
    - (A) The outer ear
    - (B) The middle ear
    - (C) The inner ear
    - (D) All of the above

21. The outer ear consists of
    - (A) The Auricle
    - (B) The acoustic meatus
    - (C) Both (A) and (B)
    - (D) None of the above

22. The different part of the outer ear is
    - (A) Tragus
    - (B) Helix
    - (C) Lobule
    - (D) All of the above

23. Which of the following is visible part of ear that projects from the side of ear?
    - (A) Malleus
    - (B) Incus
    - (C) Cochlea
    - (D) Pinna

24. Auricle is composed of
    - (A) Fibroelastic cartilage
    - (B) Hyaline cartilage
    - (C) Articular cartilage
    - (D) Heavy cartilage

25. Which of the following collect and reflects the sound waves into the external auditory canal
    - (A) Cochlea
    - (B) Pinna
    - (C) Nasopharynx
    - (D) Auditory tube

26. The outermost curvature of the ear extending from where the ear joins the head at the top where it meets the lobule
    - (A) Helix
    - (B) Malleus
    - (C) Cochlea
    - (D) Incus

27. Bottom most part of ear composed of fibrous and adipose tissue richly supplied with blood
    - (A) Malleus
    - (B) Cochlea
    - (C) Lobule
    - (D) Stapes

28. The slightly 'S' shaped tube about 2.5 cm long, extending from the auricle to the tympanic membrane

    (A) External acoustic meatus   (B) Semi-circular canal

    (C) Semilunar canal   (D) Cochlear tube

29. The external acoustic meatus also called

    (A) Semi-circular canal   (B) Auditory canal

    (C) Semilunar canal   (D) Haversian canal

30. Ceruminous gland is modified sweat gland that secretes

    (A) Cerumen   (B) Sebum

    (C) Serum   (D) Saliva

31. Cerumen is sticky material containing protective substance including

    (A) Bactericidal enzyme   (B) Lysozyme

    (C) Immunoglobulins   (D) All of the above

32. Which material prevented by cerumen from reaching the tympanic membrane

    (A) Dust   (B) Insects

    (C) Microbes   (D) All of the above

33. The cave – shaped structure with concavity directed towards the external auditory meatus

    (A) Tympanic membrane   (B) Auditory ossicles

    (C) Cochlea   (D) Semi-circular canal

34. Which of the following comes under middle ear?

    (A) Pinna   (B) Auditory ossicles

    (C) Lobule   (D) Cochlea

35. The irregular – shaped, air – filled cavity within the petrous portion of the temporal bone

    (A) Middle ear   (B) Cochlea

    (C) Lobule   (D) Auricle

36. The lateral wall of middle ear is formed by

    (A) Serous membrane   (B) Tympanic membrane

    (C) Cutaneous membrane   (D) Mucous membrane

37. The roof and floor of the middle ear are formed by the
    (A) Occipital bone
    (B) Parietal bone
    (C) Temporal bone
    (D) Sternal bone

38. The opening of the medial wall is a thin layer of temporal bone
    (A) Oval window
    (B) Round window
    (C) Both (A) and (B)
    (D) None of the above

39. Which of the following connect the middle ear cavity with the nasopharynx?
    (A) Pharyngotympanic tube
    (B) Auricle
    (C) Lobule
    (D) Cochlea

40. The length of pharyngotympanic tube is about
    (A) 10 cm
    (B) 4 cm
    (C) 12 cm
    (D) 14 cm

41. The pharyngotympanic tube is also called as
    (A) Auditory tube
    (B) Eustachian tube
    (C) Both (A) and (B)
    (D) None of the above

42. The bone of the middle ear are the auditory ossicles are
    (A) Malleus
    (B) Incus
    (C) Stapes
    (D) All of the above

43. The largest and most lateral of the ear bone attached to the tympanic membrane
    (A) Incus
    (B) Stapes
    (C) Malleus
    (D) Sternal

44. The middle anvil-shaped bone consists of a body and two limbs
    (A) Incus
    (B) Malleus
    (C) Stapes
    (D) Clavicle

45. The medial stirrup – shaped bone with a head, two limbs and a base
    (A) Incus
    (B) Stapes
    (C) Sternal
    (D) Malleus

46. The smallest bone of the human body
    (A) Stapes
    (B) Femur
    (C) Humerus
    (D) Clavicle

47. Which ear contains organ of hearing
    (A) Inner ear   (B) Middle ear
    (C) Outer ear   (D) Front ear

48. The part of inner ear
    (A) Bony labyrinth   (B) Membranous labyrinth
    (C) Both (A) and (B)   (D) None of the above

49. The inner ear divided into main regions are
    (A) The vestibule   (B) The semi-circular canals
    (C) The cochlea   (D) All of the above

50. The bony labyrinth is lined with
    (A) Periosteum   (B) Simple epithelium
    (C) Cardiac tissue   (D) Stratified epithelium

Answer Key

Peripheral Nervous System, Special Senses (Part-04)

Question	Answer	Question	Answer
01	D = All of the Above	26	A = Helix
02	A = Exocrine Glands	27	C = Lobules
03	D = All of the Above	28	A = External Acoustic Meatus
04	D = All of the Above	29	B = Auditory Canal
05	A = Macula Lutea	30	A = Cerumen
06	C = Optic Disc	31	D = All of The Above
07	D = All of the Above	32	D = All of The Above
08	D = All of the Above	33	A = Tympanic Membrane
09	A = 47 to 50 mm	34	B = Auditory Ossicles
10	C = Optic Chiasma	35	A = Middle Ear
11	A = Optic Tracts	36	B = Tympanic Membrane
12	D = All of the Above	37	C = Temporal Bone
13	D = All of the Above	38	C = Both A and B
14	A = Rhodopsin	39	A = Pharyngotympanic Tube
15	B = 493-505 nm	40	B = 3cm
16	D = All of the Above	41	C = Both A and B
17	A = Ear	42	D = All of the Above
18	A = Vestibulocochlear Nerve	43	C = Malleus
19	C = Sound Waves	44	A = Incus
20	D = All of the Above	45	B = Stapes
21	C = Both A and B	46	A = Stapes
22	D = All of the Above	47	A = Inner Ear
23	D = Pinna	48	C = Both A and B
24	A = Fibroelastic Cartilage	49	D = All of Above
25	B = Pinna	50	A = Periosteum

Part-05

1. Within the bony labyrinth, the membranous labyrinth is suspended in a watery fluid called

   (A) Saliva

   (C) Perilymph

   (B) Mucous

   (D) Cerebrospinal fluid

2. The membranous labyrinth filled with

   (A) Endolymph

   (C) Cerebrospinal fluid

   (B) Saliva

   (D) Serum

3. The middle ear contains muscles

   (A) Tensor tympani

   (C) Both (A) and (B)

   (B) Stapedius

   (D) None of the above

4. The area of the inner ear between the tympanic cavity and posterior to the cochlea that contains the otolith organs

   (A) Vestibule

   (C) Helix

   (B) Auricles

   (D) Lobule

5. The vestibule contain membranous sacs are

   (A) The utricle

   (C) Both (A) and (B)

   (B) The saccule

   (D) None of the above

6. How many semi-circular canals does each inner ear contain?

   (A) 1

   (C) 6

   (B) 3

   (D) 9

7. The three tiny, fluid – filled tubes in inner ear that help in balance is called

   (A) Auditory canal

   (C) Tympanic membrane

   (B) Semi-circular canal

   (D) Pinna

8. The border between the middle and inner ear is formed by

   (A) Incus

   (C) Oval window

   (B) Auricle

   (D) Pinna

9. Which of the following resembles a snail's shell?
   - (A) Cochlea
   - (B) Auricle
   - (C) Lobule
   - (D) Helix

10. A cross section of cochlea contains
    - (A) The scala vestibuli
    - (B) The scala media
    - (C) The scala tympani
    - (D) All of the above

11. The Scala vestibuli originates at the
    - (A) Oval window
    - (B) Round window
    - (C) Circular window
    - (D) Spherical window

12. The scala tympani originates at the
    - (A) Oval window
    - (B) Circular window
    - (C) Round window
    - (D) Spherical window

13. The organ of corti is present in
    - (A) Scala vestibuli
    - (B) Scala tympani
    - (C) Scala media
    - (D) Sclera

14. Which membrane present in between the scala media and scala tympani
    - (A) Basilar membrane
    - (B) Vascular membrane
    - (C) Medullar membrane
    - (D) Laminar membrane

15. Sound is carried out as sound wave in the air which travel at about
    - (A) 490 m/sec
    - (B) 340 m/sec
    - (C) 100 m/sec
    - (D) 120 m/sec

16. Which of the following receives sound vibration and passes to the eardrum?
    - (A) Outer ear
    - (B) Inner ear
    - (C) Middle ear
    - (D) Eustachian tube

17. Which number of cranial nerves are vestibulocochlear nerve?
    - (A) 10th
    - (B) 3rd
    - (C) 8th
    - (D) 12th

18. Which of the following have no auditory function?
    - (A) Semi-circular canals
    - (B) External acoustic meatus
    - (C) Cochlea
    - (D) Incus

19. The organ of Corti present in
    (A) Scala vestibuli
    (B) Scala tympani
    (C) Scala media
    (D) Scala medullar

20. Which of the following concerned with balance?
    (A) Vestibule
    (B) Semi-circular canals
    (C) Both (A) and (B)
    (D) None of the above

21. Which contains receptor for balance
    (A) Vestibule
    (B) Cochlea
    (C) Stapes
    (D) Auditory nerve

22. Which of the following are involved in physiology of equilibrium?
    (A) Crista
    (B) Macula
    (C) Saccule
    (D) All of the above

23. The otoliths are the crystal of
    (A) Calcium carbonate
    (B) Sodium carbonate
    (C) Potassium carbonate
    (D) Magnesium carbonate

24. The organ of smell is
    (A) Nose
    (B) Ear
    (C) Eye
    (D) Tongue

25. The sense of smell or olfaction originates in the
    (A) Lacrimal cavity
    (B) Orbital cavity
    (C) Nasal cavity
    (D) Dorsal cavity

26. Which of the following is sensory nerves of smell?
    (A) Optic nerve
    (B) Olfactory nerve
    (C) Accessory nerve
    (D) Auditory nerve

27. Which number of cranial nerves is olfactory nerve?
    (A) 4th
    (B) 5th
    (C) 9th
    (D) 1st

28. Olfactory bulb terminates at the
    (A) Olfactory bulb
    (B) Olfactory loop
    (C) Optic tract
    (D) Olfactory route

29. Olfactory nerve originates as
    (A) Cutaneous receptor
    (B) Chemoreceptors
    (C) Mechanoreceptors
    (D) Nociceptors

30. The sense of smell is detected by olfactory receptors located within the
    (A) Nasal epithelium
    (B) Nasal mucosa
    (C) Frontal sinus
    (D) Punctum

31. The olfactory bulb is an ovoid structure which contains specialised neurones called
    (A) Middle cells
    (B) Mitral cells
    (C) Lacrimal sacs
    (D) Lacrimal canaliculi

32. The olfactory nerve fibres synapse with the mitral cells, forming collections known as
    (A) Synaptic vesicle
    (B) Synaptic cleft
    (C) Synaptic knobs
    (D) Synaptic glomeruli

33. The olfactory tract travels posteriorly on the inferior surface of the
    (A) Parietal lobe
    (B) Occipital lobe
    (C) Frontal lobe
    (D) Lateral lobe

34. As the olfactory tract reaches the anterior perforated substance it can divided into
    (A) Lateral stria
    (B) Medial stria
    (C) Both (A) and (B)
    (D) None of the above

35. Which carries the axons to the primary olfactory cortex, located within the uncus of the temporal lobe
    (A) Lateral stria
    (B) Medial stria
    (C) Distal stria
    (D) Proximal stria

36. The olfactory mucosa consists of
    (A) Receptor cells
    (B) Supporting cells
    (C) Basal cells
    (D) All of the above

37. Nasal cavity is divided into
    (A) Respiratory segments
    (B) Olfactory segment
    (C) Both (A) and (B)
    (D) None of the above

38. Function of nasal cavity are
    - (A) Warms and humifies the inspired air
    - (B) Remove and traps pathogens
    - (C) Responsible of smell
    - (D) All of the above

39. The projecting out of the lateral walls of the nasal cavity curved shelves of bone. They are called
    - (A) Cornea
    - (B) Conchae
    - (C) Sclera
    - (D) Cochlea

40. The nasal conchae project into the nasal cavity creating the pathways are
    - (A) Inferior meatus
    - (B) Middle meatus
    - (C) Superior meatus
    - (D) All of the above

41. The pathway between the inferior and middle concha are
    - (A) Middle meatus
    - (B) Inferior meatus
    - (C) Superior meatus
    - (D) Distal meatus

42. The pathway between the inferior concha and floor of the nasal cavity are
    - (A) Middle meatus
    - (B) Distal meatus
    - (C) Inferior meatus
    - (D) Superior meatus

43. The middle ethmoidal sinuses empty out onto a structure called
    - (A) Temporal bulla
    - (B) Ethmoidal bulla
    - (C) Parietal bulla
    - (D) Occipital bulla

44. The nose receives blood from
    - (A) Internal carotid branches
    - (B) External carotid branches
    - (C) Both (A) and (B)
    - (D) None of the above

45. The external carotid branches are
    - (A) Superior labial artery
    - (B) Greater palatine artery
    - (C) Lateral nasal arteries
    - (D) All of the above

46. The innervation of the nose can be functionally divided into
    - (A) Special innervation
    - (B) General innervation
    - (C) Both (A) and (B)
    - (D) None of the above

47. The general sensory innervation to the septum and lateral walls is delivered by the

    (A) Nasopalatine nerve   (B) Nasociliary nerve

    (C) Trigeminal nerve   (D) All of the above

48. The branches of maxillary nerve are

    (A) Nasopalatine nerve   (B) Nasociliary nerve

    (C) Trigeminal nerve   (D) Accessory nerve

49. The branches of ophthalmic nerve are

    (A) Trigeminal nerve   (B) Accessory nerve

    (C) Nasociliary nerve   (D) Nasopalatine nerve

50. The innervation to the external skin of the nose is supplied by

    (A) Accessory nerve   (B) Nasociliary nerve

    (C) Trigeminal nerve   (D) Nasopalatine nerve

Answer Key

Peripheral Nervous System, Special Senses (Part-05)

Question	Answer	Question	Answer
01	C = Perilymph	26	B = Olfactory Nerve
02	A = Endolymph	27	D = 1st
03	C = Both A and B	28	A = Olfactory Bulb
04	A = Vestibule	29	B = Chemoreceptors
05	C = Both A and B	30	A = Nasal Epithelium
06	B = 03	31	B = Mitral Cells
07	B = Semi Circular Canal	32	D = Synaptic Glomeruli
08	C = Oval Window	33	C = Frontal Lobe
09	A = Cochlea	34	C = Both A and B
10	D = All of the Above	35	A = Lateral Stria
11	A = Oval Windows	36	D = All of the Above
12	C = Round Window	37	C = Both A and B
13	C = Scala Media	38	D = All of the Above
14	A = Basilar Membrane	39	B = Conchae
15	B = 340m/sec	40	D = All of the Above
16	A = Outer Ear	41	A = Middle Meatus
17	C = 8th	42	C = Inferior Meatus
18	A = Semi-circular Canals	43	B = Ethmoidal Bulla
19	C = Scala Media	44	C = Both A and B
20	C = Both A and B	45	D = All of the Above
21	A = Vestibules	46	C = Both A and B
22	D = All of the Above	47	D = All of the Above
23	A = Calcium Carbonate	48	A = Nasopalatine Nerve
24	A = Nose	49	C = Nasociliary Nerve
25	C = Nasal Cavity	50	C = Trigeminal Nerve

Part-06

1. The sense of smell is perceived by
   (A) Pituitary
   (B) Hypothalamus
   (C) Olfactory nerve
   (D) Cerebrum

2. The holes on the nose are called
   (A) Septum
   (B) Nostrils
   (C) Iris
   (D) Cartilage

3. Bowman's glands are found in
   (A) Olfactory epithelium
   (B) Auditory canal
   (C) Juxtamedullary
   (D) Pons

4. Which of the following enter the nose and dissolve in the olfactory epithelium?
   (A) Odorants
   (B) Colourants
   (C) Tastants
   (D) Coolants

5. Sense of smell is also called
   (A) Gustation
   (B) Olfaction
   (C) Ossification
   (D) Occipitation

6. Which type of neurons are olfactory neurons
   (A) Bipolar
   (B) Unipolar
   (C) Multipolar
   (D) Tripolar

7. The olfactory bulb is composed of
   (A) Sclera
   (B) Glomeruli
   (C) Choroid
   (D) Cornea

8. How many olfactory nerve filaments consists in olfactory neurons?
   (A) 15 – 20
   (B) 40 – 50
   (C) 80 – 90
   (D) 70 – 80

9. Olfactory cortex includes
   (A) Anterior olfactory nucleus
   (B) Prepiriform cortex
   (C) Olfactory tubercle and amygdala
   (D) All of the above

10. The factors influencing olfactory function
    (A) Threshold of olfactory receptors
    (B) Intensity of the odour
    (C) Adaptation
    (D) All of the above

11. A number of taste buds are located on the
    (A) Tongue
    (B) Ear
    (C) Nose
    (D) Eye

12. Sense of taste is also called
    (A) Olfaction
    (B) Gustation
    (C) Ossification
    (D) Occification

13. Which of the following is organ of taste?
    (A) Eye
    (B) Nose
    (C) Tongue
    (D) Ear

14. The taste buds contain
    (A) Chemoreceptors
    (B) Cutaneous receptor
    (C) Mechanoreceptors
    (D) Thermoreceptors

15. The muscular organ in the mouth is
    (A) Teeth
    (B) Tongue
    (C) Hard palate
    (D) Soft palate

16. The tongue is covered with moist, pink tissue called
    (A) Maxilla
    (B) Mandible
    (C) Mucosa
    (D) Frenum

17. The function of tongue is
    (A) Chewing food
    (B) Swallowing food
    (C) Speech
    (D) All of the above

18. The common taste is
    (A) Sour
    (B) Salty
    (C) Bitter
    (D) All of the above

19. The tongue can be divided into
    (A) Tip
    (B) Body
    (C) Base
    (D) All of the above

20. The most anterior and most mobile aspect of the tongue
    (A) Tip
    (B) Base
    (C) Band
    (D) Body

21. The most posterior part of the tongue
    (A) Band
    (B) Lobe
    (C) Base
    (D) Tip

22. The more forward surface of the tongue is covered in numerous small bumps called
    (A) Papillae
    (B) Medullar
    (C) Cuticle
    (D) Canals

23. The root of the tongue is connected to the hyoid bone via
    (A) Hyoglossus muscle
    (B) Genioglossus muscle
    (C) Both (A) and (B)
    (D) None of the above

24. The papillae of tongue are
    (A) Vallate papillae
    (B) Fungiform papillae
    (C) Filiform papillae
    (D) All of the above

25. Which is largest and visible papillae present at the base of the tongue arranged in an inverted V shape
    (A) Fungiform papillae
    (B) Filiform papillae
    (C) Vallate papillae
    (D) Circumvallate papillae

26. The number of vallate papillae are
    (A) 10
    (B) 30
    (C) 40
    (D) 50

27. Which papillae are located mainly around the tip and edges of the tongue
    (A) Fungiform papillae
    (B) Filiform papillae
    (C) Vallate papillae
    (D) Circumvallate papillae

28. Which papillae is smallest and most numerous papillae?
    (A) Fungiform papillae
    (B) Filiform papillae
    (C) Circumvallate papillae
    (D) Vallate papillae

29. The papillae which do not contain taste buds
    (A) Circumvallate papillae
    (B) Vallate papillae
    (C) Filiform papillae
    (D) Fungiform papillae

30. Which papillae located near the back of the tongue
    (A) Circumvallate papillae   (B) Fungiform papillae
    (C) Filiform papillae   (D) Vallate papillae

31. The taste buds are covered by
    (A) Simple squamous epithelium
    (B) Simple cuboidal epithelium
    (C) Stratified squamous epithelium
    (D) Simple columnar epithelium

32. The taste bud consists of
    (A) Receptor cells   (B) Basal replacement cells
    (C) Supporting cells   (D) All of the above

33. The taste receptor are also known as
    (A) Gustatory cells   (B) Olfactory cells
    (C) Optic cells   (D) Auditory cells

34. The taste receptors are present in
    (A) Upper surface of the tongue (B) Soft palate
    (C) Upper oesophagus   (D) All of the above

35. Which taste buds present on the lateral sides of the tongue
    (A) Salty   (B) Bitter
    (C) Sour   (D) Sweet

36. Which of the following dissolved in oral saliva and enter the taste pore
    (A) Coolants   (B) Tastants
    (C) Odorants   (D) Colourants

37. Taste buds consists of small sensory nerve ending of
    (A) Glossopharyngeal nerve   (B) Facial nerve
    (C) Vagus nerve   (D) All of the above

38. Which number of cranial nerves are vagus nerve?
    (A) 10th (B) 2nd
    (C) 4th (D) 6th

39. The cell bodies of second order neurons are located in the
    (A) Tractus solitarius   (B) Thalamus
    (C) Hypothalamus   (D) Fissures

40. The cell bodies of third order neurons are located in the
  - (A) Thalamus
  - (B) Fissures
  - (C) Tractus solitarius
  - (D) Medulla

41. Gustatory cells are located
  - (A) Within the taste buds
  - (B) Within the papillae
  - (C) On the surface of papillae
  - (D) Under the papillae

42. Primary taste sensations are
  - (A) Sweet sensation
  - (B) Salty sensation
  - (C) Sour sensation
  - (D) All of the above

43. Which substances produced sweet sensation
  - (A) Sugar
  - (B) Glycols
  - (C) Alcohols
  - (D) All of the above

44. Which substance produces bitter sensation
  - (A) Nicotine
  - (B) Sugars
  - (C) Alcohols
  - (D) Acids

45. Salty sensation produced by
  - (A) Nicotine
  - (B) Alcohols
  - (C) Sodium chloride
  - (D) Esters

46. Tip of the tongue are considered the area most sensitive to the
  - (A) Sweet stimuli
  - (B) Sour stimuli
  - (C) Salty stimuli
  - (D) Bitter stimuli

47. The front half of each side of the tongue area are most sensitive to
  - (A) Sour stimuli
  - (B) Salty stimuli
  - (C) Bitter stimuli
  - (D) Sweet stimuli

48. Which sensation is produced by acids?
  - (A) Sweet sensation
  - (B) Sour sensation
  - (C) Bitter sensation
  - (D) Salty sensation

49. The posterior half of each side of the tongue are considered most sensitive to
  - (A) Bitter stimuli
  - (B) Sweet stimuli
  - (C) Sour stimuli
  - (D) Salty stimuli

50. Which sensation is produced by quinine?
  - (A) Bitter sensation
  - (B) Salty sensation
  - (C) Sweet sensation
  - (D) Sour sensation

Answer Key

Peripheral Nervous System, Special Senses (Part-06)

Question	Answer	Question	Answer
01	C = Olfactory Nerve	26	A = 10
02	B = Nostrils	27	A = Fungiform Papillae
03	A = Olfactory Epithelium	28	B = Filiform Papillae
04	A = Odorants	29	C = Filiform Papillae
05	B = Olfaction	30	A = Circumvallate Papillae
06	A = Bipolar	31	C = Stratified Squamous Epithelium
07	B = Glomeruli	32	D = All of the Above
08	A = 15 to 20	33	A = Gustatory Cells
09	D = All of the Above	34	D = All of the Above
10	D = All of the Above	35	C = Sour
11	A = Tongue	36	B = Tastants
12	B = Gustation	37	D = All of the Above
13	C = Tongue	38	A = 10th
14	A = Chemoreceptors	39	A = Tractus Solitarius
15	B = Tongue	40	A = Thalamus
16	C = Mucosa	41	A = Within the Taste Buds
17	D = All of the Above	42	D = All of the Above
18	D = All of the Above	43	D = All of the Above
19	D = All of the Above	44	A = Nicotine
20	A = Tip	45	C = Sodium Chloride
21	C = Base	46	A = Sweet Stimuli
22	A = Papillae	47	B = Salty Stimuli
23	C = Both A and B	48	B = Sour Stimuli
24	D = All of the Above	49	C = Sour Stimuli
25	C = Vallate Papillae	50	A = Bitter Sensation

Part-07

1. Hearing impairment are classified into
   - (A) Conductive
   - (B) Sensorineural
   - (C) Both (A) and (B)
   - (D) None of the above

2. Which occurs due to abnormality of the outer or middle ear
   - (A) Sensorineural hearing impairment
   - (B) Conductive hearing impairment
   - (C) Presbycusis
   - (D) Cataracts

3. Example of conductive hearing impairment
   - (A) Otosclerosis
   - (B) Serous otitis media
   - (C) Both (A) and (B)
   - (D) None of the above

4. Which form hearing impairment accompanies the ageing process and therefore is common in older adults
   - (A) Presbycusis
   - (B) Cataracts
   - (C) Presbyopia
   - (D) Stye

5. The condition in which accumulation of endolymph causing distension and increased pressure within the membranous labyrinth
   - (A) Blepharitis
   - (B) Stye
   - (C) Meniere's disease
   - (D) Trachoma

6. The infection by staphylococcus aureusis the usual cause of localised inflammation in the auditory canal
   - (A) Trachoma
   - (B) External otitis
   - (C) Stye
   - (D) Presbyopia

7. The inflammation of the middle ear cavity usually caused by upward spread of microbes from an upper respiratory tract infection via the auditory tube
   - (A) Acute otitis media
   - (B) Blepharitis
   - (C) Stye
   - (D) Conjunctivitis

8. The permanent perforation of the tympanic membrane
   - (A) Chronic otitis media
   - (B) Blepharitis
   - (C) Stye
   - (D) Cataracts

9. An infection that affects the mastoid bone located behind the ear
   - (A) Glaucoma
   - (B) Presbycusis
   - (C) Mastoiditis
   - (D) Presbyopia

10. The scarring of ear drum is called
   - (A) Tympanosclerosis
   - (B) Mastoiditis
   - (C) Presbyopia
   - (D) Tinnitus

11. Which refers to ringing sensation in the ear
   - (A) Blepharitis
   - (B) Tinnitus
   - (C) Stye
   - (D) Cataracts

12. Which of the following is not an ear problem?
   - (A) Chromic otitis media
   - (B) Acute otitis media
   - (C) External otitis
   - (D) Conjunctivitis

13. Labyrinthitis accompanied by
   - (A) Vertigo
   - (B) Nausea
   - (C) Vomiting
   - (D) All of the above

14. The nausea and vomiting in some people and is usually associated with travel
   - (A) Motion sickness
   - (B) Conjunctivitis
   - (C) Blepharitis
   - (D) Stye

15. The acute and painful bacterial infection of sebaceous or tarsals glands of the eyelids margin
   - (A) Conjunctivitis
   - (B) Presbycusis
   - (C) Otosclerosis
   - (D) Stye

16. Stye is also known as
   - (A) Conjunctivitis
   - (B) Presbycusis
   - (C) Hordeolum
   - (D) Otosclerosis

17. The inflammation of the conjunctiva
   - (A) Conjunctivitis
   - (B) Blepharitis
   - (C) Presbycusis
   - (D) Hordeolum

18. Conjunctivitis may be caused by
    (A) Smoke
    (B) Dust
    (C) Microbes
    (D) All of the above

19. Infection of eye usually caused by strains of
    (A) Staphylococci
    (B) Streptococci
    (C) Haemophilus
    (D) All of the above

20. Trachoma is chronic inflammatory condition is caused by
    (A) Chlamydia trachomatis
    (B) Streptococci
    (C) Staphylococci
    (D) Haemophilus

21. Trachoma symptoms include
    (A) Mild itching
    (B) Irritation of the eyes
    (C) A discharge from the eyes
    (D) All of the above

22. Allergic conjunctivitis is caused by
    (A) Hair sprays
    (B) Fungus spores
    (C) Animal dander
    (D) All of the above

23. The conjunctival inflammation that occurs during first month of life after birth
    (A) Neonatal conjunctivitis
    (B) Glaucoma
    (C) Otosclerosis
    (D) Stye

24. Neonatal conjunctivitis may be
    (A) Septic neonatal conjunctivitis
    (B) Aseptic neonatal conjunctivitis
    (C) Both (A) and (B)
    (D) None of the above

25. Neonatal conjunctivitis is usually caused by
    (A) Chlamydia trachomatis
    (B) Neisseria gonorrhoeae
    (C) Staphylococcus aureus
    (D) All of the above

26. An open sore in the outer layer of the cornea
    (A) Corneal ulcer
    (B) Retinopathies
    (C) Glaucoma
    (D) Otosclerosis

27. The group of condition in which intraocular pressure rises and cause damage to the optic nerve
    (A) Glaucoma
    (B) Corneal ulcer
    (C) Trachoma
    (D) Conjunctivitis

28. Which of the following is type of glaucoma?
    (A) Open angle glaucoma
    (B) Closed angle glaucoma
    (C) Both (A) and (B)
    (D) None of the above

29. Normal intraocular pressure is
    (A) 1 – 2 mm Hg
    (B) 10 – 21 mm Hg
    (C) 30 – 39 mm Hg
    (D) 40 – 50 mm Hg

30. Symptoms of glaucoma
    (A) Vision loss
    (B) Redness in eye
    (C) Eye pain
    (D) All of the above

31. Which of the following is retinopathies?
    (A) Vascular retinopathies
    (B) Diabetic retinopathies
    (C) Retinopathy of prematurity
    (D) All of the above

32. The disorder in which both eyes do not line up in the same direction
    (A) Strabismus
    (B) Cataract
    (C) Presbyopia
    (D) Glaucoma

33. A white area that grows over the eye as and cause opacity of the lens
    (A) Glaucoma
    (B) Trachoma
    (C) Conjunctivitis
    (D) Cataract

34. Which abnormality is also called short sightedness?
    (A) Myopia
    (B) Hyperopia
    (C) Astigmatism
    (D) Glaucoma

35. Which lens used to correct myopia
    (A) Concave lens
    (B) Convex lens
    (C) Plano lens
    (D) Converging lens

36. Which abnormality is also called farsightedness?
    (A) Myopia
    (B) Astigmatism
    (C) Hyperopia
    (D) Glaucoma

37. Which lens is used to correct hyperopia?

    (A) Concave lens

    (B) Plano lens

    (C) Convex lens

    (D) Diverging lens

38. In which condition the close objects are focused normally bus distant vision is blurred

    (A) Astigmatism

    (B) Myopia

    (C) Hyperopia

    (D) Cataract

39. In which condition the distant objects focused normally but close objects are blurred

    (A) Astigmatism

    (B) Cataract

    (C) Hyperopia

    (D) Myopia

40. The abnormal curvature of part of the cornea or lens called

    (A) Astigmatism

    (B) Hyperopia

    (C) Longsightedness

    (D) Myopia

41. Which lens used in astigmatism

    (A) Rectangular lens

    (B) Cylindrical lens

    (C) Spherical lens

    (D) Circular lens

42. Cylindrical lens may be

    (A) Convex

    (B) Concave

    (C) Mixed

    (D) All of the above

43. Which of the following occurs when thin wall between nasal passages displaced to one side?

    (A) Sinusitis

    (B) Deviated septum

    (C) Conjunctivitis

    (D) Blepharitis

44. Inflammation of sinuses called

    (A) Sinusitis

    (B) Conjunctivitis

    (C) Arthritis

    (D) Blepharitis

45. Symptoms of sinusitis

    (A) Nasal discharge

    (B) Cough

    (C) Post nasal drip

    (D) All of the above

46. A soft, noncancerous growths on the lining of nose called
    - (A) Nasal polyps
    - (B) Labyrinthitis
    - (C) Stye
    - (D) Blepharitis

47. A condition that results in a swollen, inflamed or discoloured tongue called
    - (A) Labyrinthitis
    - (B) Stye
    - (C) Glossitis
    - (D) Blepharitis

48. An infection in which the fungus candida albicans accumulates in the mouth
    - (A) Oral thrush
    - (B) Glossitis
    - (C) Stye
    - (D) Hordeolum

49. Symptoms of hairy tongue include
    - (A) Black discolouration
    - (B) Metallic taste
    - (C) Bad breath
    - (D) All of the above

50. In which condition deep grooves can develop in the tongue
    - (A) Deviated septum
    - (B) Fissured tongue
    - (C) Stye
    - (D) Myopia

Answer Key

Peripheral Nervous System, Special Senses (Part-07)

Question	Answer	Question	Answer
01	C = Both A and B	26	A = Corneal Ulcer
02	B = Conductive Hearing Impairment	27	A = Glaucoma
03	C = Both A and B	28	C = Both A and B
04	A = Presbycusis	29	B = 10-21 mm Hg
05	C = Meniere's Disease	30	D = All of the Above
06	B = External Otitis	31	D = All of the Above
07	A = Acute Otitis Media	32	A = Strabismus
08	A = Chronic Otitis Media	33	D = Cataract
09	C = Mastoiditis	34	A = Myopia
10	A = Tympanosclerosis	35	A = Concave Lens
11	B = Tinnitus	36	C = Hyperopia
12	D = Conjunctivitis	37	C = Convex Lens
13	D = All of the Above	38	B = Myopia
14	A = Motion Sickness	39	C = Hyperopia
15	D = Stye	40	A = Astigmatism
16	C = Hordeolum	41	B = Cylindrical Lens
17	A = Conjunctivitis	42	D = All of the Above
18	D = All of the Above	43	B = Deviated Septum
19	D = All of the Above	44	A = Sinusitis
20	A = Chlamydia Trachomatis	45	D = All of the Above
21	D = All of the Above	46	A = Nasal Polyps
22	D = All of the Above	47	C = Glossitis
23	A = Neonatal Conjunctivitis	48	A = Oral Thrush
24	C = Both A and B	49	D = All of the Above
25	D = All of the Above	50	B = Fissured Tongue

Unit - V

Endocrine System

Part-01

1. The endocrine system releases mediator molecules called
   - (A) Hormone
   - (C) Fluids
   - (B) Neurotransmitter
   - (D) Toxins

2. The study of endocrine glands and role of their secretions is called
   - (A) Ophthalmology
   - (C) Neurology
   - (B) Endocrinology
   - (D) Nephrology

3. Type of glands are
   - (A) Endocrine gland
   - (C) Both (A) and (B)
   - (B) Exocrine gland
   - (D) None of the above

4. Which gland are also called "ductless gland"?
   - (A) Endocrine gland
   - (C) Merocrine gland
   - (B) Exocrine gland
   - (D) Holocrine gland

5. Example of unicellular exocrine gland are
   - (A) Goblet cells
   - (C) Salivary gland
   - (B) Sweat gland
   - (D) Pancreas

6. Example of multicellular exocrine glands are
   - (A) Salivary gland
   - (C) Sweat gland
   - (B) Pancreas
   - (D) All of the above

7. Which gland form the secretion and release it from the cells
   - (A) Merocrine gland
   - (C) Holocrine gland
   - (B) Apocrine gland
   - (D) Endocrine gland

8. Example of merocrine gland
   - (A) Salivary gland
   - (C) Pituitary gland
   - (B) Sebaceous gland
   - (D) Thyroid gland

9. Multicellular exocrine gland can be functionally classified into
   - (A) Merocrine gland
   - (B) Apocrine gland
   - (C) Holocrine gland
   - (D) All of the above

10. Which gland accumulate the secretion at the apical surface of the cell
   - (A) Holocrine gland
   - (B) Apocrine gland
   - (C) Merocrine gland
   - (D) Adrenal gland

11. Which gland accumulate the secretion in the cytosol of the skin
   - (A) Holocrine gland
   - (B) Apocrine gland
   - (C) Merocrine gland
   - (D) Pituitary gland

12. Sebaceous gland of skin is example of
   - (A) Apocrine gland
   - (B) Merocrine gland
   - (C) Holocrine gland
   - (D) Pituitary gland

13. Which gland present ducts at the surface of covering
   - (A) Exocrine gland
   - (B) Endocrine gland
   - (C) Pituitary gland
   - (D) Thyroid gland

14. Which of the following is not a secretion of exocrine gland?
   - (A) Sebaceous
   - (B) Saliva
   - (C) Sweat
   - (D) Growth hormone

15. Endocrine gland includes
   - (A) Thyroid gland
   - (B) Pituitary gland
   - (C) Adrenal gland
   - (D) All of the above

16. The hormone can be classified into
   - (A) Steroid hormones
   - (B) Nonsteroid hormones
   - (C) Both (A) and (B)
   - (D) All of the above

17. Steroid hormone derived from
   - (A) Cholesterol
   - (B) Peptides
   - (C) Amino acid
   - (D) Water

18. The steroid hormones are synthesized in
   - (A) Adrenal cortex
   - (B) Gonads
   - (C) Placenta
   - (D) All of the above

19. Example of steroid hormone are
    (A) Oestrogen
    (B) Aldosterone
    (C) Hydrocortisone
    (D) All of the above

20. The nonsteroid hormones may be
    (A) Proteins
    (B) Peptides
    (C) Amino acids
    (D) All of the above

21. Which of the following is protein hormone?
    (A) Insulin
    (B) Aldosterone
    (C) Hydrocortisone
    (D) Glucocorticoids

22. Protein hormone include
    (A) Calcitonin
    (B) Insulin
    (C) Glucagon
    (D) All of the above

23. Example of peptides hormone is
    (A) Oxytocin
    (B) Somatostatin
    (C) Antidiuretic hormones
    (D) All of the above

24. Which of the following is not a protein hormone?
    (A) Calcitonin
    (B) Glucagon
    (C) Mineralocorticoids
    (D) Prolactin

25. Which of the following is amino acid hormone?
    (A) Epinephrine
    (B) Norepinephrine
    (C) Melatonin
    (D) All of the above

26. Which of the following is not a peptide hormone?
    (A) Oxytocin
    (B) Somatostatin
    (C) Hydrocortisone
    (D) Antidiuretic hormone

27. Example of glycoprotein is
    (A) Luteinizing hormone
    (B) Chorionic gonadotropin
    (C) Follicle – stimulating hormone
    (D) All of the above

28. Hormones that are secreted into the blood and act on distant target cells are called
    (A) Circulating hormones
    (B) Non circulating hormones
    (C) Local hormones
    (D) Flowing hormones

29. Lipid insoluble hormones are
- (A) Adrenaline
- (B) Noradrenaline
- (C) Both (A) and (B)
- (D) None of the above

30. Lipid soluble hormones are
- (A) Glucocorticoids
- (B) Mineralocorticoids
- (C) Hydrocortisone
- (D) All of the above

31. Example of second messenger is
- (A) Cyclic adenosine monophosphate (cAMP)
- (B) Inositol triphosphate (I_3)
- (C) Diacyl glycerol (DAG)
- (D) All of the above

32. The hormone – receptor complex activates a membrane protein called
- (A) G protein
- (B) P protein
- (C) S protein
- (D) T protein

33. G protein cause the release of an enzyme
- (A) Amylase
- (B) Lipases
- (C) Adenylate cyclase
- (D) Ribonuclease

34. When the effects of two hormones acting together is greater than the effect of each hormone acting alone. The two hormones are said to have the
- (A) Synergistic effect
- (B) Antagonistic effect
- (C) Agonistic effect
- (D) Inverse agonistic effect

35. When one hormone opposes the action of the other, the hormones are said to have the
- (A) Agonistic effect
- (B) Reverse antagonistic effect
- (C) Antagonistic effect
- (D) Synergistic effect

36. Which of the following situated below and in front of the thalamus and immediately above the pituitary gland
- (A) Medulla oblongata
- (B) Spinal cord
- (C) Cerebrum
- (D) Hypothalamus

37. Hypothalamus is connected to the pituitary gland through a funnel – shaped stalk called
    (A) Infundibulum
    (B) Pons
    (C) Meninges
    (D) Medulla oblongata

38. The hypothalamus controls release of hormones from
    (A) Anterior pituitary
    (B) Posterior pituitary
    (C) Both (A) and (B)
    (D) None of the above

39. The hypothalamus contains specialized nerve cells called
    (A) Alpha secretory cells
    (B) Neurosecretory cells
    (C) Distal secretory cells
    (D) Lateral secretory cells

40. The network of vessels transports blood from the hypothalamus to the anterior pituitary called
    (A) Pituitary portal system
    (B) Hepatic portal system
    (C) Renal portal system
    (D) Pulmonary portal system

41. Function of pituitary portal system
    (A) Permit easy passage of hormones into bloodstream
    (B) Providing nutrients
    (C) Providing oxygen
    (D) All of the above

42. The anterior lobe of the pituitary gland also known as
    (A) Neurohypophysis
    (B) Adenohypophysis
    (C) Renohypophysis
    (D) Pulmohypophysis

43. The posterior lobe of the pituitary gland also known as
    (A) Pulmohypophysis
    (B) Renohypophysis
    (C) Neurohypophysis
    (D) Adenohypophysis

44. Pituitary gland is connected to hypothalamus by the stalk that contains
    (A) Neurosecretory fibres
    (B) Capillaries
    (C) Hypophyseal portal system
    (D) All of the above

45. Which hormones is secreted by anterior pituitary?
    (A) Growth hormones
    (B) Prolactin
    (C) Luteinizing hormone
    (D) All of the above

46. Which hormone is not secreted by anterior pituitary?
   (A) Prolactin
   (B) Follicle stimulating hormone
   (C) Oxytocin
   (D) Growth hormones

47. Types of secretory cells of anterior pituitary
   (A) Somatotrophs
   (B) Thyrotrophs
   (C) Corticotrophs
   (D) All of the above

48. Which secretory cells secrete GH or somatotropin
   (A) Corticotrophs
   (B) Gonadotrophs
   (C) Somatotrophs
   (D) Lactotrophs

49. Which secretory cells secrete TSH or Thyrotropin
   (A) Thyrotrophs
   (B) Somatotrophs
   (C) Gonadotrophs
   (D) Lactotrophs

50. Which secretory cells secrete prolactin
   (A) Thyrotrophs
   (B) Lactotrophs
   (C) Gonadotrophs
   (D) Somatotrophs

Answer Key

Endorcrine System (Part-01)

Question	Answer	Question	Answer
01	A = Hormone	26	C = Hydrocortisone
02	B = Endocrinology	27	D = All of the above
03	C = Both A and B	28	A = Circulating Hormones
04	A = Endocrine Gland	29	C = Both A and B
05	A = Goblet Cells	30	D = All of the Above
06	D = All of the Above	31	D = All of the above
07	A = Merocrine Gland	32	A = G-Protein
08	A = Salivary Gland	33	C = Adenylate Cyclase
09	D = All of the Above	34	A = Synergistic Effect
10	B = Apocrine Gland	35	C = Antagonistic Effects
11	A = Holocrine Gland	36	D = Hypothalamus
12	C = Holocrine Gland	37	A = Infundibulum
13	A = Exocrine Gland	38	C = Both A and B
14	D = Growth Hormone	39	B = Neurosecretory cells
15	D = All of the Above	40	A = Pituitary Portal System
16	C = Both A and B	41	D = All of the Above
17	A = Cholesterol	42	B = Adenohypophysis
18	D = All of the Above	43	C = Neurohypophysis
19	D = All of the Above	44	D = All of the Above
20	D = All of the Above	45	D = All of the Above
21	A = Insulin	46	C = Oxytocin
22	D = All of the Above	47	D = All of the Above
23	D = All of the Above	48	C = Somatotrophs
24	C = Mineralocorticoids	49	A = Thyrotrophs
25	D = All of the Above	50	B = Lactotrophs

Part-02

1. Gonadotrophs cells secrete hormone
   - (A) Follicle stimulating hormone
   - (B) Luteinizing hormone
   - (C) Both (A) and (B)
   - (D) None of the above

2. The FSH and LH are collectively called
   - (A) Gonadotropins
   - (B) Lactotropins
   - (C) Corticotrophs
   - (D) Thyrotropins

3. Thyrotropin stimulates
   - (A) Adrenal gland
   - (B) Thyroid gland
   - (C) Gonadotrophs
   - (D) Lactotrophs

4. The most abundant hormone synthesized by anterior pituitary
   - (A) Growth hormone
   - (B) Vasopressin
   - (C) Oxytocin
   - (D) Prolactin

5. Which hormone is responsible for growth of the body?
   - (A) Oxytocin
   - (B) Vasopressin
   - (C) Growth hormone
   - (D) Follicle stimulating hormone

6. How many amino acids present in growth hormone?
   - (A) 400
   - (B) 590
   - (C) 191
   - (D) 391

7. Growth hormone essential for
   - (A) Protein metabolism
   - (B) Lipid metabolism
   - (C) Carbohydrate metabolism
   - (D) All of the above

8. The secretion of growth hormone is highest in
   - (A) Childhood
   - (B) Adolescence
   - (C) Both (A) and (B)
   - (D) None of the above

9. Growth hormone stimulates the liver to secrete small protein hormones called
   - (A) Insulin – like growth factors
   - (B) Oestrogen – like growth factors
   - (C) Hydrocortisone – like growth factors
   - (D) Aldosterone – like growth factors

10. Growth hormone regulates aspects of metabolism in
    - (A) Liver
    - (B) Intestine
    - (C) Pancreas
    - (D) All of the above

11. Types of growth hormone are
    - (A) Somatropin
    - (B) Somatotropin
    - (C) Both (A) and (B)
    - (D) None of the above

12. The release of growth hormone stimulated by
    - (A) Growth hormone releasing hormone
    - (B) Growth hormone inhibiting hormone
    - (C) Growth hormone depressing hormone
    - (D) Growth hormone suppressing hormone

13. The release of growth hormone suppressed by
    - (A) Growth hormone releasing hormone
    - (B) Growth hormone release inhibiting hormone
    - (C) Thyroid hormone increasing hormone
    - (D) Follicle stimulating hormone

14. Growth hormone release inhibiting hormone also called
    - (A) Somatocrinin
    - (B) Somatostatin
    - (C) Lactotrophs
    - (D) Gonadotropin

15. Growth hormone releasing hormone also called
    - (A) Somatocrinin
    - (B) Thyrotrophs
    - (C) Somatostatin
    - (D) Gonadotrophs

16. Prolactin is also known as
    - (A) Somatocrinin
    - (B) Gonadotropic
    - (C) Luteotropic
    - (D) Thyrotropin

17. Prolactin promotes
    (A) Development of mammary glands during pregnancy
    (B) Stimulates lactation after parturition
    (C) Both (A) and (B)
    (D) None of the above

18. The release of prolactin is stimulated by
    (A) Prolactin – releasing hormone
    (B) Growth – releasing hormone
    (C) Prolactin – inhibiting hormone
    (D) Growth hormone inhibiting hormone

19. The secretion of prolactin is lowered by
    (A) Growth hormone inhibiting hormone
    (B) Prolactin – inhibiting hormone
    (C) Thyroid releasing hormone
    (D) Growth – releasing hormone

20. The target gland of prolactin releasing hormone
    (A) Adrenal cortex
    (B) Thyroid gland
    (C) Breast
    (D) Ovaries

21. The main regulator of production of prolactin from the pituitary gland is
    (A) Acetylcholine
    (B) Dopamine
    (C) Serotonin
    (D) Melanin

22. How many amino acids composed prolactin?
    (A) 199
    (B) 578
    (C) 489
    (D) 345

23. Which type of hormone is thyroid stimulating hormone
    (A) Peptide
    (B) Protein
    (C) Glycoprotein
    (D) Steroid

24. Thyroid - stimulating hormone stimulate the thyroid gland to secretes
    (A) Thyroxine
    (B) Tri – iodothyronine
    (C) Both (A) and (B)
    (D) None of the above

25. The thyroid – stimulating hormone is stimulated by
    (A) Thyrotropin – releasing hormone
    (B) Somatotropin – releasing hormone
    (C) Prolactin – releasing hormone
    (D) Prolactin – inhibiting hormone

26. The target gland of thyrotropin – releasing hormone
    (A) Thyroid gland
    (B) Breast
    (C) Ovaries
    (D) Adrenal cortex

27. Function of thyroid stimulating hormone
    (A) Controls production of thyroid hormones
    (B) Controls releasing of thyroid hormones
    (C) Both (A) and (B)
    (D) None of the above

28. The secretion of adrenocorticotropic hormone is stimulated by
    (A) Growth hormone releasing hormone
    (B) Corticotrophin – releasing hormone
    (C) Thyroid stimulating hormone
    (D) Prolactin – releasing hormone

29. The Adrenocorticotropic hormone stimulates the adrenal cortex to release
    (A) Glucocorticoids
    (B) Mineralocorticoids
    (C) Both (A) and (B)
    (D) None of the above

30. Which type of hormone is glucocorticoids
    (A) Amino acid
    (B) Glycoprotein
    (C) Protein
    (D) Steroids

31. The target gland of corticotropin releasing hormone
    (A) Adrenal cortex
    (B) Breast
    (C) Ovaries
    (D) Thyroid gland

32. Adrenocorticotropic hormone promotes and maintain the
    (A) Growth of the adrenal cortex
    (B) Stimulates the adrenal gland to secrete hormones
    (C) Both (A) and (B)
    (D) None of the above

33. Cortisol helps in
    (A) Control blood pressure
    (B) Fight infection
    (C) Respond to stress
    (D) All of the above

34. The gonadotrophins hormone is
    (A) Follicle stimulating hormone
    (B) Luteinizing hormone
    (C) Both (A) and (B)
    (D) None of the above

35. Function of follicle stimulating hormone in females
    (A) Control secretion of oestrogen and progesterone
    (B) Development of follicles in ovaries
    (C) Both (A) and (B)
    (D) None of the above

36. Follicle stimulating hormone is stimulated by
    (A) Gonadotropin – releasing hormone
    (B) Corticotrophin – releasing hormone
    (C) Thyroid stimulating hormone
    (D) Growth - hormone releasing hormone

37. Which hormone is also known as interstitial cell – stimulating hormone?
    (A) Prolactin hormone
    (B) Growth hormone
    (C) Oxytocin
    (D) Luteinizing hormone

38. The production of Luteinizing hormone is regulated by
    (A) Growth - hormone releasing hormone
    (B) Gonadotropin – releasing hormone
    (C) Thyroid stimulating hormone
    (D) Corticotrophin – releasing hormone

39. The target tissue of gonadotropin – releasing hormone is
    (A) Ovaries in females
    (B) Testis in males
    (C) Both (A) and (B)
    (D) None of the above

40. The major male sex hormone is
    (A) Testosterone
    (B) Serotonin
    (C) Thyronine
    (D) Oxytocin

41. In both males and females sex hormones involved in
    (A) Reproduction
    (B) Promoting hair growth
    (C) Sexual desire
    (D) All of the above

42. The major female sex hormone is
    (A) Oestrogen and progesterone
    (B) Serotonin
    (C) Cortisol
    (D) Thyroxine

43. The posterior pituitary consists primarily of nerve cells surrounded by specialized neuroglial cells called
    (A) Osteocytes
    (B) Osteoblast
    (C) Monocytes
    (D) Pituicytes

44. The pituicytes neurones have their cell bodies in the
    (A) Supraoptic nuclei
    (B) Paraventricular nuclei
    (C) Both (A) and (B)
    (D) None of the above

45. The hormone released from posterior pituitary is
    (A) Vasopressin
    (B) Oxytocin
    (C) Both (A) and (B)
    (D) None of the above

46. Vasopressin is also called as
    (A) Antidiabetic hormone
    (B) Antidiuretic hormone
    (C) Antiemetic hormone
    (D) Antiulcer hormone

47. Posterior pituitary hormones are synthesized in the nerve cell bodies of the
    (A) Cerebrum
    (B) Spinal cord
    (C) Hypothalamus
    (D) Cerebellum

48. Which hormone maintains the water balance of the body
    (A) Vasopressin
    (B) Oxytocin
    (C) Melanin
    (D) Prolactin

49. Antidiuretic hormone acts on
    (A) Distal convoluted tubules
    (B) Collecting ducts
    (C) Both (A) and (B)
    (D) None of the above

50. Which hormone increased water reabsorption from nephrons of the kidneys
    (A) Oxytocin
    (B) Growth hormone
    (C) Thyroxine
    (D) Vasopressin

Answer Key

Endorcrine System (Part-02)

Question	Answer	Question	Answer
01	C = Both A and B	26	A = Thyroid Gland
02	A = Gonadotropins	27	C = Both A and B
03	B = Thyroid Gland	28	B = Corticotropin Releasing Hormone
04	A = Growth Hormone	29	C = Both A and B
05	C = Growth Hormone	30	D = Steroids
06	C = 191	31	A = Adrenal Gland
07	D = All of the Above	32	C = Both A and B
08	C = Both A and B	33	D = All of the Above
09	A = Insulin like Growth Factor	34	C = Both A and B
10	D = All of the Above	35	C = Both A and B
11	C = Both A and B	36	A = Gonadotropin Releasing Hormone
12	A = Growth Hormone Releasing Hormone	37	D =Luteinizing Hormone
13	B = Growth Hormone Releasing Hormone Inhibitors	38	B = Gonadotropin-Releasing Hormone
14	B = Somatostatin	39	C = Both A and B
15	A = Somatostatin	40	A = Testosterone
16	C = Luteotropic Hormone	41	D = All of the Above
17	C = Both A and B	42	A = Oestrogen and Progesterone
18	A = Prolactin Releasing Hormone	43	D = Pituicytes
19	B = Prolactin releasing Hormone	44	C = Both A and B
20	C = Breast	45	C = Both A and B
21	B = Dopamine	46	B = Antidiuretic Hormone
22	A = 199	47	C = Hypothalamus
23	C = Glycoprotein	48	A = Both A and B
24	C = Both A and B	49	C = Both A and B
25	A = Thyrotropin-Releasing Hormone	50	D = Vasopressin

Part-03

1. The hypothalamus regulates ADH secretion through

    (A) Chemoreceptors
    (B) Osmoreceptors
    (C) Cutaneous receptors
    (D) Nociceptors

2. The high osmotic pressure due to

    (A) Diarrhoea
    (B) Excessive sweating
    (C) Stimulate osmoreceptors in the hypothalamus
    (D) All of the above

3. Oxytocin stimulates target tissues during and after childbirth are

    (A) Uterine smooth muscle
    (B) Muscle cells of the lactating breast
    (C) Both (A) and (B)
    (D) None of the above

4. Which hormone is called birth hormone?

    (A) Oxytocin
    (B) Thyronine
    (C) Vasopressin
    (D) Serotonin

5. Release of oxytocin hormone during child birth is an example

    (A) Negative feedback mechanism
    (B) Positive feedback mechanism
    (C) Alpha feedback mechanism
    (D) Gamma feedback mechanism

6. Oxytocin hormone enhances the

    (A) Contractions of uterus muscle
    (B) Relaxation of uterus muscle
    (C) Contraction of cardiac muscle
    (D) Relaxation of cardiac muscle

7. A small, pine – shaped gland attached to the roof of the third ventricle and is present between the two cerebral hemispheres of the brain
   (A) Adrenal gland
   (B) Thyroid gland
   (C) Pineal gland
   (D) Pancreas

8. Pineal gland is also called as
   (A) Pineal body
   (B) Adrenal gland
   (C) Pineal organ
   (D) Pineal tract

9. The hormone secretes by the pineal gland is
   (A) Mineralocorticoids
   (B) Insulin
   (C) Thyronine
   (D) Melatonin

10. Pineal gland has hormone producing cells called
    (A) Pituicytes
    (B) Pinealocytes
    (C) Osteocytes
    (D) Osteoblast

11. Function of pineal gland is
    (A) Regulates sleep pattern
    (B) Regulates circadian rhythm
    (C) Both (A) and (B)
    (D) None of the above

12. The largest endocrine gland is
    (A) Adrenal gland
    (B) Thyroid gland
    (C) Pineal gland
    (D) Pancreas

13. The weight of thyroid gland is about
    (A) 20 – 40 gm
    (B) 1 – 2 gm
    (C) 80 – 90 gm
    (D) 120 – 150 gm

14. Which gland situated in the neck just inferior to the larynx and consists of two lobes
    (A) Adrenal gland
    (B) Pineal gland
    (C) Thyroid gland
    (D) Pancreas

15. The wall of each follicle of thyroid gland consists primarily of cuboidal epithelial cells called
    (A) Follicular cells
    (B) Mast cells
    (C) Medullar cells
    (D) Schwann cells

16. Which hormone is produced by follicular cells?
    (A) Tetraiodothyronine
    (B) Tri – iodothyronine
    (C) Both (A) and (B)
    (D) None of the above

17. How many iodine atoms contains in tri – iodothyronine
    (A) 2
    (B) 3
    (C) 1
    (D) 6

18. How many iodine atoms contains in tetraiodothyronine?
    (A) 6
    (B) 7
    (C) 3
    (D) 4

19. Between the follicles there are other cells called
    (A) Parafollicular cells
    (B) Paramodular cells
    (C) Schwann cells
    (D) Oligodendrocytes

20. Parafollicular cells is also called
    (A) T cells
    (B) H cells
    (C) C cells
    (D) B cells

21. The parafollicular cells secretes
    (A) Melatonin
    (B) Serotonin
    (C) Calcitonin
    (D) Insulin

22. The thyroid gland secrete hormones are
    (A) Thyroxine
    (B) Thyronine
    (C) Calcitonin
    (D) All of the above

23. The arterial blood supply to the thyroid gland is through the
    (A) Superior thyroid arteries
    (B) Inferior thyroid arteries
    (C) Both (A) and (B)
    (D) None of the above

24. Which of the following is essential for formation of thyroid hormones?
    (A) Iron
    (B) Iodine
    (C) Potassium
    (D) Chloride

25. The thyroid gland selectively takes up iodine from the blood a process is called
    (A) Iodine trapping
    (B) Iodine tracking
    (C) Iodine gaining
    (D) Iodine receiving

26. Thyroid hormone is synthesized as large precursor molecules called
   - (A) Epinine
   - (B) Tryptophane
   - (C) Tyrosine
   - (D) Thyroglobulin

27. The thyroid–stimulating hormone stimulates thyroid to release the thyroid hormones in condition of
   - (A) Stress
   - (B) Malnutrition
   - (C) Cold
   - (D) All of the above

28. T_3 and T_4 affect most cells of the body by
   - (A) Increasing the metabolic rate and heat production
   - (B) Regulating metabolism of carbohydrates, proteins and fats
   - (C) Both (A) and (B)
   - (D) None of the above

29. Function of thyroid hormone is
   - (A) Normal growth of bones
   - (B) Increase basal metabolic rate
   - (C) Thermal regulation
   - (D) All of the above

30. Which hormone lowers blood calcium levels
   - (A) Calcitonin
   - (B) Melatonin
   - (C) Serotonin
   - (D) Melanin

31. Calcitonin works by acting on
   - (A) Bone cells by promoting storage of calcium
   - (B) Kidney tubules by inhibiting the reabsorption of calcium
   - (C) Both (A) and (B)
   - (D) None of the above

32. How many amino acids present on calcitonin?
   - (A) 32
   - (B) 56
   - (C) 89
   - (D) 78

33. Which gland located behind the thyroid gland
   - (A) Parathyroid gland
   - (B) Adrenal gland
   - (C) Pancreas
   - (D) Pineal gland

34. How many parathyroid glands are there?
    (A) One   (B) Six
    (C) Four   (D) Two

35. Which hormone is secreted by parathyroid gland?
    (A) Parathormone   (B) Mineralocorticoids
    (C) Insulin   (D) Oxytocin

36. Which hormone increase blood calcium levels
    (A) Oxytocin   (B) Vasopressin
    (C) Insulin   (D) Parathormone

37. Calcium is essential for
    (A) Muscle contraction   (B) Blood clotting
    (C) Transmission of nerve impulses   (D) All of the above

38. Which hormone enhances active reabsorption of calcium and magnesium from kidney
    (A) Oxytocin   (B) Prolactin
    (C) Parathormone   (D) Thyronine

39. Which glands situated on the upper pole of kidney
    (A) Thyroid gland   (B) Parathyroid gland
    (C) Adrenal gland   (D) Pineal gland

40. Adrenal gland is also called
    (A) Suprarenal gland   (B) Pineal gland
    (C) Pineal body   (D) Parathyroid gland

41. The parts of adrenal gland are
    (A) Adrenal cortex   (B) Adrenal medulla
    (C) Both (A) and (B)   (D) None of the above

42. Which of the following is outer part of adrenal gland?
    (A) Adrenal medulla   (B) Adrenal cortex
    (C) Adrenal compact   (D) Adrenal cisternae

43. Which of the following is inner part of adrenal gland?
    (A) Adrenal compact   (B) Adrenal cisternae
    (C) Adrenal medulla   (D) Adrenal cortex

44. The adrenal cortex is subdivided into zone are
    (A) Zona glomerulosa
    (B) Zona fasciculata
    (C) Zona reticulata
    (D) All of the above

45. The outer zone of adrenal cortex is
    (A) Zona reticulata
    (B) Zona glomerulosa
    (C) Zona fasciculata
    (D) Zona cisternae

46. The middle zone of adrenal cortex is
    (A) Zona fasciculata
    (B) Zona reticulata
    (C) Zona cisternae
    (D) Zona glomerulosa

47. The inner zone of adrenal cortex is
    (A) Zona cisternae
    (B) Zona glomerulosa
    (C) Zona reticulata
    (D) Zona fasciculata

48. The zona glomerulosa (outer zone) of adrenal cortex secretes
    (A) Mineralocorticoids
    (B) Glucocorticoids
    (C) Gonadocorticoids
    (D) Melatonin

49. The zona fasciculata (middle zone) of adrenal cortex secretes
    (A) Gonadocorticoids
    (B) Melatonin
    (C) Mineralocorticoids
    (D) Glucocorticoids

50. The zona reticulata (inner zone) of adrenal cortex
    (A) Melatonin
    (B) Gonadocorticoids
    (C) Mineralocorticoids
    (D) Glucocorticoids

Answer Key

Endorcrine System (Part-03)

Question	Answer	Question	Answer
01	B = Osmoreceptors	26	D = Thyroglobulin
02	D = All of the Above	27	D = All of the Above
03	C = Both A and B	28	C = Both A and B
04	A = Oxytocin	29	D = All of the Above
05	B = Positive Feedback Mechanism	30	A = Calcitonin
06	A = Contraction of Uterus Muscle	31	C = Both A and B
07	C = Pineal Gland	32	A = 32
08	A = Pineal Body	33	A = Parathyroid Gland
09	D = Melatonin	34	C = Four
10	B = Pinealocytes	35	A = Parathormone
11	C = Both A and B	36	D = Parathormone
12	B = Thyroid Gland	37	D = All of the Above
13	A = 20-40 gm	38	C = Parathormone
14	C = Thyroid Gland	39	C = Adrenal Gland
15	A = Follicular Cells	40	A = Suprarenal Gland
16	C = Both A and B	41	C = Both A and B
17	B = 03	42	B = Adrenal Cortex
18	D = 04	43	C = Adrenal Medulla
19	A = Parafollicular Cells	44	D = All of the Above
20	C = C Cells	45	B = Zona Glomerulosa
21	C = Calcitonin	46	A = Zona Fasciculata
22	D = All of the Above	47	C = Zona Reticulata
23	C = Both A and B	48	A = Mineralocorticoids
24	B = Iodine	49	D = Glucocorticoids
25	A = Iodine Trapping	50	B = Gonadocorticoids

Part-04

1. Cortisol helps in control of
   - (A) Suppresses inflammation
   - (B) Regulates blood pressure
   - (C) Increase blood sugar
   - (D) All of the above

2. When extensive sympathetic nerve supply stimulates the adrenal gland release
   - (A) Epinephrine (80 %)
   - (B) Norepinephrine (20 %)
   - (C) Both (A) and (B)
   - (D) None of the above

3. Together epinephrine and norepinephrine potentiate the fight or flight response by
   - (A) Increasing blood pressure
   - (B) Increasing heart rate
   - (C) Dilating the pupils
   - (D) All of the above

4. The hormones of adrenal cortex are collectively known as
   - (A) Corticosteroids
   - (B) Adrenaline
   - (C) Noradrenaline
   - (D) Melatonin

5. All adrenocortical hormones are
   - (A) Glycoproteins
   - (B) Amino acids
   - (C) Steroids
   - (D) Peptides

6. The adrenocortical hormones are mainly synthesized from the
   - (A) Protein
   - (B) Vitamin
   - (C) Cholesterol
   - (D) Carbohydrate

7. The adrenocortical hormones include
   - (A) Mineralocorticoids
   - (B) Glucocorticoids
   - (C) Gonadocorticoids
   - (D) All of the above

8. The major mineralocorticoids are
   - (A) Melatonin
   - (B) Aldosterone
   - (C) Melanin
   - (D) Histamine

9. The major function of aldosterone involves
    - (A) Water balance
    - (B) Electrolyte balance
    - (C) Regulates blood volume in body
    - (D) All of the above

10. By negative feedback mechanism aldosterone stimulates
    - (A) Reabsorption of sodium by renal tubules
    - (B) Excretion of potassium in the urine
    - (C) Both (A) and (B)
    - (D) None of the above

11. Which cells of kidney stimulate when decrease in the sodium ion concentration or blood volume
    - (A) Juxtaglomerular cells
    - (B) Schwann cells
    - (C) Osteocytes
    - (D) Oligodendrocytes

12. The juxtaglomerular cells of kidney secrete
    - (A) Melanin
    - (B) Renin
    - (C) Melatonin
    - (D) Thyronine

13. Angiotensinogen produced in
    - (A) Liver
    - (B) Lungs
    - (C) Brain
    - (D) Stomach

14. Angiotensin I is converted into angiotensin II in the presence of enzyme
    - (A) Acetyl Cholinesterase
    - (B) Angiotensin converting enzyme
    - (C) Pyruvate kinase
    - (D) Phosphoglycerate kinase

15. Angiotensin II stimulates the adrenal cortex to secrete
    - (A) Melatonin
    - (B) Melanin
    - (C) Aldosterone
    - (D) Thyronine

16. Aldosterone causes
    - (A) Vasoconstriction
    - (B) Vasodilation
    - (C) Bronchodilation
    - (D) Bronchoconstriction

17. Which of the following is stressful conditions?
    - (A) Infection
    - (B) Emotional disturbance
    - (C) Fasting
    - (D) All of the above

18. The major glucocorticoids are
    - (A) Melatonin
    - (B) Thyronine
    - (C) Cortisol
    - (D) Melanin

19. Glucocorticoids are essential for
    - (A) Regulating metabolism
    - (B) Inflammatory response
    - (C) Response to stress
    - (D) All of the above

20. The secretion of glucocorticoids controlled by through a negative feedback system involving the
    - (A) Hypothalamus
    - (B) Anterior pituitary
    - (C) Both (A) and (B)
    - (D) None of the above

21. Adrenal medulla mainly consists of hormone – producing cells called
    - (A) Schwann cells
    - (B) Osteocytes
    - (C) Chromaffin cells
    - (D) Mast cells

22. The major hormone synthesised by adrenal medulla is
    - (A) Epinephrine
    - (B) Norepinephrine
    - (C) Both (A) and (B)
    - (D) None of the above

23. Epinephrine is also called
    - (A) Adrenaline
    - (B) Noradrenaline
    - (C) Norepinephrine
    - (D) Melanin

24. Noradrenaline is also called
    - (A) Adrenaline
    - (B) Norepinephrine
    - (C) Melanin
    - (D) Epinephrine

25. Eptinephrine and norepinephrine prepare the body for stressful situations include
    - (A) Injury
    - (B) Exercise
    - (C) Trauma
    - (D) All of the above

26. Adrenaline and noradrenaline increased blood flow to essential organs include
    - (A) Heart
    - (B) Liver
    - (C) Brain
    - (D) All of the above

27. Precursor of adrenaline and noradrenaline
    (A) Amino acid tyrosine   (B) Acetyl CoA
    (C) UDP glucose   (D) Tryptophane

28. Function of adrenaline and noradrenaline
    (A) Produces vasoconstriction   (B) Increased heart rate
    (C) Increased blood pressure   (D) All of the above

29. The flattened, elongated organ located in the epigastric and hypochondriac regions of the abdomen
    (A) Pineal gland   (B) Thyroid gland
    (C) Pancreas   (D) Adrenal gland

30. The pancreatic juice is composed of
    (A) Digestive enzyme   (B) Bicarbonate
    (C) Both (A) and (B)   (D) None of the above

31. The enzyme presents in pancreatic juice
    (A) Trypsin   (B) Lipase
    (C) Amylase   (D) All of the above

32. In pancreas the digestive enzymes are synthesized and secreted from
    (A) Acinar cells   (B) Schwann cells
    (C) Goblet cells   (D) Paneth cells

33. Pancreas mainly consists of lobules or acini that secrete the
    (A) Bile juice   (B) Pancreatic juice
    (C) Saliva   (D) Intestinal juice

34. The secretion of pancreatic juice is stimulated by
    (A) Gastrin   (B) Secretin
    (C) Cytokinin   (D) Enterokinase

35. In pancreas tiny clusters of endocrine tissues called
    (A) Pancreatic islets   (B) Adrenal islets
    (C) Adrenal medulla   (D) Adrenal cortex

36. Pancreatic islets are also called
    (A) Islets of Schwann   (B) Islets of Langerhans
    (C) Loop of Henle   (D) Islets of glomerulus

37. How many pancreatic islets are there?
   (A) 1 – 2 million
   (B) 5 – 6 million
   (C) 10 – 11 million
   (D) 13 – 14 million

38. Which cells present in islets of Langerhans
   (A) Alpha cells
   (B) Beta cells
   (C) Delta cells
   (D) All of the above

39. Alpha cells of pancreas secrete
   (A) Glucagon
   (B) Insulin
   (C) Somatostatin
   (D) Melanin

40. Beta cells of pancreas secrete
   (A) Melanin
   (B) Somatostatin
   (C) Insulin
   (D) Glucagon

41. Delta cells of pancreas secrete
   (A) Insulin
   (B) Glucagon
   (C) Somatostatin
   (D) Melatonin

42. Which of the following hormone increase blood glucose level?
   (A) Melatonin
   (B) Calcitonin
   (C) Insulin
   (D) Glucagon

43. Which of the following hormone lower the blood glucose levels?
   (A) Calcitonin
   (B) Insulin
   (C) Glucagon
   (D) Melatonin

44. How many amino acids present in insulin?
   (A) 90
   (B) 70
   (C) 32
   (D) 50

45. Which hormone prevents the breakdown of proteins and fats and inhibits gluconeogenesis
   (A) Insulin
   (B) Melanin
   (C) Histamine
   (D) Serotonin

46. Which promotes the rapid conversion of glucose into glycogen
   (A) Serotonin
   (B) Thyronine
   (C) Insulin
   (D) Melanin

47. Function of insulin
    (A) Uptake of glucose by tissue
    (B) Utilization of glucose
    (C) Lipogenesis
    (D) All of the above

48. PP cells of pancreas secrete
    (A) Insulin
    (B) Pancreatic polypeptide
    (C) Glucagon
    (D) Melatonin

49. How many amino acids present in glucagon?
    (A) 56
    (B) 90
    (C) 29
    (D) 60

50. Function of glucagon is
    (A) Conversion of glycogen to glucose
    (B) Gluconeogenesis
    (C) Increase blood sugar level
    (D) All of the above

Answer Key

Endorcrine System (Part-04)

Question	Answer	Question	Answer
01	D = All of the Above	26	D = All of the Above
02	C = Both A and B	27	A = Amino Acid Tyrosine
03	D = All of the Above	28	D = All of the Above
04	A = Corticosteroids	29	C = Pancreas
05	C = Steroids	30	C = Both A and B
06	C = Cholesterol	31	D = All of the Above
07	D = All of the Above	32	A = Acinar Cells
08	B = Aldosterone	33	B = Pancreatic Juice
09	D = All of the Above	34	B = Secretin
10	C = Both A and B	35	A = Pancreatic Islet
11	A = Juxtaglomerular Cells	36	B = Islet of Langerhans
12	B = Renin	37	A = 1-2 Million
13	A = Liver	38	D = All of the Above
14	B = Angiotensin Converting Enzyme	39	A = Glucagon
15	C = Aldosterone	40	C = Insulin
16	A = Vasoconstriction	41	C = Somatostatin
17	D = All of the Above	42	D = Glucagon
18	C = Cortisol	43	B = Insulin
19	D = All of the Above	44	D = 50
20	C = Both A and B	45	A = Insulin
21	C = Chromaffin Cells	46	C = Insulin
22	C = Both A and B	47	D = All of the Above
23	A = Adrenaline	48	B = Pancreatic Polypeptides
24	B = Norepinephrine	49	C = 29
25	D = All of the Above	50	D = All of the Above

Part-05

1. The hormone secreted by gonads include
   - (A) Oestrogen
   - (B) Testosterone
   - (C) Progesterone
   - (D) All of the above

2. Which hormone responsible for the development of male reproductive structures
   - (A) Serotonin
   - (B) Oestrogen
   - (C) Testosterone
   - (D) Melatonin

3. Testosterone promotes the development of accessory male sexual characters such as
   - (A) Growth of facial and chest hair
   - (B) Deepening of the voice
   - (C) Muscular development
   - (D) All of the above

4. Which hormone responsible for the development of female reproductive structures
   - (A) Testosterone
   - (B) Melatonin
   - (C) Oestrogen
   - (D) Thyroxine

5. Oestrogen hormone promotes the development of accessory female sexual characters such as
   - (A) Enlargement of breasts
   - (B) Onset of menstrual cycle
   - (C) Growth of pubic and axillary hair
   - (D) All of the above

6. Which hormone is also called 'hormone of pregnancy'
   - (A) Melatonin
   - (B) Thyronine
   - (C) Progesterone
   - (D) Testosterone

7. Progesterone plays major role in
   - (A) Implanting foetus to the uterine wall
   - (B) Forming of placenta
   - (C) Regulating development of foetus in the uterus
   - (D) All of the above

8. Relaxin hormone secreted by
 (A) Pancreas
 (B) Ovary
 (C) Stomach
 (D) Liver

9. Which of the following is local hormone?
 (A) Histamine
 (B) Serotonin
 (C) Prostaglandins
 (D) All of the above

10. Histamine is synthesised and stored in
 (A) Mast cells
 (B) Schwann cells
 (C) Astrocytes
 (D) Osteocytes

11. Which of the following present in histamine?
 (A) Amine
 (B) Aldehydes
 (C) Ketone
 (D) Alcohol

12. In allergies mast cells release chemicals called
 (A) Hormones
 (B) Mediators
 (C) Saliva
 (D) Lacrimal fluid

13. The allergens may be
 (A) Pet dander
 (B) Dust
 (C) Pollen
 (D) All of the above

14. Histamine causes allergic symptoms are
 (A) Expanding blood vessels
 (B) Itchy skin
 (C) Tightening airways
 (D) All of the above

15. Which hormone is called 5 – hydroxy tryptamine
 (A) Melatonin
 (B) Serotonin
 (C) Oxytocin
 (D) Vasopressin

16. Serotonin present in
 (A) Platelets
 (B) Brain
 (C) Intestinal wall
 (D) All of the above

17. Serotonin plays a key role in
 (A) Wound healing
 (B) Mood and sleep
 (C) Blood clotting
 (D) All of the above

18. Prostaglandins have potent and wide – ranging physiological effects in
    (A) Inflammatory response   (B) Potentiation of pain
    (C) Fever   (D) All of the above

19. A disease in which growth hormone is hyper secreted usually by the
    hormone secreting pituitary gland
    (A) Gigantism   (B) Graves' disease
    (C) Exophthalmos   (D) Goitre

20. The effect of excess growth hormone includes
    (A) Excessive growth of bone
    (B) Enlargement of internal organs
    (C) Formations of excessive connective tissue
    (D) All of the above

21. Which occurs in adults when there is excessive growth hormone secretion
    after ossification is complete
    (A) Tetany   (B) Hypocalcaemia
    (C) Acromegaly   (D) Goitre

22. Which body parts are mostly affecting acromegaly?
    (A) Face   (B) Enlarged tongue
    (C) Excessive large hands and feet   (D) All of the above

23. Treatment of acromegaly include
    (A) Irradiation   (B) Radioisotope implantation
    (C) Surgical removal of the tumour   (D) All of the above

24. Which changes noticed in acromegaly
    (A) Coarse facial features   (B) Enlarged tongue
    (C) Large hands and feet   (D) All of the above

25. Which condition characterized by hyposecretion of growth hormone during
    growth years
    (A) Pituitary dwarfism   (B) Cretinism
    (C) Myxoedema   (D) Grave's disease

26. Which of the following caused by a tumour that secretes large amounts
    of prolactin?
    (A) Hypercalcaemia   (B) Hypocalcaemia
    (C) Hyperprolactinaemia   (D) Exophthalmos

27. The hyposecretion of anterior pituitary hormones causes
    (A) Tumours of hypothalamus or pituitary
    (B) Ischaemic necrosis
    (C) Infections
    (D) All of the above

28. Which of the following also called postpartum necrosis?
    (A) Graves' disease
    (B) Pituitary necrosis
    (C) Hyperthyroidism
    (D) Diabetes insipidus

29. Pituitary necrosis can be caused by
    (A) Bleeding into the pituitary
    (B) Blocked blood flow to the pituitary
    (C) Both (A) and (B)
    (D) None of the above

30. A chronic endocrine disorder in which the adrenal gland produce insufficient steroid hormones is called
    (A) Diabetes mellitus
    (B) Addison's disease
    (C) Pituitary necrosis
    (D) Grave disease

31. The most common symptoms of Addison's disease are
    (A) Fatigue
    (B) Mental lethargy
    (C) Anorexia
    (D) All of the above

32. A very common disorder manifested by high blood glucose
    (A) Diabetes mellitus
    (B) Addison's disease
    (C) Grave disease
    (D) Pituitary necrosis

33. The main type of diabetes is
    (A) Type 1 diabetes
    (B) Type 2 diabetes
    (C) Both (A) and (B)
    (D) None of the above

34. Which of the following is insulin dependent diabetes mellitus?
    (A) Type 1 diabetes
    (B) Type 2 diabetes
    (C) Type 3 diabetes
    (D) Type 4 diabetes

35. Which diabetes occurs due to the absence of insulin
    (A) Type 3 diabetes
    (B) Type 1 diabetes
    (C) Type 2 diabetes
    (D) Type 4 diabetes

36. Which of the following diabetes is non – insulin dependent diabetes mellitus?
    - (A) Type 3 diabetes
    - (B) Type 4diabetes
    - (C) Type 2 diabetes
    - (D) Type 1 diabetes

37. Symptoms of diabetes is
    - (A) Excessive thirst
    - (B) Excessive urination
    - (C) Fatigue and weight loss
    - (D) All of the above

38. Which of the following mainly occurs due to deficiency of antidiuretic hormone?
    - (A) Diabetes insipidus
    - (B) Goitre
    - (C) Hyperthyroidism
    - (D) Grave disease

39. The enlargement of thyroid gland that leads to the swelling of the neck or larynx
    - (A) Diabetes insipidus
    - (B) Diabetes mellitus
    - (C) Goitre
    - (D) Acromegaly

40. Which hormone reduced in goitre
    - (A) Thyroxine
    - (B) Tri – iodothyronine
    - (C) Both (A) and (B)
    - (D) None of the above

41. Which of the following refers to the increased thyroid hormones?
    - (A) Hyperthyroidism
    - (B) Hypothyroidism
    - (C) Exophthalmos
    - (D) Diabetes insipidus

42. Hyperthyroidism also called as
    - (A) Exophthalmos
    - (B) Pituitary necrosis
    - (C) Thyrotoxicosis
    - (D) Cushing's syndrome

43. The symptoms of hyperthyroidism include
    - (A) Nervousness
    - (B) Irritability
    - (C) Anxiety
    - (D) All of the above

44. Which of the following refers to deficiency of thyroid hormone?
    - (A) Hyperthyroidism
    - (B) Hypothyroidism
    - (C) Acromegaly
    - (D) Cushing's syndrome

45. Which disease is characterized by the increased secretion of ACTH from the anterior pituitary?

    (A) Acromegaly

    (B) Cushing's syndrome

    (C) Grave's disease

    (D) Myxoedema

46. Symptoms of Cushing's syndrome

    (A) Weight gain

    (B) Moon – like face

    (C) Hyperhidrosis

    (D) All of the above

47. Which disease is characterised by hyperthyroidism?

    (A) Grave's disease

    (B) Glaucoma

    (C) Pituitary necrosis

    (D) Acromegaly

48. Treatment of grave's disease include

    (A) Removal of a portion of the thyroid gland

    (B) Radioiodine

    (C) Antithyroid drugs

    (D) All of the above

49. The symptoms of myxoedema are

    (A) Slow pulse

    (B) Dry and brittle hair

    (C) Sensation of coldness

    (D) All of the above

50. Which of the following is not a disorder of thyroid gland?

    (A) Myxoedema

    (B) Cretinism

    (C) Glaucoma

    (D) Grave's disease

Answer Key

Endorcrine System (Part-05)

Question	Answer	Question	Answer
01	D = All of the Above	26	C = Hyperprolactinemia
02	C = Testosterone	27	D = All of the Above
03	D = All of the Above	28	B = Pituitary Necrosis
04	C = Oestrogen	29	C = Both A and B
05	D = All of the Above	30	B = Addison's Disease
06	C = Progesterone	31	D = All of the Above
07	D = All of the Above	32	A = Diabetes Mellitus
08	B = Ovary	33	C = Both A and B
09	D = All of the Above	34	A = Type 1 Diabetes
10	A = Mast Cells	35	B = Type 1 Diabetes
11	A = Amine	36	C = Type 2 Diabetes
12	B = Mediators	37	D = All of the Above
13	D = All of the Above	38	A = Diabetes Insipidus
14	D = All of the Above	39	C = Goitre
15	B = Serotonin	40	C = Both A and B
16	D = All of the Above	41	A = Hyperthyroidism
17	D = All of the Above	42	C = Thyrotoxicosis
18	D = All of the Above	43	D = All of the Above
19	A = Gigantism	44	B = Hypothyroidism
20	D = All of the Above	45	B = Cushing's Syndrome
21	C = Acromegaly	46	D = All of the Above
22	D = All of the Above	47	A = Grave's Disease
23	D = All of the Above	48	D = All of the Above
24	D = All of the Above	49	D = All of the Above
25	A = Pituitary Dwarfism	50	C = Glaucoma

Notes

Unit - VI

Body Fluids and Blood, Lymphatic System

Part-01

1. Which of the following is fluid connective tissue?
   - (A) Bone
   - (B) Blood
   - (C) Cartilage
   - (D) Tendons

2. Blood is considered as the
   - (A) Fluid of life
   - (B) Fluid of health
   - (C) Fluid of growth
   - (D) All of the above

3. The branch of science concerned with the study of blood
   - (A) Haematology
   - (B) Neurology
   - (C) Osteology
   - (D) Nephrology

4. Blood accounts total body weight is about
   - (A) 30 %
   - (B) 7 %
   - (C) 49 %
   - (D) 60 %

5. Blood has pH is
   - (A) 1.5 to 2.7
   - (B) 3.1 to 4.1
   - (C) 8.2 to 9.4
   - (D) 7.2 to 7.4

6. Blood has specific gravity is
   - (A) 2.09
   - (B) 3.03
   - (C) 1.06
   - (D) 2.04

7. Blood transports
   - (A) Oxygen
   - (B) Nutrients
   - (C) Hormones
   - (D) All of the above

8. Blood carries nutrients like
   - (A) Glucose
   - (B) Amino acids
   - (C) Lipids
   - (D) All of the above

9. Blood consists components are
   (A) Plasma
   (B) Blood cells
   (C) Both (A) and (B)
   (D) None of the above

10. Plasma proteins play a vital role in maintaining normal osmotic pressure of the blood is
    (A) 10 mm Hg
    (B) 80 mm Hg
    (C) 25 mm Hg
    (D) 5 mm Hg

11. Which constituent present in plasma in large amount
    (A) Water
    (B) Salts
    (C) Hormones
    (D) Gases

12. The percentage of water present in plasma
    (A) 20 – 30 %
    (B) 10 – 20 %
    (C) 90 – 92 %
    (D) 20 – 25 %

13. Plasma carries a range of dissolved and suspended substances including
    (A) Plasma proteins
    (B) Hormones
    (C) Nutrients
    (D) All of the above

14. Plasma contains plasma proteins about
    (A) 40 %
    (B) 50 %v
    (C) 7 %
    (D) 30 %

15. The protein contains in blood are
    (A) Albumin
    (B) Fibrinogens
    (C) Globulins
    (D) All of the above

16. The most abundant plasma proteins are
    (A) Albumin
    (B) Alanine
    (C) Collagen
    (D) Myosin

17. The molecular weight of plasma albumin is
    (A) 90,000
    (B) 89,000
    (C) 23,000
    (D) 69,000

18. The percentage of albumins present in plasma
    (A) 10 %
    (B) 12 %
    (C) 65 %
    (D) 18 %

19. Albumin act as carrier of molecules is
    (A) Free fatty acids
    (B) Drugs
    (C) Steroid hormones
    (D) All of the above

20. The globulin is a mixture of several proteins are
    - (A) á globulin
    - (B) ® globulin
    - (C) ã globulin
    - (D) All of the above

21. The globulins transport and stored proteins are
    - (A) Transferrin
    - (B) Ferritin
    - (C) Both (A) and (B)
    - (D) None of the above

22. The molecular weight of fibrinogens is
    - (A) 3,45,000
    - (B) 20,000
    - (C) 56,000
    - (D) 1,23,000

23. Which of the following is clotting proteins?
    - (A) Actin
    - (B) Fibrinogens
    - (C) Alanine
    - (D) Myosin

24. Amount of blood contains in adult human body
    - (A) 5 – 6 litres
    - (B) 1 – 2 litres
    - (C) 2 – 3 litres
    - (D) 1.5 – 2.0 litres

25. The main function of globulins is
    - (A) Transport hormone
    - (B) Inhibition of some proteolytic enzymes
    - (C) Neutralize foreign materials
    - (D) All of the above

26. Electrolytes present in plasma that have functions are
    - (A) Muscle contraction
    - (B) Transmission of nerve impulses
    - (C) Maintenance acid – base balance
    - (D) All of the above

27. Which electrolyte present in plasma
    - (A) Ca^{2+}
    - (B) Na^+
    - (C) K^+
    - (D) All of the above

28. How many oxygens carries blood?
    - (A) 40 %
    - (B) 98 %
    - (C) 10 %
    - (D) 20 %

29. Nutrients in essential for cellular growth and metabolism include
    - (A) Glucose
    - (B) Amino acids
    - (C) Vitamins
    - (D) All of the above

30. Waste products of protein metabolism

(A) Urea

(B) Creatinine

(C) Uric acid

(D) All of the above

31. How many blood cells present in blood?

(A) 45 %

(B) 10 %

(C) 90 %

(D) 20 %

32. Which proteins play an important role in defence mechanism of the body

(A) Alanine

(B) Actin

(C) Immunoglobulin

(D) Collagen

33. During conditions like fasting or inadequate food intake, plasma proteins are utilized by body tissues for their routine activities and thus the plasma proteins are also referred to as

(A) Reserve proteins

(B) Stored proteins

(C) Target proteins

(D) Balanced proteins

34. Function of blood

(A) Transportation

(B) Defence

(C) Blood coagulation

(D) All of the above

35. Types of blood cells are

(A) Red blood cells

(B) White blood cells

(C) Platelets

(D) All of the above

36. Red blood cells are also called

(A) Leukocytes

(B) Erythrocytes

(C) Thrombocytes

(D) Platelets

37. White blood cells are also called

(A) Platelets

(B) Thrombocytes

(C) Leukocytes

(D) Thrombocytes

38. Platelets are also called

(A) Red blood cells

(B) Thrombocytes

(C) Erythrocytes

(D) Leukocytes

39. Red blood cells make up the volume of blood cells

(A) 20 %

(B) 40 %

(C) 95 %

(D) 35%

40. The leukocytes are divided into

(A) Granular leukocytes

(B) Agranular leukocytes

(C) Both (A) and (B)

(D) None of the above

41. Types of granular leukocytes are
    - (A) Neutrophils
    - (B) Basophils
    - (C) Eosinophils
    - (D) All of the above

42. The percentage of WBCs make up neutrophils
    - (A) 20 – 30 %
    - (B) 60 – 70 %
    - (C) 10 – 20 %
    - (D) 30 – 35 %

43. The percentage of WBCs make up eosinophils
    - (A) 60 – 70 %
    - (B) 20 – 30 %
    - (C) 2 – 4 %
    - (D) 50 – 60 %

44. The percentage of WBCs make up basophils
    - (A) 30 – 40 %
    - (B) 50 – 60 %
    - (C) 60 – 65 %
    - (D) 0.5 – 1 %

45. Which of the following have granules in their cytoplasm?
    - (A) Monocytes
    - (B) Lymphocytes
    - (C) Agranulocytes
    - (D) Neutrophils

46. Types of Agranulocytes is
    - (A) Monocytes
    - (B) Lymphocytes
    - (C) Both (A) and (B)
    - (D) None of the above

47. Which of the following do not have granules in their cytoplasm?
    - (A) Neutrophils
    - (B) Monocytes
    - (C) Basophils
    - (D) Eosinophils

48. The process of development of blood cells called
    - (A) Haemopoiesis
    - (B) Haemolysis
    - (C) Ossification
    - (D) Osteogenesis

49. Haemopoiesis also called as
    - (A) Ossification
    - (B) Osteogenesis
    - (C) Haematopoiesis
    - (D) Haemolysis

50. The percentage of total blood volume occupied by RBCs is called
    - (A) Haematocrit value
    - (B) Triglycerides value
    - (C) Urea value
    - (D) Bilirubin value

Answer Key

Body Fluids and Blood, Lymphatic System (Part-01)

Question	Answer	Question	Answer
01	B = Blood	26	D = All of the Above
02	D = All of the Above	27	D = All of the Above
03	A = Haematology	28	B = 98%
04	B = 07%	29	D = All of the Above
05	D = 7.2 to 7.4	30	D = All of the Above
06	C = 1.06	31	A = 45%
07	D = All of the Above	32	C = Immunoglobulin
08	D = All of the Above	33	A = Reverse Proteins
09	C = Both A and B	34	D = All of the Above
10	C = 25 mm Hg	35	D = All of the Above
11	A = Water	36	B = Erythrocytes
12	C = 90 to 92 %	37	C = Leukocytes
13	D = All of the Above	38	B = Thrombocytes
14	C = 07%	39	C = 95%
15	D = All of the Above	40	C = Both A and B
16	A = Albumin	41	D = All of the Above
17	D = 69,000	42	B = 60 to 70%
18	C = 65%	43	C = 2-4 %
19	D = All of the Above	44	D = 0.5-1%
20	D = All of the Above	45	D = Neutrophils
21	C = Both A and B	46	C = Both A and B
22	A = 3,45,000	47	B = Monocytes
23	B = Fibrinogens	48	A = Haemopoiesis
24	A = 5-6 Litres	49	C = Haematopoiesis
25	D = All of the Above	50	A = Haematocrit Value

Part-02

1. Before birth haemopoiesis first takes place in
   - (A) Liver
   - (B) Spleen
   - (C) Egg yolk of embryo
   - (D) Thymus

2. In which part of fetus haemopoiesis takes place after birth
   - (A) Liver
   - (B) Spleen
   - (C) Lymph nodes
   - (D) All of the above

3. The blood cells develop from the primitive cells in the bone marrow. These primitive cells are called
   - (A) Root cells
   - (B) Stem cells
   - (C) Node cells
   - (D) Mast cells

4. Stem cells possess fundamental properties
   - (A) Self – replication
   - (B) Differentiation and commitment
   - (C) Both (A) and (B)
   - (D) None of the above

5. The stem cells have capacity to develop into different types of blood cells they called
   - (A) Pluripotent haemopoietic stem cells
   - (B) Pluripotent ossification bone cells
   - (C) Pluripotent haemolysis root cells
   - (D) Pluripotent ossification root cells

6. The pluripotent haemopoietic stem cells are developed into
   - (A) Lymphoid stem cells
   - (B) Myeloid stem cells
   - (C) Both (A) and (B)
   - (D) None of the above

7. The cells give rise to lymphocytes
   - (A) Lymphoid stem cells
   - (B) Monocytes stem cells
   - (C) Neutrophils stem cells
   - (D) Myeloid stem cells

8. The cells give rise to the blood cells other than lymphocytes by forming different colony - forming units
   - (A) Bone stem cells
   - (B) Myeloid stem cells
   - (C) Astrocytes cells
   - (D) Schwann cells

9. Types of colonies – forming cells (CFUs) are
   - (A) CFU – erythrocytes
   - (B) CFU – monocytes
   - (C) CFU – megakaryocytes
   - (D) All of the above

10. Which colony – forming cells develop into erythrocytes
    - (A) CFU – monocytes
    - (B) CFU – erythrocytes
    - (C) CFU – megakaryocytes
    - (D) CFU – granulocytes

11. Which colony – forming cells develop into platelets
    - (A) CFU – granulocytes
    - (B) CFU – megakaryocytes
    - (C) CFU – monocytes
    - (D) CFU – erythrocytes

12. The diameter of RBC is about
    - (A) 50 μm
    - (B) 40 μm
    - (C) 7 μm
    - (D) 35 μm

13. Surface area of each RBC
    - (A) $200 - 400$ μm²
    - (B) $120 - 140$ μm²
    - (C) $300 - 400$ μm²
    - (D) $250 - 300$ μm²

14. Which cells do not have nucleus
    - (A) Red blood cells
    - (B) Nerve cells
    - (C) Mast cells
    - (D) Osteocytes

15. The main function of RBC
    - (A) Transport of oxygen
    - (B) Acid base balance
    - (C) Maintain viscosity
    - (D) All of the above

16. The lifespan of RBC is about
    - (A) 200 days
    - (B) 120 days
    - (C) 190 days
    - (D) 210 days

17. The composition of RBC present
    - (A) Water
    - (B) Hemoglobulin
    - (C) Lipid
    - (D) All of the above

18. RBCs present a red oxygen carrying pigment called
    - (A) Haemoglobin
    - (B) Haemoalbumin
    - (C) Hemeoglobulin
    - (D) Haemolytes

19. Haemoglobin is
    - (A) Lipid
    - (B) Protein
    - (C) Vitamin
    - (D) Carbohydrate

20. Main function of haemoglobin

    (A) Transport of oxygen

    (B) Transport of waste product

    (C) Maintain acid base balance

    (D) Defence mechanism

21. How many bindings site has haemoglobin for oxygen?

    (A) 7   (B) 9

    (C) 4   (D) 5

22. What is oxyhaemoglobin

    (A) Carbon dioxide binds to haemoglobin

    (B) Oxygen binds to haemoglobin

    (C) Carbon monoxide binds to haemoglobin

    (D) Nitrogen binds to haemoglobin

23. The subunit of haemoglobin is

    (A) Alpha – globins   (B) Beta – globins

    (C) Both (A) and (B)   (D) None of the above

24. The average range of haemoglobin in male is

    (A) 14 – 18 g/dL   (B) 7 – 8 g/dL

    (C) 10 – 11 g/dL   (D) 6 – 7 h/dL

25. The average range of haemoglobin in female is

    (A) 6 – 7 g/dL   (B) 10 – 10.5 g/dL

    (C) 12 – 15.5 g/dL   (D) 9 – 10 g/dL

26. Haemoglobin level in new born is

    (A) 10 g/dL   (B) 11 g/dL

    (C) 8g/dL   (D) 23 g/dL

27. What is haem in haemoglobin

    (A) Iron – containing complex

    (B) Calcium – containing complex

    (C) Chloride – containing complex

    (D) Phosphate – containing complex

28. An average red blood cell carries haemoglobin molecules about

    (A) 120 million   (B) 280 million

    (C) 100 million   (D) 130 million

29. How many iron ions contains in each haem molecule?
    (A) Six
    (B) Seven
    (C) Four
    (D) Five

30. The process of development of RBC is called
    (A) Erythropoiesis
    (B) Leucopoiesis
    (C) Thrombopoiesis
    (D) Ossification

31. Erythropoiesis occur in
    (A) Red bone marrow
    (B) Lungs
    (C) Liver
    (D) Pancreas

32. Which hormone regulates the process of erythropoiesis
    (A) Melatonin
    (B) Thyroxine
    (C) Erythropoietin
    (D) Melanin

33. Erythropoietin is produced by
    (A) Lungs
    (B) Kidney
    (C) Liver
    (D) Stomach

34. Other than kidney erythropoietin is produced by
    (A) Spleen
    (B) Stomach
    (C) Hepatocytes
    (D) Pancreas

35. The earliest recognizable cell of the erythroid series seen in the red bone marrow is
    (A) Sporoblast
    (B) Trophoblast
    (C) Macroblast
    (D) Pronormoblast

36. The pronormoblast progresses into the early
    (A) Normoblast
    (B) Trophoblast
    (C) Macroblast
    (D) Sporoblast

37. In which stage of erythropoiesis haemoglobin appears
    (A) Pronormoblast
    (B) Early normoblast
    (C) Intermediate normoblast
    (D) Reticulocytes

38. In which stage of RBC production nucleus is disappears
    (A) Trophoblast
    (B) Normoblast
    (C) Pronormoblast
    (D) Sporoblast

39. The last stage in the formation of erythrocytes is
    (A) Ribocytes
    (B) Reticulocytes
    (C) Oocyte
    (D) Osteocyte

40. Which component is essential for erythropoiesis?
    (A) Vitamin B12   (B) Folate
    (C) Iron   (D) All of the above

41. Vitamin B12 is also called
    (A) Cobalamin   (B) Retinol
    (C) Tocopherol   (D) Ascorbic acid

42. The destruction of red blood cells is called
    (A) Hemolysis   (B) Sacrolysis
    (C) Fibrinolysis   (D) Mucolysis

43. Destruction of RBC takes place in
    (A) Kidney   (B) Spleen
    (C) Lungs   (D) Pancreas

44. Which of the following called graveyard of RBCs?
    (A) Pancreas   (B) Lungs
    (C) Spleen   (D) Stomach

45. Hypoxia can result from
    (A) Anaemia   (B) Low blood volume
    (C) Poor blood flow   (D) All of the above

46. A condition in which have low number of healthy RBCs
    (A) Anaemia   (B) Glaucoma
    (C) Goitre   (D) Grave's disease

47. Types of anaemia is
    (A) Iron deficiency anaemia   (B) Pernicious anaemia
    (C) Aplastic anaemia   (D) All of the above

48. Symptoms of anaemia is
    (A) Weakness   (B) Fatigue
    (C) Shortness of breath   (D) All of the above

49. An inherited disease in which the red blood cells have an abnormal crescent
    shape called
    (A) Sickle cell anaemia   (B) Pernicious anaemia
    (C) Iron deficiency anaemia   (D) Aplastic anaemia

50. Causes of anaemia is
    (A) Blood loss   (B) Lack of RBC production
    (C) Higher RBC destruction   (D) All of the above

Answer Key

Body Fluids and Blood, Lymphatic System (Part-02)

Question	Answer	Question	Answer
01	C = Egg Yolk of Embryo	26	D = 23g/dL
02	D = All of the Above	27	A = Iron-Containing Complex
03	B = Stem Cells	28	B = 280 Million
04	C = Both A and B	29	C = Four
05	A = Pluripotent Haemopoietic Stem Cells	30	A = Erythropoiesis
06	C = Both A and B	31	A = Red Bone Marrow
07	A = Lymphoid Stem Cells	32	C = Erythropoietin
08	B = Myeloid Stem Cells	33	B = Kidney
09	D = All of the Above	34	C = Hepatocytes
10	B = CFU-Erythrocytes	35	D = Pronormoblast
11	B = CFU-Megakaryocytes	36	A = Normoblast
12	C = 7μm	37	C = Intermediate Normoblast
13	B = 120-140 μm^2	38	B = Normoblast
14	A = Red Blood Cells	39	B = Reticulocytes
15	D = All of the Above	40	D = All of the Above
16	B = 120 Days	41	A = Cobalamin
17	D = All of the Above	42	A =Hemolysis
18	A = Haemoglobin	43	B = Spleen
19	B = Protein	44	C = Spleen
20	A = Transport of Oxygen	45	D = All of the Above
21	C = 04	46	A = Anaemia
22	B = Oxygen Binds to Haemoglobin	47	D = All of the Above
23	C = Both A and B	48	D = All of the Above
24	A = 14-18g/dL	49	A = Sickle Cell Anaemia
25	C = 12-15.5g/dL	50	D = All of the Above

Part-03

1. Anaemia may be cause due to less intake of
   - (A) Fats
   - (B) Sugar
   - (C) Iron
   - (D) Salts

2. Iron is absorbed in the
   - (A) Stomach
   - (B) Duodenum
   - (C) Pancreas
   - (D) Kidney

3. Iron absorption enhance due to
   - (A) Citric acid
   - (B) Calcium
   - (C) Vitamin C
   - (D) Carbohydrate

4. Identify the pathological condition associated with normocytic anaemia
   - (A) Sickle cell anaemia
   - (B) G6PD deficiency
   - (C) Aplastic anaemia
   - (D) All of the above

5. What are the conditions with increased erythropoietin production?
   - (A) Exogenous hypoxia
   - (B) Arterial hypertension
   - (C) Acidosis
   - (D) Polyurea

6. In which anaemia bone marrow damaged and unable to make enough red blood cells
   - (A) Pernicious anaemia
   - (B) Iron deficiency anaemia
   - (C) Aplastic anaemia
   - (D) Sickle cells anaemia

7. Anaemia caused by blood loss occur due to
   - (A) Peptic ulcers
   - (B) Use of NSAIDs drugs
   - (C) Heavy menstruation
   - (D) All of the above

8. The cells that have important function in defence and immunity
   - (A) White blood cells
   - (B) Bone cells
   - (C) Nerve cells
   - (D) Hepatic cells

9. Which of the following is largest blood cells?
   - (A) Erythrocytes
   - (B) Leucocytes
   - (C) Red blood cells
   - (D) Platelets

10. How many percentages WBCs account of blood
    - (A) 1 %
    - (B) 7 %
    - (C) 90 %
    - (D) 50 %

11. Abnormal increase in WBC count is called
    - (A) Leukopenia
    - (B) Leukocytosis
    - (C) Leukomia
    - (D) Leukaemia

12. Abnormal decrease in WBC count is called
    - (A) Leukomia
    - (B) Leukocytosis
    - (C) Leukopenia
    - (D) Leukaemia

13. Abnormal uncontrolled increase in leukocyte counts up to
    - (A) $10,00,000\,/m^3$
    - (B) $20,000\,/m^3$
    - (C) $11,000\,/m^3$
    - (D) $5,00,000\,/m^3$

14. The abnormal uncontrolled increase in leukocyte counts up to $10,00,000\,/m^3$ is termed as
    - (A) Leukopenia
    - (B) Leukopemia
    - (C) Leukaemia
    - (D) Leukocytosis

15. WBC are nucleated cells containing organelles are
    - (A) Golgi apparatus
    - (B) Mitochondria
    - (C) Centrioles
    - (D) All of the above

16. The lifespan of WBC is
    - (A) 120 – 125 days
    - (B) 30 – 40 days
    - (C) 2 – 6 days
    - (D) 60 – 70 days

17. Dead WBCs are phagocytized in
    - (A) Blood
    - (B) Liver
    - (C) Lymph nodes
    - (D) All of the above

18. Properties of WBCs is
    - (A) Diapedesis
    - (B) Chemotaxis
    - (C) Phagocytosis
    - (D) All of the above

19. The ability of WBCs to squeeze out of the capillaries to reach the area of infection is called
    - (A) Diapedesis
    - (B) Chemotaxis
    - (C) Adhere
    - (D) Cohesion

20. Diapedesis is also called
    - (A) Chemotaxis
    - (B) Adhesion
    - (C) Cohesion
    - (D) Emigration

21. Diapedesis can occur at
    (A) Paracellular
    (B) Transcellular
    (C) Both (A) and (B)
    (D) None of the above

22. Which process mainly engulf and destroy foreign substances and protect the body from disease
    (A) Pinocytosis
    (B) Phagocytosis
    (C) Facilitate diffusion
    (D) Receptor – mediated endocytosis

23. The cells in the body show phagocytosis and the cells is termed as
    (A) Phagocytes
    (B) Lipocyte
    (C) Adipocyte
    (D) Osteocyte

24. Which process is also called "cell eating"?
    (A) Pinocytosis
    (B) Phagocytosis
    (C) Receptor mediated endocytosis
    (D) Simple diffusion

25. The cells that are active in phagocytosis is
    (A) Neutrophils
    (B) Monocytes
    (C) Both (A) and (B)
    (D) None of the above

26. DLC stands for
    (A) Differential leukocyte count
    (B) Differential leukocyte content
    (C) Double leukocyte content
    (D) Double lymphocyte content

27. Which test measure the percentage of every single type of WBC present in the blood
    (A) TLC test
    (B) DLC test
    (C) HLC test
    (D) WLC test

28. Granulocytes cells are produced in the red bone marrow and the process of their formation is called
    (A) Erythropoiesis
    (B) Ossification
    (C) Granulopoiesis
    (D) Osteogenesis

29. WBCs flow through bloodstream to fight against
    (A) Viruses
    (B) Bacteria
    (C) Foreign invaders
    (D) All of the above

30. Which of the following is type of WBCs?
    - (A) Monocytes
    - (B) Neutrophils
    - (C) Basophils
    - (D) All of the above

31. Neutrophils makes up percent of white blood cells
    - (A) 30 – 35 %
    - (B) 55 – 70 %
    - (C) 10 – 20 %
    - (D) 3 – 5 %

32. The most abundant white blood cells are
    - (A) Neutrophils
    - (B) Monocytes
    - (C) Eosinophils
    - (D) Basophils

33. The diameter of neutrophils is
    - (A) 1 – 2 μm
    - (B) 2 – 2.5 μm
    - (C) 12 – 15 μm
    - (D) 30 – 40 μm

34. Which WBC cells is first line of defence is
    - (A) Neutrophils
    - (B) Eosinophils
    - (C) Monocytes
    - (D) Lymphocytes

35. Neutrophils are attracted to the site of infection mostly by
    - (A) Chemotaxis
    - (B) Adhesion
    - (C) Cohesion
    - (D) Dispersion

36. Neutrophils remove microbes by
    - (A) Pinocytosis
    - (B) Phagocytosis
    - (C) Lysocytosis
    - (D) Elliptocytosis

37. Neutrophils may increase physiologically
    - (A) After exercise
    - (B) In emotional conditions
    - (C) In later stages of pregnancy
    - (D) All of the above

38. The abnormal increase in neutrophils count in pathological condition is called
    - (A) Neutrophilic leukocytosis
    - (B) Neutrophilic leukomenia
    - (C) Neutrophilic leukopenia
    - (D) Neutrophilic leukaemia

39. When uncontrolled, excessive accumulation of activated neutrophils into tissue leads to tissue damage during hyperinflammatory disorders includes
    - (A) Acute lung injury
    - (B) Vascular inflammation
    - (C) Arthritis
    - (D) All of the above

40. Major function of eosinophils
    - (A) Elimination of parasites
    - (B) Role in allergic conditions
    - (C) Both (A) and (B)
    - (D) None of the above

41. Eosinophil's granules contain certain cytotoxic substances
    (A) Eosinophil peroxidase
    (B) Eosinophilic cationic protein
    (C) Both (A) and (B)
    (D) None of the above

42. Eosinophils contain the enzymes
    (A) Amylase
    (B) Lipase
    (C) Histaminase
    (D) Ligase

43. Histaminase enzyme breakdown the
    (A) Histamine
    (B) Prostaglandins
    (C) Serotonin
    (D) Melanin

44. The abnormal increase of eosinophils count is called
    (A) Eosinophimia
    (B) Eosinophilia
    (C) Eosinomenia
    (D) Eosinaemia

45. Eosinophilia mainly occurs in
    (A) Allergic conditions
    (B) Asthma
    (C) Blood parasitism
    (D) All of the above

46. The basophilic are the granules of
    (A) Basophils
    (B) Neutrophils
    (C) Monocytes
    (D) Eosinophils

47. Basophils ply an important role in
    (A) Inflammation
    (B) Allergic reaction
    (C) Both (A) and (B)
    (D) None of the above

48. Basophils bind to allergen and release granules that contain
    (A) Histamine
    (B) Heparin
    (C) Both (A) and (B)
    (D) None of the above

49. The abnormal increase in basophils count called
    (A) Basophilia
    (B) Eosinophilia
    (C) Neutroemia
    (D) Basophiemia

50. The condition is which abnormal increase in basophils count is
    (A) Small pox
    (B) Chicken pox
    (C) Both (A) and (B)
    (D) None of the above

Answer Key

Body Fluids and Blood, Lymphatic System (Part-03)

Question	Answer	Question	Answer
01	C = Iron	26	A = Differential Leukocytes Count
02	B = Duodenum	27	B = DLC Test
03	C = Vitamin C	28	C = Granulopoiesis
04	D = All of the Above	29	D = All of the Above
05	A = Exogenous Hypoxia	30	D = All of the Above
06	C = Aplastic Anaemia	31	B = 55 to 70 %
07	D = All of the Above	32	A = Neutrophils
08	A = White Blood Cells	33	C = 12 to 15 μm
09	B = Leukocytes	34	A = Neutrophils
10	A = 01%	35	A = Chemotaxis
11	B = Leukocytosis	36	B = Phagocytosis
12	C = Leukopenia	37	D = All of the Above
13	A = $10,00,000/m^3$	38	A = Neutrophilic Leukocytosis
14	C = Leukaemia	39	D = All of the Above
15	D = All of the Above	40	C = Both A and B
16	C = 02 to 06 Days	41	C = Both A and B
17	D = All of the Above	42	C = Histaminase
18	D = All of the Above	43	A = Histamine
19	A = Diapedesis	44	B = Eosinophilia
20	D = Emigration	45	D = All of the Above
21	C = Both A and B	46	A = Basophils
22	B = Phagocytosis	47	C = Both A and B
23	A = Phagocytes	48	C = Both A and B
24	B = Phagocytosis	49	A = Basophils
25	C = Both A and B	50	C = Both A and B f

Part-04

1. Monocytes produced in
   - (A) Liver
   - (B) Stomach
   - (C) Bone marrow
   - (D) Lungs
2. The process of formation of agranulocytes is called
   - (A) Granulopoiesis
   - (B) Agranulopoiesis
   - (C) Erythropoiesis
   - (D) Osteogenesis
3. The largest cells of the leukocyte are
   - (A) Monocytes
   - (B) Neutrophils
   - (C) Basophils
   - (D) Lymphocytes
4. The diameter of monocytes is
   - (A) $10 - 11\ \mu m$
   - (B) $1 - 2\ \mu m$
   - (C) $3 - 4\ \mu m$
   - (D) $15 - 18\ \mu m$
5. Monocytes make up the percent of volume
   - (A) 70 %
   - (B) 44 %
   - (C) 7 %
   - (D) 67 %
6. The monocyte – macrophage system is called
   - (A) Reticuloendothelial system
   - (B) Endoplasmic reticulum system
   - (C) Reticuloexothelial system
   - (D) Retinocular interstitial system
7. The abnormal increase in monocytes count is called
   - (A) Endocytosis
   - (B) Monocytosis
   - (C) Basophilia
   - (D) Monomenia
8. Causes of Monocytosis
   - (A) Bacterial infection
   - (B) Glandular fever
   - (C) Viral infection
   - (D) All of the above
9. Monocytosis occur in microbial infection are
   - (A) Tuberculosis
   - (B) Syphilis
   - (C) Malaria
   - (D) All of the above

10. Monocyte macrophage series include
    (A) Monoblast
    (B) Promonocytes
    (C) Monocyte
    (D) All of the above

11. The smallest leukocyte are
    (A) Lymphocytes
    (B) Monocytes
    (C) Neutrophils
    (D) Basophils

12. Lymphocytes circulate in the blood and are present mainly in lymphatic tissues are
    (A) Lymph node
    (B) Spleen
    (C) Both (A) and (B)
    (D) None of the above

13. The diameter of large lymphocyte is
    (A) $2 - 3\ \mu m$
    (B) $1 - 2\ \mu m$
    (C) $4 - 5\ \mu m$
    (D) $14 - 20\ \mu m$

14. The diameter of small lymphocyte is
    (A) $30 - 40\ \mu m$
    (B) $14 - 20\ \mu m$
    (C) $7 - 10\ \mu m$
    (D) $20 - 30\ \mu m$

15. Normal lymphocyte range in adult is
    (A) 1,000 – 4,800 per microliter of blood
    (B) 10,000 – 12,000 per microliter of blood
    (C) 6,000 – 7,000 per microliter of blood
    (D) 13,000 – 14,000 per microliter of blood

16. Lymphocytes make up percentage of WBC
    (A) 80 – 90 %
    (B) 20 – 30 %
    (C) 50 – 60 %
    (D) 70 – 80 %

17. Lymphocytes are classified into
    (A) B lymphocytes
    (B) T lymphocytes
    (C) Both (A) and (B)
    (D) None of the above

18. The T – cells produce by
    (A) Thymus
    (B) Adrenal gland
    (C) Pancreas
    (D) Pineal gland

19. In thymus T – cells multiply and differentiate into
    (A) Helper T – cells
    (B) Memory T – cells
    (C) Cytotoxic T – cells
    (D) All of the above

20. The helper T – cells secrete chemical messenger called
    (A) Melatonin
    (B) Cytokines
    (C) Melanin
    (D) Thyroxine
21. Which hormone stimulate the development of T – cells
    (A) Melanin
    (B) Serotonin
    (C) Thymosin
    (D) Thyroxine
22. The main role of cytotoxic T – cells is
    (A) Destruction of body cells infected by microbes
    (B) Destruction of some tumour cells
    (C) Cells of tissue transplant
    (D) All of the above
23. Function of suppressor T – cells is
    (A) Modulate the immune system
    (B) Maintain tolerance to self-antigens
    (C) Prevent autoimmune disease
    (D) All of the above
24. Function of helper T – cells is
    (A) Production of cytokines
    (B) Corporation with B – cells to produce antibodies
    (C) Both (A) and (B)
    (D) None of the above
25. The B – lymphocytes produced and mature in
    (A) Kidney
    (B) Bone marrow
    (C) Pancreas
    (D) Lungs
26. Types of B – lymphocytes are
    (A) Plasma cells
    (B) Memory B – cells
    (C) Both (A) and (B)
    (D) None of the above
27. B – lymphocytes migrate and stay in the lymphoid tissue present in the '
    (A) Lymph nodes
    (B) Spleen
    (C) Bone marrow
    (D) All of the above
28. Which cells produce antibodies
    (A) T – cells
    (B) B – cells
    (C) L – cells
    (D) D – cells

29. Immunoglobulins is also called
    (A) Antibodies
    (B) Antibiotics
    (C) Antigens
    (D) Pathogens
30. Each plasma cell produce molecules of antibodies is
    (A) 100 molecules
    (B) 2000 molecules
    (C) 10 molecules
    (D) 50 molecules
31. Which of the following is antibody?
    (A) Immunoglobulin A
    (B) Immunoglobulin D
    (C) Immunoglobulin E
    (D) All of the above
32. Which immunoglobulin found in body secretion like breast milk and saliva
    (A) Immunoglobulin D
    (B) Immunoglobulin E
    (C) Immunoglobulin A
    (D) Immunoglobulin M
33. Which immunoglobulin found in excess allergy
    (A) Immunoglobulin A
    (B) Immunoglobulin E
    (C) Immunoglobulin M
    (D) Immunoglobulin G
34. The largest, longest – lived and most common type of antibody is
    (A) Immunoglobulin G
    (B) Immunoglobulin M
    (C) Immunoglobulin A
    (D) Immunoglobulin E
35. The decrease in lymphocyte count is called
    (A) Lymphopenia
    (B) Monocytosis
    (C) Lymphocytosis
    (D) Lymphoemia
36. Causes of lymphopenia is
    (A) Patient with immunosuppressive therapy
    (B) Hypoplastic bone marrow
    (C) Acquired immunodeficiency syndrome
    (D) All of the above
37. Increase in lymphocytes count called
    (A) Monocytosis
    (B) Lymphocytosis
    (C) Lymphopenia
    (D) Lymphoemia
38. The process of development of WBCs is called
    (A) Erythropoiesis
    (B) Leukopoiesis
    (C) Thrombopoiesis
    (D) Osteogenesis
39. Leukopoiesis occurs in
    (A) Lymph nodes
    (B) Spleen
    (C) Thymus
    (D) All of the above

40. The major form of leukopoiesis is
    (A) Myelopoiesis
    (B) Lymphopoiesis
    (C) Both (A) and (B)
    (D) None of the above

41. The cells of myeloid series include
    (A) Myeloblast
    (B) Promyeloblast
    (C) Myelocytes
    (D) All of the above

42. The process of formation of lymphocytes is called
    (A) Lymphopoiesis
    (B) Erythropoiesis
    (C) Thrombopoiesis
    (D) Osteogenesis

43. The lymphocytes are formed from
    (A) Lymphocyte root cells
    (B) Lymphocyte stem cells
    (C) Lymphocyte myeloid cells
    (D) Lymphocyte adipocytes

44. Which of the following is smallest blood cells?
    (A) Platelets
    (B) Red blood cells
    (C) White blood cells
    (D) Leukocytes

45. The diameter of platelets is
    (A) $20 - 30$ μm
    (B) $15 - 20$ μm
    (C) $2 - 5$ μm
    (D) $40 - 50$ μm

46. Platelets is also called as
    (A) Erythrocytes
    (B) Leukocytes
    (C) Thrombocytes
    (D) White blood cells

47. The increase in number of platelets is called
    (A) Thrombocytosis
    (B) Thromboemia
    (C) Thrombocytopenia
    (D) Thrombopenia

48. The decrease in number of platelets is called
    (A) Thromboemia
    (B) Thrombocytosis
    (C) Thrombonia
    (D) Thrombocytopenia

49. The cytoplasm of platelets contains
    (A) Proteins
    (B) Enzymes
    (C) Hormones
    (D) All of the above

50. Lifespan of platelets is
    (A) $120 - 125$ days
    (B) $8 - 10$ days
    (C) $60 - 70$ days
    (D) $45 - 50$ days

Answer Key

Body Fluids and Blood, Lymphatic System (Part-04)

Question	Answer	Question	Answer
01	C = Bone Marrow	26	C = Both A and B
02	B = Agranulopoiesis	27	D = All of the Above
03	A = Monocytes	28	B = B-Cells
04	D = 15-18μm	29	A = Antibodies
05	C = 07 %	30	B = 2000 Molecules
06	A = Reticuloendothelial System	31	D = All of the Above
07	B = Monocytosis	32	C = Immunoglobulin A
08	D = All of the Above	33	B = Immunoglobulin E
09	D = All of the Above	34	A = Immunoglobulin G
10	D = All of the Above	35	A = Lymphopenia
11	A = Lymphocytes	36	D = All of the Above
12	C = Both A and B	37	B = Lymphocytosis
13	D = 14-20μm	38	B = Leukopoiesis
14	C = 07 to 10 μm	39	D = All of the Above
15	A = 1000-4000 per μl of Blood	40	C = Both A and b
16	B = 20-30 %	41	D = All of the Above
17	C = Both A and B	42	A = Lymphopoiesis
18	A = Thymus	43	B = Lymphocytes Stem cells
19	D = All of the Above	44	A = Platelet
20	B = Cytokines	45	C = 02 to 05 μm
21	C = Thymosin	46	C = Thrombocytes
22	D = All of the Above	47	A = Thrombocytosis
23	D = All of the Above	48	D = Thrombocytopenia
24	C = Both A and B	49	D = All of the Above
25	B = Bone Marrow	50	B = 08 to 10 Days

Part-05

1. Properties of platelets are
   - (A) Adhesiveness
   - (B) Platelet agglutination
   - (C) Both (A) and (B)
   - (D) None of the above

2. The property of platelets to get activated to the rough surface of the ruptured blood vessel is termed as
   - (A) Emigration
   - (B) Adhesiveness
   - (C) Cohesiveness
   - (D) Chemotaxis

3. The clumping together of platelets at the site of injury is called
   - (A) Platelet agglutination
   - (B) Platelet cohesiveness
   - (C) Platelet chemotaxis
   - (D) Platelet emigration

4. Function of platelets is
   - (A) Blood clotting
   - (B) Prevention of blood loss
   - (C) Repair of ruptures blood vessel
   - (D) All of the above

5. Platelets secrete
   - (A) Melatonin
   - (B) Thyroxine
   - (C) Prolactin
   - (D) Serotonin

6. Platelets secrete serotonin which cause
   - (A) Vasoconstriction
   - (B) Vasodilation
   - (C) Bronchodilation
   - (D) Nasal dilation

7. PDGF present in the cytoplasm of platelets are
   - (A) Platelet – divert growth factor
   - (B) Platelet – derived growth factor
   - (C) Platelet – divert gain factor
   - (D) Platelet – diffusion gain factor

8. The process of formation of platelets is called
   - (A) Leukopoiesis
   - (B) Erythropoiesis
   - (C) Thrombopoiesis
   - (D) Osteogenesis

9. Thrombopoiesis mainly regulated by a hormone
   - (A) Erythropoietin
   - (B) Leukopoietin
   - (C) Thrombopoietin
   - (D) Melatonin

10. Thrombopoietin hormone released by
    - (A) Liver
    - (B) Lungs
    - (C) Pancreas
    - (D) Kidney

11. A large cell found in bone marrow that is responsible for the production of platelets
    - (A) Osteocyte
    - (B) Megakaryocyte
    - (C) Osteoblast
    - (D) Osteoclast

12. Megakaryocyte are produced from stem cell in bone marrow by a process called
    - (A) Thrombopoiesis
    - (B) Erythropoiesis
    - (C) Leukopoiesis
    - (D) Osteogenesis

13. Thrombocytes are derived from
    - (A) Multipotential myeloma stem cells
    - (B) Multinucleated myoma root cells
    - (C) Multipotential myeloid stem cells
    - (D) Multinucleated myeloid stem cells

14. The sequence of reactions to prevent blood loss is referred to as
    - (A) Haemophilia
    - (B) Haemostasis
    - (C) Homeostasis
    - (D) Homogeneous

15. Stages of haemostasis is
    - (A) Vasoconstriction
    - (B) Formation of platelet plug
    - (C) Blood coagulation
    - (D) All of the above

16. The platelets first adhere to the damaged blood vessel by a process called
    - (A) Platelet cohesion
    - (B) Platelet emigration
    - (C) Platelet adhesion
    - (D) Platelet collision

17. Platelets is responsible for vasoconstriction by releasing a vasoconstrictor substance is
    - (A) Thromboxane A_2
    - (B) Thyroxine
    - (C) Thyronine
    - (D) Melatonin

18. The ADP and thromboxane A_2 attract more platelets to the site of injury, this process is called
    - (A) Platelet repeat stage
    - (B) Platelet release reaction
    - (C) Platelet retention phase
    - (D) Platelet retention stage

19. The adherent platelets clump to each other by a process called
    (A) Platelet retention
    (B) Platelet arrangement
    (C) Platelet aggregation
    (D) Platelet repetition

20. Accumulation and attachment of large numbers of platelets form a temporary seal called
    (A) Platelet plug
    (B) Platelet band
    (C) Platelet disc
    (D) Platelet coiling

21. Platelet plug formation are usually complete within
    (A) 15 minutes
    (B) 20 minutes
    (C) 25 minutes
    (D) 6 minutes

22. Major work of platelet plug is
    (A) Closes the vessel
    (B) Prevents blood loss
    (C) Both (A) and (B)
    (D) None of the above

23. The process by which liquid blood changes into semisolid blood clots called
    (A) Coagulation of blood
    (B) Emigration of blood
    (C) Aggression of blood
    (D) Cohesion of blood

24. Coagulation of blood several substances called
    (A) Adhesive factors
    (B) Clotting factors
    (C) Clotting section
    (D) Cohesion factors

25. Blood coagulation process requires
    (A) Coagulation factors
    (B) Calcium
    (C) Phospholipids
    (D) All of the above

26. Which vitamin plays an important role in blood clotting
    (A) Vitamin A
    (B) Vitamin E
    (C) Vitamin D
    (D) Vitamin K

27. Vitamin K is essential for synthesis of
    (A) Factors II
    (B) Factors VII
    (C) Factors IX
    (D) All of the above

28. Which of the following is clotting factor I
    (A) Hageman factor
    (B) Stuart – Prower factor
    (C) Labile factor
    (D) Fibrinogen

29. Which number of clotting factors is stable factor?
    (A) Factor VII
    (B) Factor IX
    (C) Factor X
    (D) Factor XII

30. Which of the following factor is clotting factor IX
    - (A) Fibrinogen
    - (B) Prothrombin
    - (C) Christmas factor
    - (D) Hageman factor

31. Which clotting factor is unassigned or missing
    - (A) Factor IX
    - (B) Factor XIII
    - (C) Factor VI
    - (D) Factor I

32. Clotting factor is made up of
    - (A) Proteins
    - (B) Steroids
    - (C) Carbohydrates
    - (D) Fats

33. Which clotting factor precursor of fibrin
    - (A) Factor III
    - (B) Factor I
    - (C) Factor V
    - (D) Factor XII

34. Which of the following is responsible for formation of clotting factor II
    - (A) Liver
    - (B) Kidney
    - (C) Pancreas
    - (D) Stomach

35. Liver is responsible for formation of clotting factors
    - (A) Factor I
    - (B) Factor II
    - (C) Factor V
    - (D) All of the above

36. Which of the following is calcium ions (Ca^{2+}) clotting factor
    - (A) Factor XIII
    - (B) Factor X
    - (C) Factor IV
    - (D) Factor IX

37. Prothrombin activator can be formed by pathways are
    - (A) Extrinsic pathways
    - (B) Intrinsic pathways
    - (C) Both (A) and (B)
    - (D) None of the above

38. Which pathway occurs rapidly when there is tissue damage outside the circulation
    - (A) Intrinsic pathway
    - (B) Extrinsic pathway
    - (C) Intracellular pathway
    - (D) Interstitial pathway

39. Which pathway triggered by damage to endothelium
    - (A) Intracellular pathway
    - (B) Extrinsic pathway
    - (C) Interstitial pathway
    - (D) Intrinsic pathway

40. Intrinsic pathway is slower and take time of
    - (A) 10 – 15 minutes
    - (B) 3 – 6 minutes
    - (C) 20 – 25 minutes
    - (D) 30 – 40 minutes

41. Extrinsic pathway named as because of tissue protein called
    (A) Thromboplastin   (B) Actin
    (C) Myosin   (D) Alanine

42. The component of blood which prevent its coagulation in the blood vessels is
    (A) Haemoglobin   (B) Plasma
    (C) Thrombin   (D) Heparin

43. Which plasma protein is involved in coagulation of blood?
    (A) Albumin   (B) Myosin
    (C) Fibrinogen   (D) Actin

44. Damaged tissue releases a complex of chemicals called
    (A) Thromboplastin   (B) Melanin
    (C) Histamine   (D) Melatonin

45. After a time, the clot shrinks because the
    (A) Platelets contract   (B) Squeezing out serum
    (C) A clear sticky fluid   (D) All of the above

46. The fibrin strands have trapped
    (A) Red blood cells   (B) White blood cells
    (C) Platelets   (D) All of the above

47. Prothrombin activates the enzyme
    (A) Thrombin   (B) Amylase
    (C) Lipase   (D) Ligase

48. Which enzyme converts inactive fibrinogen to insoluble threads of fibrin
    (A) Amylase   (B) Ligase
    (C) Thrombin   (D) Lipase

49. Platelets are removed by macrophage in
    (A) Kidney   (B) Pancreas
    (C) Lungs   (D) Spleen

50. The breakdown of fibrin is called
    (A) Fibrinolysis   (B) Mucolysis
    (C) Sacrolysis   (D) Dermolysis

Answer Key

Body Fluids and Blood, Lymphatic System (Part-05)

Question	Answer	Question	Answer
01	C = Both A and B	26	D = Vitamin K
02	B = Adhesiveness	27	D = All of the Above
03	A = Platelet Agglutination	28	D = Fibrinogen
04	D = All of the Above	29	A = Factor VII
05	D = Serotonin	30	C = Christmas Factor
06	A = Vasoconstriction	31	C = Factor VI
07	B = Platelet Derived Growth Factors	32	A = Proteins
08	C = Thrombopoiesis	33	B = Factor I
09	C = Thrombopoietin	34	A = Liver
10	D = Kidney	35	D = All of the Above
11	B = Megakaryocytes	36	C = Factor IV
12	A = Thrombopoiesis	37	C = Both A and B
13	C = Multipotential Myeloid Stem cells	38	B = Extrinsic Pathway
14	B = Haemostasis	39	D = Intrinsic Pathway
15	D = All of the Above	40	B = 03 to 06 Minutes
16	C = Platelet Adhesion	41	A = Thromboplastin
17	A = Thromboxane A_2	42	D = Heparin
18	B = Platelet Release reaction	43	C = Fibrinogen
19	C = Platelet Aggregation	44	A = Thromboplastin
20	A = Platelet Plug	45	D = All of the Above
21	D = 06 Minutes	46	D = All of the Above
22	C = Both A and B	47	A = Thrombin
23	A = Coagulation of Blood	48	C = Thrombin
24	B = Clotting Factors	49	D = Spleen
25	D = All of the Above	50	A = Fibrinolysis

Part-06

1. How many bloods group are there?
   (A) 1
   (B) 2
   (C) 3
   (D) 4

2. Who discovered the blood groups?
   (A) Alexander Fleming
   (B) Karl Landsteiner
   (C) Robert Koch
   (D) Louis Pasteur

3. How many blood types exist including positive and negative factors?
   (A) 3
   (B) 6
   (C) 8
   (D) 10

4. Which blood group is universal donor?
   (A) O group
   (B) AB group
   (C) A group
   (D) B group

5. Karl Landsteiner discovered the ABO blood group system in
   (A) 1931
   (B) 1901
   (C) 1940
   (D) 1951

6. Which blood group is universal recipient?
   (A) AB group
   (B) O group
   (C) A group
   (D) Bgroup

7. Blood having antigen A belong to
   (A) AB group
   (B) B group
   (C) A group
   (D) O group

8. Which antibody present in the serum of A blood group's blood
   (A) α antibody
   (B) β antibody
   (C) γ antibody
   (D) δ antibody

9. Blood having antigen B belong to
   (A) B group
   (B) A group
   (C) AB group
   (D) O group

10. Which antibody present in the serum of B blood group's blood
    (A) δ antibody
    (B) γ antibody
    (C) α antibody
    (D) β antibody

11. If both the antigen A and antigen B are present, then the blood group is called
    (A) A group
    (B) B group
    (C) AB group
    (D) O group

12. Which group does not contain any antibody in the serum?
    (A) B group
    (B) A group
    (C) AB group
    (D) O group

13. If both antigen A and antigen B are absent in the blood group the it is called
    (A) O group
    (B) AB group
    (C) A group
    (D) B group

14. In which group both á antibody and â antibody are present in the serum
    (A) A group
    (B) B group
    (C) AB group
    (D) O group

15. RBCs possess another antigen called
    (A) Rs factor
    (B) Rm factor
    (C) Rh factor
    (D) Rf factor

16. The Rh blood group system was discovered by
    (A) Landsteiner and wiener
    (B) Watson and crick
    (C) Singer and Nicolson
    (D) David Robertson

17. Rh factor discovered in
    (A) 1954
    (B) 1965
    (C) 1940
    (D) 1966

18. Individual having D (Rh) antigen on their RBC are designated as
    (A) Rh positive
    (B) Rh negative
    (C) Rh neutral
    (D) None of the above

19. Individual have lacking D (Rh) antigen on their RBC are designated as
    (A) Rh neutral
    (B) Rh negative
    (C) Rh positive
    (D) None of the above

20. Rh factor was first found in
    (A) Rats
    (B) Mice
    (C) Rhesus monkey
    (D) Guinea pig

21. The antigens for ABO and Rh blood group are present on
    (A) Plasma
    (B) White blood cells
    (C) Red blood cells
    (D) Platelets

22. What is the process of transfer of human blood called?
    (A) Transfusion
    (B) Transduction
    (C) Transmission
    (D) Processing

23. Which is the rarest blood group
    (A) AB negative
    (B) A positive
    (C) B positive
    (D) O positive

24. Types of blood transfusions
    (A) Red blood cell transfusions
    (B) Platelet transfusions
    (C) Plasma transfusions
    (D) All of the above

25. A person may receive a red blood cell transfusions in condition of
    (A) Blood loss
    (B) Anaemia
    (C) Both (A) and (B)
    (D) None of the above

26. A platelet transfusion can help those who have
    (A) Lower platelet count
    (B) Higher platelet count
    (C) Low RBC count
    (D) Low WBC count

27. A person may receive a plasma transfusion in condition of
    (A) Severe burn
    (B) Infections
    (C) Liver failure
    (D) All of the above

28. The abnormal increase in number of red blood cells is called
    (A) Anaemia
    (B) Polycythaemia
    (C) Polyurea
    (D) Glaucoma

29. The increase in number of red blood cells cause
    (A) Increase blood viscosity
    (B) Slows blood flow
    (C) Blood to be thicker
    (D) All of the above

30. The type of polycythaemia is
    (A) Primary polycythaemia
    (B) Secondary polycythaemia
    (C) Both (A) and (B)
    (D) None of the above

31. Causes of secondary polycythaemia include
    (A) Being at a very altitude
    (B) Certain types of tumours
    (C) Heart and lungs disease
    (D) All of the above

32. Symptoms of polycythaemia
    (A) Blurred vision
    (B) Fatigue
    (C) Excessive sweating
    (D) All of the above

33. The inherited condition in which RBCs are destroyed at a faster rate than normal
    - (A) Pernicious anaemia
    - (B) Haemolytic anaemia
    - (C) Iron deficiency anaemia
    - (D) Megaloblastic anaemia

34. Inadequate granulopoiesis may be caused by
    - (A) Irradiation of the bone marrow
    - (B) Red bone marrow disorders
    - (C) Severe infection
    - (D) All of the above

35. Which of the following is not a disorder of white blood cells?
    - (A) Leukopenia
    - (B) Leukocytosis
    - (C) Leukaemia
    - (D) Otosclerosis

36. The proliferating immature leukemic blast cells crowd out other blood cells formed in bone marrow causing
    - (A) Anaemia
    - (B) Thrombocytopenia
    - (C) Leukopenia
    - (D) All of the above

37. Causes of leukopenia is
    - (A) Ionising radiation
    - (B) Chemicals
    - (C) Genetic factors
    - (D) All of the above

38. Leukaemia symptoms include
    - (A) Frequent infection
    - (B) Shortness of breath
    - (C) Pale skin
    - (D) All of the above

39. An inherited bleeding disorder where blood doesn't clot properly
    - (A) Haemophilia
    - (B) Giantism
    - (C) Gingivitis
    - (D) Osteoporosis

40. Type of haemophilia are
    - (A) Haemophilia A
    - (B) Haemophilia B
    - (C) Both (A) and (B)
    - (D) None of the above

41. Haemophilia A is caused by reduced levels of clotting factor
    - (A) Factor I
    - (B) Factor VIII
    - (C) Factor II
    - (D) Factor III

42. Haemophilia B is caused by reduced levels of clotting factor
    - (A) Factor V
    - (B) Factor XI
    - (C) Factor IX
    - (D) Factor X

43. Which haemophilia called Christmas disease
    (A) Haemophilia A   (B) Haemophilia B
    (C) Haemophilia C   (D) Haemophilia D

44. Which haemophilia called classic haemophilia
    (A) Haemophilia C   (B) Haemophilia D
    (C) Haemophilia A   (D) Haemophilia B

45. Symptoms of haemophilia include
    (A) Blood in stool
    (B) Heavy and prolonged periods
    (C) Joint pain and swelling   (D) All of the above

46. The blood clotting in an unbroken blood vessel is called
    (A) Thrombosis   (B) Cataracts
    (C) Presbyopia   (D) Acromegaly

47. Thalassemia associated with abnormal
    (A) Lysosomal enzyme   (B) Haemoglobin
    (C) Plasmin   (D) Fibrinogen

48. Thrombosis may cause due to
    (A) Atherosclerosis   (B) Trauma
    (C) Infection   (D) All of the above

49. Reticuloendothelial system found in
    (A) Spleen   (B) Liver
    (C) Bone marrow   (D) All of the above

50. The reticuloendothelial cells located in the blood cavities of the liver are
    called
    (A) Cupper cells   (B) Kupffer cells
    (C) Bone cells   (D) Osteocytes

Answer Key

Body Fluids and Blood, Lymphatic System (Part-06)

Question	Answer	Question	Answer
01	D = 04	26	A = Lower Platelet Count
02	B = Karl Landsteiner	27	D = All of the Above
03	C = 08	28	B = Polycythaemia
04	A = O Group	29	D = All of the Above
05	B = 1901	30	C = Both A and B
06	A = AB Group	31	D = All of the Above
07	C = A Group	32	D = All of the Above
08	B = β Antibody	33	B = Haemolytic Anaemia
09	A = B Group	34	D = All of the Above
10	C = α Antibody	35	D = Otosclerosis
11	C = AB Group	36	D = All of the Above
12	C = AB Group	37	D = All of the Above
13	A = O Group	38	D = All of the Above
14	D = O Group	39	A = Haemophilia
15	C = Rh Factors	40	C = Both A and B
16	A = Landsteiner and Wiener	41	B = Factor VIII
17	C = 1940	42	C = Factor IX
18	A = Rh Positive	43	B = Haemophilia B
19	B = Rh Negative	44	C = Haemophilia A
20	C = Rhesus Monkey	45	D = All of the Above
21	C = Red Blood Cells	46	A = Thrombosis
22	A = Transformation	47	B = Haemoglobin
23	A = AB Negative	48	D = All of the Above
24	D = All of the Above	49	D = All of the Above
25	C = Both A and B	50	B = Kupffer Cells

Part-07

1. The network of vessels, nodes and duct that collect and circulate excess fluid in the body is called
   - (A) Lymphatic system
   - (B) Digestive system
   - (C) Skeletal system
   - (D) Nervous system

2. The study of lymphatic system is called
   - (A) Cardiology
   - (B) Nephrology
   - (C) Hepatology
   - (D) Lymphology

3. Lymphatic system consists of
   - (A) Lymph
   - (B) Lymph vessels
   - (C) Lymph node
   - (D) All of the above

4. Which of the following is lymph organ?
   - (A) Spleen
   - (B) Thymus
   - (C) Both (A) and (B)
   - (D) None of the above

5. The lymphatic system consist of fluid called
   - (A) Lacrimal fluid
   - (B) Lymph
   - (C) Cerebrospinal fluid
   - (D) Synovial fluid

6. Lymph consists of
   - (A) Proteins
   - (B) Water
   - (C) Lipid
   - (D) All of the above

7. How many lymph nodes throughout the body?
   - (A) $500 - 600$
   - (B) $1000 - 2000$
   - (C) $100 - 150$
   - (D) $10 - 20$

8. Function of lymphatic system
   - (A) Drainage of excessive interstitial fluid
   - (B) Immunity
   - (C) Transport of dietary fats
   - (D) All of the above

9. The lymphatic capillaries of the small intestine which absorb digested fats
   - (A) Lacteals
   - (B) Collecting duct
   - (C) Fissures
   - (D) Culcus

10. The absorbs fats and fat – soluble vitamins to form a milky fluid called
    - (A) Chyme
    - (B) Chyle
    - (C) Saliva
    - (D) Mucous

11. The body's first line of defence involves
    - (A) Physical barriers
    - (B) Toxic barriers
    - (C) "friendly" bacteria in the body
    - (D) All of the above

12. Which of the following acts as physical barrier?
    - (A) Antibacterial substances
    - (B) Mucous
    - (C) Stomach acid
    - (D) All of the above

13. The lymphatic system produces white blood cells called
    - (A) Lymphocytes
    - (B) Monocytes
    - (C) Neutrophils
    - (D) Basophils

14. The lymphatic organs are divided into
    - (A) Primary lymphatic organs
    - (B) Secondary lymphatic organs
    - (C) Both (A) and (B)
    - (D) None of the above

15. The primary lymphatic organs consist of
    - (A) Red bone marrow
    - (B) Thymus gland
    - (C) Both (A) and (B)
    - (D) None of the above

16. The secondary lymphatic organs consist of
    - (A) Spleen
    - (B) Lymph nodes
    - (C) Both (A) and (B)
    - (D) None of the above

17. Where lymphocytes are generated from immature progenitor cells
    - (A) Primary lymphatic organs
    - (B) Secondary lymphatic organs
    - (C) Tertiary lymphatic organs
    - (D) Quaternary lymphatic organs

18. Where the lymphocytes reside and positioned to mount immune responses
    - (A) Tertiary lymphatic organs
    - (B) Primary lymphatic organs
    - (C) Secondary lymphatic organs
    - (D) Quaternary lymphatic organs

19. What is the amount of fluid return by lymphatic system in each day from the tissue to the circulatory system?

    (A) 10 litres

    (B) 20 litres

    (C) 7 litres

    (D) 30 litres

20. When the lymphatic system is blocked, the human body defenceless against

    (A) Viruses

    (B) Bacteria

    (C) Fungi

    (D) All of the above

21. Lymph is a fluid connective tissue that contains

    (A) Proteins

    (B) Fats

    (C) Hormones

    (D) All of the above

22. The amount of water contains in lymph

    (A) 9 %

    (B) 14 %

    (C) 96 %

    (D) 19 %

23. The amount of protein contains in lymph

    (A) 90 – 92 %

    (B) 2 – 6 %

    (C) 70 – 80 %

    (D) 55 – 60 %

24. Which protein contain in lymph

    (A) Albumin

    (B) Globulin

    (C) Prothrombin

    (D) All of the above

25. Lymph contain electrolytes are

    (A) Calcium

    (B) Sodium

    (C) Potassium

    (D) All of the above

26. The cellular content of lymph is

    (A) Macrophages

    (B) Monocytes

    (C) Lymphocytes

    (D) All of the above

27. Lymphatic system consists of all except

    (A) Lymph

    (B) Yellow bone marrow

    (C) Lymph node

    (D) Lymph vessel

28. The amount of non – protein nitrogenous substance contains in lymph

    (A) 600 mg %

    (B) 34 mg %

    (C) 1000 mg %

    (D) 500 mg %

29. The non – protein nitrogenous substance contain in lymph are

    (A) Urea

    (B) Creatinine

    (C) Both (A) and (B)

    (D) None of the above

30. All the lymph from the body is collected into channels are
   - (A) Thoracic duct
   - (B) Right lymphatic duct
   - (C) Both (A) and (B)
   - (D) None of the above

31. Thoracic duct begins at the
   - (A) Cisterna chyli
   - (B) Compact chyli
   - (C) Crucial chyli
   - (D) Fissures chyli

32. How long the thoracic duct
   - (A) 1 – 2 cm
   - (B) 5 – 10 cm
   - (C) 38 – 45 cm
   - (D) 90 – 98 cm

33. The diameter of thoracic duct
   - (A) 20 – 25 mm
   - (B) 2 – 6 mm
   - (C) 40 – 50 mm
   - (D) 50 – 60 mm

34. Which duct open into the left subclavian vein in the root of the neck
   - (A) Thoracic duct
   - (B) Collecting duct
   - (C) Bile duct
   - (D) Cystic duct

35. The thoracic duct drains lymph from
   - (A) Legs
   - (B) Pelvic
   - (C) Abdominal cavities
   - (D) All of the above

36. The right lymphatic duct is a dilated lymph vessel about
   - (A) 20 cm long
   - (B) 1 cm long
   - (C) 30 cm long
   - (D) 15 cm long

37. Which duct lies in the root of the neck and opens into the right subclavian vein
   - (A) Right lymphatic duct
   - (B) Cystic duct
   - (C) Distal lymphatic duct
   - (D) Left lymphatic duct

38. The right lymphatic duct drains lymph from
   - (A) Right half of the thorax
   - (B) Head
   - (C) Right arm
   - (D) All of the above

39. The lymph capillaries originate as blind – ended tubes in the
   - (A) Interstitial space
   - (B) Extracellular space
   - (C) Lacrimal space
   - (D) Intracellular space

40. Lymph vessels become
   - (A) Larger as they join together
   - (B) Eventually forming two large ducts
   - (C) Both (A) and (B)
   - (D) None of the above

41. Small lymph vessel is celled
    (A) Lymph capillaries
    (B) Lymph canal
    (C) Blood vessels
    (D) Lymph conduit

42. Rate of flow of lymph highest in
    (A) Gastrointestinal tract
    (B) Liver
    (C) Both (A) and (B)
    (D) None of the above

43. Which of the following originate as closed endothelial tubes that are permeable to fluid and high – molecular weight compounds
    (A) Lymph conduits
    (B) Lymph canal
    (C) Lymph capillaries
    (D) Lymph tube

44. The lymphatic capillaries are present in most of the tissues of body except
    (A) Brain
    (B) Cartilage
    (C) Splenic pulp
    (D) All of the above

45. Avascular tissue involves
    (A) Cornea
    (B) Hairs
    (C) Nails
    (D) All of the above

46. The endothelial cells of lymph capillaries are attached to the surrounding tissues by
    (A) Anchoring filament
    (B) Transitional filament
    (C) Keratin filament
    (D) Underlying filament

47. The factors are responsible for lymph formation
    (A) Capillary pressure
    (B) Permeability of the capillary wall
    (C) Both (A) and (B)
    (D) None of the above

48. If capillary pressure is raised, the rate of lymph formation is
    (A) Increases
    (B) Decreases
    (C) No change
    (D) None of the above

49. The factors that affect the capillary permeability
    (A) Temperature
    (B) Oxygen supply
    (C) Both (A) and (B)
    (D) None of the above

50. If rise in temperature the capillary permeability will
    (A) Increases
    (B) Decreases
    (C) No change
    (D) None of the above

Answer Key

Body Fluids and Blood, Lymphatic System (Part-07)

Question	Answer	Question	Answer
01	A = Lymphatic System	26	D = All of the Above
02	D = Lymphology	27	B = Yellow Bone Marrow
03	D = All of the Above	28	B = 34 mg%
04	C = Both A and B	29	C = Both A and B
05	B = Lymph	30	C = Both A and B
06	D = All of the Above	31	A = Cisterna Chyli
07	A = 500-600	32	C = 38-45 cm
08	D = All of the Above	33	B = 2-6 mm
09	A = Lacteals	34	A = Thoracic Duct
10	B = Chyle	35	D = All of the Above
11	D = All of the Above	36	B = 1 cm long
12	D = All of the Above	37	A = Right Lymphatic Duct
13	A = Lymphocytes	38	D = All of the Above
14	C = Both A and B	39	A = Interstitial Space
15	C = Both A and B	40	C = Both A and B
16	C = Both A and B	41	A = Lymph Capillaries
17	A = Primary Lymphatic Organ	42	C = Both A and B
18	C = Secondary Lymphatic Organ	43	C = Lymph Capillaries
19	C = 07 Litre	44	D = All of the Above
20	D = All of the Above	45	D = All of the Above
21	D = All of the Above	46	A = Anchoring Filaments
22	C = 96%	47	C = Both A and B
23	B = 2-6%	48	A = Increases
24	D = All of the Above	49	C = Both A and B
25	D = All of the Above	50	A = Increases

Part-08

1. The principle lymphatic trunks of the body are
   - (A) Lumbar trunk
   - (B) Intestinal trunk
   - (C) Subclavian trunk
   - (D) All of the above

2. Lumbar trunk drains the lymph from the
   - (A) Lower limbs
   - (B) Viscera of pelvis
   - (C) Kidney
   - (D) All of the above

3. Intestinal trunk drains lymph from the
   - (A) Stomach
   - (B) Intestine
   - (C) Pancreas
   - (D) All of the above

4. Which trunk drains lymph from the thorax, lungs and heart
   - (A) Broncho mediastinal trunk
   - (B) Lumbar trunk
   - (C) Intestinal trunk
   - (D) Subclavian trunk

5. Which trunk drains lymph from upper limbs
   - (A) Lumbar trunk
   - (B) Subclavian trunk
   - (C) Intestinal trunk
   - (D) Intercoastal trunk

6. Jugular trunk drains lymph from
   - (A) Head
   - (B) Neck
   - (C) Both (A) and (B)
   - (D) None of the above

7. Which trunk drains lymph from the portions of the thorax
   - (A) Intercoastal trunk
   - (B) Lumbar trunk
   - (C) Intestinal trunk
   - (D) Broncho mediastinal trunk

8. The lymphatic capillaries join to form larger lymphatic vessels called
   - (A) Lymphatism
   - (B) Lymphonoid
   - (C) Lymphatics
   - (D) Lymphotism

9. At internals along the length of lymphatic vessels, lymph flows through
   - (A) Lymph root
   - (B) Lymph node
   - (C) Lymph band
   - (D) Lymph shoot

10. Specialized lymphatic tissue consisting of masses of
    - (A) B cells
    - (B) T cells
    - (C) Both (A) and (B)
    - (D) None of the above

11. The oval or bean – shaped organs that lie along the length of lymph vessels, often in group

  (A) Lymph shoot   (B) Lymph band

  (C) Lymph root   (D) Lymph node

12. How long is Lymph nodes

  (A) 1 – 25 mm   (B) 40 – 50 mm

  (C) 60 – 70 mm   (D) 80 -90 mm

13. The lymph drains through a number of nodes usually

  (A) 20 – 30   (B) 8 – 10

  (C) 30 – 35   (D) 40 – 50

14. Lymph nodes are scattered throughout the body, whereas large groups of lymph nodes aggregated in the

  (A) Groin   (B) Armpits

  (C) Neck   (D) All of the above

15. The main substance of the node consists of

  (A) Reticular cells   (B) Lymphatic tissue

  (C) Both (A) and (B)   (D) None of the above

16. Which cells produce the network of fibres that provide internal structure with in the lymph node

  (A) Medullar cells   (B) Reticular cells

  (C) Compact cells   (D) Schwann cells

17. Which tissue is packed with immune and defence cells in the lymph node?

  (A) Medullar tissue   (B) Schwann cells

  (C) Lymphatic tissue   (D) Lacrimal tissue

18. The lymphatic tissue is packed with immune and defence cells including

  (A) Lymphocytes   (B) Macrophages

  (C) Both (A) and (B)   (D) None of the above

19. The parenchyma of the lymph node is divided into

  (A) Cortex   (B) Paracortex

  (C) Medulla   (D) All of the above

20. The cortex of the lymph node consists of

  (A) Primary lymphatic nodules

  (B) Secondary lymphatic nodules

  (C) Both (A) and (B)

  (D) None of the above

21. The primary and secondary lymphatic nodules of the cortex of the lymph node contain aggregates of

   (A) B lymphocytes
   (B) Macrophages
   (C) Both (A) and (B)
   (D) None of the above

22. The active proliferation of the cells occurs in a particular area of the nodule called

   (A) Germinal centre
   (B) Cortical centre
   (C) Thermal centre
   (D) Crucial centre

23. The lymph node is enclosed in a capsule and has an indentation on one surface known as

   (A) Cristae
   (B) Hilum
   (C) Hyline
   (D) Matrix

24. Which of the following present in between the cortex and medulla of lymph nodes

   (A) metacortex
   (B) Paracortex
   (C) Temporal cortex
   (D) Cortical

25. Which parenchyma of the lymph node does not contain lymphatic nodule?

   (A) Cortex
   (B) Medulla
   (C) Paracortex
   (D) Compact

26. Which parenchyma of the lymph node main consist of T – lymphocytes

   (A) Medulla
   (B) Paracortex
   (C) Cortex
   (D) Compact

27. The medulla of lymph nodes contains

   (A) B lymphocytes
   (B) T lymphocytes
   (C) Macrophages
   (D) All of the above

28. The cervical lymph nodes can be divided into

   (A) Superficial cervical nodes
   (B) Deep cervical nodes
   (C) Both (A) and (B)
   (D) None of the above

29. The superficial cervical nodes are divided into

   (A) Pre – auricle nodes
   (B) Mastoid nodes
   (C) Occipital nodes
   (D) All of the above

30. Which of the following is not a superficial lymph node?

   (A) Occipital lymph node
   (B) Parotid lymph node
   (C) Coeliac lymph node
   (D) Submental lymph node

31. Which lymph node present nearest the front of the neck
    (A) Anterior cervical lymph node
    (B) Posterior cervical lymph node
    (C) Occipital lymph node
    (D) Parietal lymph node

32. Which lymph node located behind the band of the muscles on the side of the neck
    (A) Anterior cervical lymph node
    (B) Posterior cervical lymph node
    (C) Occipital lymph node
    (D) Temporal lymph node

33. Which lymph node located at the back of the neck at the base of the skull
    (A) Posterior cervical lymph node
    (B) Anterior cervical lymph node
    (C) Occipital lymph node
    (D) Temporal lymph node

34. How many lymph nodespresents in axilla?
    (A) 10 – 40
    (B) 100 – 200
    (C) 2 – 3
    (D) 80 – 90

35. Axillary lymph node located in the axilla are the chief lymph nodes draining the
    (A) Upper limbs
    (B) Skin
    (C) Muscle of chest
    (D) All of the above

36. Which lymph node lying just above the medial epicondyle of humerus
    (A) Supratrochlear lymph node
    (B) Supraclavicular lymph node
    (C) Occipital lymph node
    (D) Parietal lymph node

37. Which lymph node located just above the collarbone
    (A) Supraclavicular lymph node
    (B) Mediastinal lymph node
    (C) Occipital lymph node
    (D) Temporal lymph node

38. The lymph nodes of thorax divided into
    (A) Parietal nodes of thoracic region
    (B) Visceral sets of thoracic lymph nodes
    (C) Both (A) and (B)
    (D) None of the above

39. The parietal nodes of thoracic region which drains the thoracic wall include

    (A) Parasternal lymph nodes   (B) Intercoastal lymph nodes

    (C) Diaphragmatic lymph nodes   (D) All of the above

40. Which of the following is not lymph nodes of abdominal and pelvic region?

    (A) Coeliac lymph nodes

    (B) Common iliac lymph nodes

    (C) Internal iliac lymph nodes

    (D) Occipital lymph nodes

41. Which lymph node located reside in the centre of the chest cavity between the lungs

    (A) Supraclavicular lymph node   (B) Occipital lymph node

    (C) Parietal lymph node   (D) Mediastinal lymph node

42. Which lymph node located in the groin

    (A) Inguinal lymph node   (B) Occipital lymph node

    (C) Lacrimal lymph node   (D) Parietal lymph node

43. Which lymph node located at the back of the abdominal wall

    (A) Occipital lymph node

    (B) Temporal lymph node

    (C) Lacrimal lymph node

    (D) Retroperitoneal lymph node

44. Pelvic lymph node situated in the lower abdomen in the area that contain the

    (A) Hip bone   (B) Bladder

    (C) Rectum   (D) All of the above

45. Lymphoid follicles without a germinal centre are

    (A) Primary lymphatic follicles

    (B) Secondary lymphatic follicles

    (C) Tertiary lymphatic nodules

    (D) Quaternary lymphatic follicle

46. The nodes are covered by a capsule of dense connective tissue and have capsular extension of connective tissue called

    (A) Medullae   (B) Trabeculae

    (C) Lamillnae   (D) Tubulinae

47. Function of lymph node is
    (A) Filtration
    (B) Phagocytosis
    (C) Destruction of cancer cells
    (D) All of the above
48. The lymph node filtering the
    (A) Bacteria
    (B) Viruses
    (C) Foreign matter
    (D) All of the above
49. The function of macrophages of the lymph nodes
    (A) Destroy microorganisms
    (B) Engulf cellular debris
    (C) Engulf toxic substance
    (D) All of the above
50. The coats of lymph vessels are
    (A) Tunica intima
    (B) Tunica media
    (C) Tunica adventitia
    (D) All of the above

Answer Key

Body Fluids and Blood, Lymphatic System (Part-08)

Question	Answer	Question	Answer
01	D = All of the Above	26	B = paracortex
02	D = All of the Above	27	D = All of the Above
03	D = All of the Above	28	C = Both A and B
04	A = Broncho Mediastinal Trunk	29	D = All of the Above
05	B = Subclavian Trunk	30	C = Coeliac Lymph Node
06	C = Both A and B	31	A = Anterior Cervical Lymph Node
07	A = Intercoastal Trunk	32	B = Posterior Cervical Lymph Node
08	C = Lymphatics	33	C = Occipital Lymph Node
09	B = Lymph Node	34	A = 10-40
10	C = Both A and B	35	D = All of the Above
11	D = Lymph Node	36	A = Supratrochlear Lymph Node
12	A = 1-25 mm	37	A = Supraclavicular Lymph Node
13	B = 08-10	38	C = Both A and B
14	D = All of the Above	39	D = All of the Above
15	C = Both A and B	40	D = Occipital Lymph Nodes
16	B = Reticular Cells	41	D = Mediastinal Lymph Node
17	C = Lymphatic Tissue	42	A = Inguinal Lymph Node
18	C = Both A and B	43	D = Retroperitoneal Lymph Node
19	D = All of the Above	44	D = All of the Above
20	C = Both A and B	45	A = Primary Lymphatic Follicles
21	C = Both A and B	46	B = Trabeculae
22	A = Germinal Centre	47	D = All of the Above
23	B = Hilum	48	D = All of the Above
24	B = Paracortex	49	D = All of the Above
25	C = Paracortex	50	D = All of the Above

Part-09

1. The largest lymphatic organ in the body is
   (A) Spleen
   (B) Tonsils
   (C) Thymus
   (D) Kidney
2. The weight of spleen in adults is about
   (A) 400 gm
   (B) 500 gm
   (C) 200 gm
   (D) 1000 gm
3. Which organ located in the left hypochondrial region of the abdominal cavity between the stomach and the diaphragm
   (A) Liver
   (B) Lungs
   (C) Pancreas
   (D) Spleen
4. What a long spleen in adults
   (A) 40 cm
   (B) 10 cm
   (C) 60 cm
   (D) 50 cm
5. The parenchyma of spleen is composed of tissue are
   (A) White pulp
   (B) Red pulp
   (C) Both (A) and (B)
   (D) None of the above
6. Red pulp contains
   (A) Venous sinuses
   (B) Splenic cords
   (C) Both (A) and (B)
   (D) None of the above
7. White pulp mostly consists of immune cells are
   (A) T cells
   (B) B cells
   (C) Both (A) and (B)
   (D) None of the above
8. Function of spleen is
   (A) Immune surveillance
   (B) Proliferation and maturation of lymphocytes
   (C) Destruction of RBCs
   (D) All of the above
9. The ligaments originating from the surrounding structures attach to the spleen are
   (A) Gastrosplenic ligament
   (B) Splenorenal ligament
   (C) Phrenicocolic ligament
   (D) All of the above

10. Which connects the hilum with the greater curvature of the stomach
    (A) Splenorenal ligament
    (B) Phrenicocolic ligament
    (C) Gastrosplenic ligament
    (D) Hepatosplenic ligament

11. Which connects the hilum of the spleen with left kidney
    (A) Splenorenal ligament
    (B) Hepatosplenic ligament
    (C) Gastrosplenic ligament
    (D) Phrenicocolic ligament

12. Which ligament of spleen originates from the colon
    (A) Hepatosplenic ligament
    (B) Splenorenal ligament
    (C) Phrenicocolic ligament
    (D) Gastrosplenic ligament

13. The outer surface of spleen can be divided into
    (A) Diaphragmatic surface
    (B) Visceral surface
    (C) Both (A) and (B)
    (D) None of the above

14. Diaphragmatic surface of spleen is in contact with
    (A) Diaphragm
    (B) Ribcage
    (C) Both (A) and (B)
    (D) None of the above

15. Spleen receives most of its arterial supply from
    (A) Splenic artery
    (B) Hepatic artery
    (C) Renal artery
    (D) Gastric artery

16. Venous drainage in spleen occurs through the
    (A) Renal vein
    (B) Pulmonary vein
    (C) Splenic vein
    (D) Temporal vein

17. The splenic vein of spleen combines with the superior mesenteric vein to form
    (A) Hepatic portal vein
    (B) Pulmonary vein
    (C) Pulmonary artery
    (D) Patella vein

18. The lymphatic vessels of the spleen follow the splenic vessels and drain into the
    (A) Pancreatic splenic lymph nodes
    (B) Occipital lymph nodes
    (C) Cervical lymph nodes
    (D) Temporal lymph nodes

19. Spleen contains blood up to
    (A) 10 mL
    (B) 30 mL
    (C) 350 mL
    (D) 1000 ML

20. Which organ located medially to the spleen
    (A) Pancreas
    (B) Left kidney
    (C) Both (A) and (B)
    (D) None of the above

21. Which of the following located superiorly and posteriorly to the spleen?
    (A) Diaphragm
    (B) Kidney
    (C) Stomach
    (D) Pancreas

22. Which of the following is a bilobed organ located in the mediastinum between the sternum and the arota
    (A) Thymus gland
    (B) Thyroid gland
    (C) Adrenal gland
    (D) Pineal gland

23. The weight of thymus gland at birth is about
    (A) 10 – 15 gm
    (B) 80 – 90 gm
    (C) 70 – 80 gm
    (D) 65 – 70 gm

24. The maximum weight of thymus gland at puberty is about
    (A) 10 – 12 gm
    (B) 90 – 95 gm
    (C) 30 – 40 gm
    (D) 80 – 90 gm

25. Which organ located at the lateral of the thymus gland
    (A) Lungs
    (B) Kidney
    (C) Brain
    (D) Stomach

26. Which of the following located at the posterior of the thymus gland
    (A) Aortic arches and its branched
    (B) Branchiocepalic veins
    (C) Trachea
    (D) All of the above

27. Which organ located at the inferior of the thymus gland
    (A) Stomach
    (B) Thyroid gland
    (C) Heart
    (D) Kidney

28. The thymus consists of two lobes joined by
    (A) Areolar connective tissue
    (B) Simple squamous epithelium
    (C) Simple cuboidal epithelium
    (D) Stratified columnar epithelium

29. The lobes of thymus are enclosed by a capsule of fibrous connective tissue and the capsular extensions called
    (A) Trabeculae
    (B) Medullae
    (C) Lamillnae
    (D) Tubularae

30. Each lobule of the thymus consists of the
    (A) Outer cortex
    (B) Inner medulla
    (C) Both (A) and (B)
    (D) None of the above

31. The cortex of thymus consists of
    (A) T lymphocytes
    (B) Dendritic cells
    (C) Macrophages
    (D) All of the above

32. The medulla of thymus consists of
    (A) T cells
    (B) Epithelial cells
    (C) Dendritic cells
    (D) All of the above

33. The thymus gland have venous blood drains into
    (A) Left brachiocephalic
    (B) Internal thoracic veins
    (C) Both (A) and (B)
    (D) None of the above

34. The arterial supply to the thymus gland is mainly from the branches of
    (A) Internal thoracic arteries
    (B) Inferior thyroid arteries
    (C) Both (A) and (B)
    (D) None of the above

35. The cellular component of the thymus is
    (A) Lymphocytes
    (B) Epithelial reticular cells
    (C) Macrophages
    (D) All of the above

36. Function of tonsils are
    (A) Production of T lymphocytes
    (B) Maturation of T lymphocytes
    (C) Specification of T lymphocytes
    (D) All of the above

37. Which of the following are egg – shaped small masses of lymphoid tissue that are not enclosed by a capsule
    (A) Lymphatic nodules
    (B) Lymphatic medullar
    (C) Lymphatic tubular
    (D) Lymphatic modules

38. Lymphatic nodules are present throughout the mucous membrane that lies the
    (A) Gastrointestinal tract
    (B) Urinary tract
    (C) Respiratory tract
    (D) All of the above

39. The lymphatic nodules present in large aggregation in specific body parts include
    (A) Tonsils
    (B) Peyer's patches
    (C) Both (A) and (B)
    (D) None of the above

40. The groups of tonsils are
    (A) Adenoid tonsils
    (B) Palatine tonsils
    (C) Lingual tonsils
    (D) All of the above

41. Which tonsils located in the posterior wall of the nasopharynx
    (A) Adenoid tonsils
    (B) Palatine tonsils
    (C) Lingual tonsils
    (D) Temporal tonsils

42. The adenoid tonsils are also called
    (A) Palatine tonsils
    (B) Lingual tonsils
    (C) Pharyngeal tonsils
    (D) Temporal tonsils

43. Which tonsils located at the posterior region of the oral cavity one on either side
    (A) Lingual tonsils
    (B) Palatine tonsils
    (C) Pharyngeal tonsils
    (D) Parietal tonsils

44. Which tonsils located on the back surface of the base of the tongue
    (A) Lingual tonsils
    (B) Palatine tonsils
    (C) Adenoid tonsils
    (D) Pharyngeal tonsils

45. Which of the following aggregated lymphoid tissues located in the wall of the small intestine?
    (A) Peyer's patches
    (B) Pineal gland
    (C) Thymus gland
    (D) Adrenal gland

46. Which of the following is characterized by the inflammation of tonsils?
    (A) Arthritis
    (B) Tonsillitis
    (C) Gastritis
    (D) Neuritis

47. Which of the following characterized by enlargement of the spleen?
    (A) Splenomegaly
    (B) Presbycusis
    (C) Labyrinthitis
    (D) Otosclerosis

48. The enlargement of spleen occurs due to
    (A) Infections
    (B) Circulatory disorders
    (C) Blood disease
    (D) All of the above

49. Which of the following disease is a group of diseases that almost always present with painless enlargement of the lymph nodes throughout the body?
    (A) Hodgkin's disease
    (B) Cushing syndrome
    (C) Cholelithiasis
    (D) Cholangitis

50. Which organ is not major organ of the lymphatic system?
    (A) Lymph nodes
    (B) Thymus
    (C) Kidney
    (D) Spleen

Answer Key

Body Fluids and Blood, Lymphatic System **(Part-09)**

Question	Answer	Question	Answer
01	A = Spleen	26	D = All of the Above
02	C = 200 gm	27	C = Heart
03	D = Spleen	28	A = Areolar Connective Tissue
04	B = 10 cm	29	A = Trabeculae
05	C = Both A and B	30	C = Both A and B
06	C = Both A and B	31	D = All of the Above
07	C = Both A and B	32	D = All of the Above
08	D = All of the Above	33	C = Both A and B
09	D = All of the Above	34	C = Both A and B
10	C = Gastrosplenic Ligament	35	D = All of the Above
11	A = Splenorenal Ligament	36	D = All of the Above
12	C = Phrenicocolic Ligament	37	A = Lymphatic Nodules
13	C = Both A and B	38	D = All of the Above
14	C = Both A and B	39	C = Both A and B
15	A = Splenic Artery	40	D = All of the Above
16	C = Splenic Artery	41	A = Adenoid Tonsil
17	A = Hepatic Portal Vein	42	C = Pharyngeal Tonsil
18	A = Pancreatic splenic Lymph Nodes	43	B = Palatine Tonsil
19	C = 350 ml	44	A = Lingual Tonsil
20	C = Both A and B	45	A = Peyer's Patches
21	A = Diaphragm	46	B = Tonsilitis
22	A = Thymus Gland	47	A = Splenomegaly
23	A = 10 – 15 gm	48	D = All of the Above
24	C = 30 – 40 gm	49	A = Hodgkin's Disease
25	A = Lungs	50	C = Kidney

Notes

Unit - VII

Cardiovascular System

Part-01

1. The study of cardiovascular system is known as
   (A) Cardiology
   (B) Arthrology
   (C) Neurology
   (D) Nephrology

2. Cardiovascular system is also called as
   (A) Circulatory system
   (B) Nervous system
   (C) Digestive system
   (D) Respiratory system

3. Cardiovascular system consists of
   (A) Heart
   (B) Blood vessels
   (C) Blood
   (D) All of the above

4. Primary function of cardiovascular system is
   (A) Distribution of nutrients and oxygen to all body cells
   (B) Collection of waste products and CO_2 from different body cells
   (C) Both (A) and (B)
   (D) None of the above

5. Secondary function of cardiovascular system is
   (A) Thermoregulation
   (B) Distribution of hormones to the target tissues
   (C) Delivery of antibodies, platelets and leucocytes
   (D) All of the above

6. The pumping organ of circulatory system is
   (A) Heart
   (B) Kidney
   (C) Liver
   (D) Brain

7. The cone – shaped, hollow muscular pump designed to ensure the circulation of blood through the tissues of the body
   (A) Liver
   (B) Brain
   (C) Heart
   (D) Stomach

8. Which organ lies in the mediastinal area of thoracic cavity between the lungs
   (A) Heart
   (B) Kidney
   (C) Brain
   (D) Spleen

9. How long the heart
   (A) 40 cm
   (B) 10 cm
   (C) 50 cm
   (D) 30 cm

10. The weight of heart of women is
    (A) 225 gm
    (B) 800 gm
    (C) 400 gm
    (D) 458 gm

11. The weight of heart of men is
    (A) 450 gm
    (B) 600 gm
    (C) 310 gm
    (D) 700 gm

12. The heart pumps blood into two separate blood vessels are
    (A) The pulmonary circulation
    (B) Systemic circulation
    (C) Both (A) and (B)
    (D) None of the above

13. Which of the following located superior to the heart?
    (A) Aorta
    (B) Superior vena cava
    (C) Pulmonary artery
    (D) All of the above

14. Which of the following located anterior to the heart?
    (A) Sternum
    (B) Ribs
    (C) Intercoastal muscles
    (D) All of the above

15. The posterior surface of the heart is associated with the
    (A) Esophagus
    (B) Trachea
    (C) Inferior vena cava
    (D) All of the above

16. The heart is made up of layer of tissue are
    (A) Pericardium
    (B) Myocardium
    (C) Endocardium
    (D) All of the above

17. The outer covering of heart is
    (A) Pericardium
    (B) Endocardium
    (C) Endometrium
    (D) Myocardium

18. The pericardium is made up of layer are
    (A) Fibrous layer
    (B) Serous layer
    (C) Both (A) and (B)
    (D) None of the above

19. The outer layer of pericardium is
    (A) Serous layer
    (B) Fibrous layer
    (C) Tendon layer
    (D) Fissure layer

20. The fibrous pericardium has number of attachments to the
    (A) Diaphragm
    (B) Sternum
    (C) Vertebral column
    (D) All of the above

21. The inner layer of pericardium is
    (A) Fissure layer
    (B) Fibrous layer
    (C) Serous layer
    (D) Tendon layer

22. The outer layer of pericardium is
    (A) Tough
    (B) Inelastic
    (C) Fibrous
    (D) All of the above

23. The serous pericardium is a thin delicate membrane made up of layer are
    (A) Parietal layer
    (B) Visceral layer
    (C) Both (A) and (B)
    (D) None of the above

24. The outer layer of serous pericardium is
    (A) Parietal layer
    (B) Visceral layer
    (C) Medullar layer
    (D) Tubular layer

25. The inner layer of serous pericardium is
    (A) Medullar layer
    (B) Tubular layer
    (C) Visceral layer
    (D) Parietal layer

26. The serous pericardium is also called
    (A) Epicardium
    (B) Exocardium
    (C) Endometrium
    (D) Epimetrium

27. The pericardial fluid secreted by
    (A) Fibrous pericardium
    (B) Serous pericardium
    (C) Myometrium
    (D) Endometrium

28. The space present between the parietal and visceral layers of serous pericardium is
    (A) Pericardial cavity
    (B) Perimetrium cavity
    (C) Endometrium cavity
    (D) Endocardium cavity

29. The pericardial cavity is filled with fluid called
    (A) Cerebrospinal fluid
    (B) Pericardial fluid
    (C) Lacrimal fluid
    (D) Synovial fluid

30. The pericardium cavity contain pericardial fluid is about
    (A) 80 – 90 mL
    (B) 100 – 200 mL
    (C) 15 – 50 mL
    (D) 200 – 250 mL

31. Function of pericardial fluid
    (A) Helps to decrease friction
    (B) Allows smooth movement of the heart
    (C) Both (A) and (B)
    (D) None of the above

32. The arterial supply to the pericardium of heart through
    (A) Pericardiacophrenic artery
    (B) Bronchial artery
    (C) Superior phrenic artery
    (D) All of the above

33. The venous drainage to the pericardium of heart involves
    (A) Azygous system
    (B) Pericardiacophrenic veins
    (C) Both (A) and (B)
    (D) None of the above

34. Function of pericardium of heart is
    (A) Protect the heart
    (B) Prevents friction during heart contractions
    (C) Both (A) and (B)
    (D) None of the above

35. The inflammation of serous pericardium of heart is called
    (A) Pericarditis
    (B) Endocarditis
    (C) Endometritis
    (D) Perimetritis

36. The buildup of too much fluid between the pericardium of heart called
    (A) Pericardium effusion
    (B) Pericardium transfusion
    (C) Pericardium infusion
    (D) Pericarditis

37. Causes of pericardial effusion include
    (A) Hypothyroidism
    (B) Infections
    (C) Recent heart surgery
    (D) All of the above

38. Symptoms of pericardial effusion
    (A) Chest pain
    (B) Nausea
    (C) Shortness of breath
    (D) All of the above

39. The middle layer of wall of heart is
    (A) Myocardium
    (B) Pericardium
    (C) Epicardium
    (D) Endometrium

40. The myocardium is composed of

    (A) Epithelial tissue
    (B) Stratified epithelial tissue
    (C) Cardiac muscle tissue
    (D) Connective tissue

41. The cardiac muscle fibers are

    (A) Involuntary
    (B) Striated
    (C) Branched
    (D) All of the above

42. Which tissue found only in the heart wall

    (A) Skeletal muscle tissue
    (B) Cardiac muscle tissue
    (C) Smooth muscle tissue
    (D) Loose connective tissue

43. Which muscle fibers are cylindrical branched and usually have only one nucleus?

    (A) Skeletal muscle fibers
    (B) Cardiac muscle fibers
    (C) Smooth muscle fibers
    (D) Areolar muscle fibers

44. In which muscle tissue intercalated disc are present

    (A) Smooth muscle tissue
    (B) Cardiac muscle tissue
    (C) Skeletal muscle tissue
    (D) Areolar muscle tissue

45. The intercalated disc comprised components of

    (A) Adherents' junction
    (B) Desmosomes
    (C) Gap junction
    (D) All of the above

46. The intercellular junctions of epithelia and cardiac muscle are

    (A) Liposomes
    (B) Niosomes
    (C) Desmosomes
    (D) Liosomes

47. Which junction play an important role in impulse conduction in heart

    (A) Gap junctions
    (B) Hollow junctions
    (C) Loose junction
    (D) Empty junction

48. The ribbon – like protein structures that function as a connector and binder of cardiac muscle cells are called

    (A) Fascia adherens
    (B) Fissure adherens
    (C) Liposomes
    (D) Niosomes

49. The thickest layer of heart is

    (A) Myocardium
    (B) Myometrium
    (C) Pericardium
    (D) Endocardium

50. Which layer of heart is made up of cardiomyocytes?

    (A) Epicardium
    (B) Myocardium
    (C) Endometrium
    (D) Perimetrium

Answer Key

Cardiovascular System (Part-01)

Question	Answer	Question	Answer
01	A = Cardiology	26	A = Epicardium
02	A = Circulatory System	27	B = Serous Pericardium
03	D = All of the Above	28	A = Pericardial Cavity
04	C = Both A and B	29	B = Pericardial Fluid
05	D = All of the Above	30	C = 15-50 ml
06	A = Heart	31	C = Both A and B
07	C = Heart	32	D = All of the Above
08	A = Heart	33	C = Both A and B
09	B = 10 cm	34	C = Both A and B
10	A = 225 gm	35	A = Pericarditis
11	C = 310 gm	36	A = Pericardium Effusion
12	C = Both A and B	37	D = All of the Above
13	D = All of the Above	38	D = All of the Above
14	D = All of the Above	39	A = Myocardium
15	D = All of the Above	40	C = Cardiac Muscle Tissue
16	D = All of the Above	41	D = All of the Above
17	A = Pericardium	42	B = Cardiac Muscle Tissue
18	C = Both A and B	43	B = cardiac Muscle Fibres
19	B = Fibrous Layer	44	B = Cardiac Muscle Tissue
20	D = All of the Above	45	D = All of the Above
21	C = Serous Layer	46	C = Desmosomes
22	D = All of the Above	47	A = Gap Junction
23	C = Both A and B	48	A = Fascia Adherens
24	A = Parietal Layer	49	A = Myocardium
25	C = Visceral Layer	50	B = Myocardium

Part-02

1. The innermost layer of the heart wall
   - (A) Endocardium
   - (B) Endometrium
   - (C) Myocardium
   - (D) Pericardium
2. Which layer of heart make up the lining of the chambers and valves of the heart
   - (A) Perimetrium
   - (B) Endocardium
   - (C) Endometrium
   - (D) Myometrium
3. The inner most layer of heart serves as important function are
   - (A) Anatomic function
   - (B) Conduction system
   - (C) Both (A) and (B)
   - (D) None of the above
4. The endocardium is composed of layers are
   - (A) Endothelium
   - (B) Elastic tissue layer
   - (C) Subendocardial layer
   - (D) All of the above
5. The innermost layer of endocardium which controls the exchange of any materials between bloodstream and the heart muscles are
   - (A) Endothelium
   - (B) Perithelium
   - (C) Myothelium
   - (D) Exothelium
6. The outermost sub – layer of endometrium that serves as a connecting tissue to the cardiac muscle
   - (A) Subexometrial layer
   - (B) Subpericardial layer
   - (C) Subendocardial layer
   - (D) Submyocardial layer
7. Endocardium is comprised of
   - (A) Loose connective tissue
   - (B) Simple squamous epithelial tissue
   - (C) Both (A) and (B)
   - (D) None of the above
8. Which layer lies between and joins the endocardium and myocardium
   - (A) Subendocardial layer
   - (B) Endothelial
   - (C) Pericardium
   - (D) Perimetrium

9. How many chambers present in heart?
   - (A) One
   - (B) Two
   - (C) Three
   - (D) Four

10. The upper chamber of heart is known as
    - (A) Atrium
    - (B) Ventricle
    - (C) Fundus
    - (D) Villi

11. The lower chamber of heart is known as
    - (A) Villi
    - (B) Atrium
    - (C) Ventricle
    - (D) Fundus

12. The atrium is divided into
    - (A) Right atrium
    - (B) Left atrium
    - (C) Both (A) and (B)
    - (D) None of the above

13. The ventricle is divided into
    - (A) Right ventricle
    - (B) Left ventricle
    - (C) Both (A) and (B)
    - (D) None of the above

14. The septum between two atria is called
    - (A) Interatrial septum
    - (B) Intercoastal septum
    - (C) Intervertebral septum
    - (D) Interventricle septum

15. The septum between the ventricle is called
    - (A) Intercoastal septum
    - (B) Intervertebral septum
    - (C) Interventricular septum
    - (D) Interatrial septum

16. Each atrium has pouch – like structure on its anterior surface called
    - (A) Cisternae
    - (B) Auricle
    - (C) Fissures
    - (D) Cristae

17. The surface of heart also comprise a series of grooves called
    - (A) Sulci
    - (B) Myosin
    - (C) Chromatin
    - (D) Tetrad

18. How many atrium present in heart?
    - (A) Three
    - (B) Four
    - (C) Two
    - (D) Six

19. How many ventricles present in the heart?
    - (A) Four
    - (B) Two
    - (C) Three
    - (D) Five

20. Which atrium receives deoxygenated blood
    (A) Left ventricle
    (B) Right atrium
    (C) Left atrium
    (D) Coronary artery

21. Right atrium receives deoxygenated blood from tissues of the entire body through
    (A) Superior vena cava
    (B) Inferior vena cava
    (C) Both (A) and (B)
    (D) None of the above

22. The blood passes into right ventricle through
    (A) Right atrioventricular orifice
    (B) Left atrioventricular orifice
    (C) Intercoastal orifice
    (D) Intervertebral orifice

23. The right atrium has got the pacemaker known as
    (A) SN node
    (B) SE node
    (C) AN node
    (D) SA node

24. Which valves allow deoxygenated blood from right atrium to the right ventricle
    (A) Unicuspid valve
    (B) Tricuspid valve
    (C) Bicuspid valve
    (D) Tetracupsid valve

25. Which valve is located between the left atrium and left ventricle?
    (A) Tetracupsid valve
    (B) Tricuspid valve
    (C) Bicuspid valve
    (D) Unicuspid valve

26. Which atrium receive oxygenated blood from lungs
    (A) Left atrium
    (B) Right atrium
    (C) Right ventricle
    (D) None of the above

27. The left atrium receives oxygenated blood from the lungs through
    (A) Pulmonary artery
    (B) Pulmonary vein
    (C) Renal vein
    (D) Gastric vein

28. Which of the following passes deoxygenated blood from right ventricle to the lungs?
    (A) Pulmonary artery
    (B) Renal vein
    (C) Gastric artery
    (D) Pulmonary vein

29. The oxygenated blood passes into left ventricle through
    (A) Right atrioventricular orifice
    (B) Intercoastal orifice
    (C) Intervertebral orifice
    (D) Left atrioventricular orifice

30. How many valve present in human heart?
    (A) Six
    (B) Four
    (C) Ten
    (D) Seven

31. The valve present in heart is
    (A) Atrioventricular valves
    (B) Semilunar valve
    (C) Both (A) and (B)
    (D) None of the above

32. How many atrioventricular valves are present in heart?
    (A) One
    (B) Two
    (C) Four
    (D) Five

33. How may semilunar valves be present in heart
    (A) Five
    (B) Three
    (C) Two
    (D) Six

34. Which valves separate the atrium and the ventricle
    (A) AV valves
    (B) AN valves
    (C) AE valves
    (D) AT valves

35. Which valves consists of three flaps or cusps
    (A) Bicuspid valve
    (B) Tricuspid valve
    (C) Tetracuspid valve
    (D) Unicuspid valve

36. Which valves consists two flaps or cusps
    (A) Mitral valve
    (B) Tricuspid valve
    (C) Tetracuspid valve
    (D) Unicaspid valve

37. The cusps of AV valves are connected to tendon – like cords the
    (A) Chordate tendinae
    (B) Chordate tubular
    (C) Chordate medullae
    (D) Chordate tenoblast

38. The semilunar valves are present at the opening of
    (A) Systemic aorta
    (B) Pulmonary artery
    (C) Both (A) and (B)
    (D) None of the above

39. The pulmonary valve guards the orifice between the
    (A) Right ventricle
    (B) Pulmonary artery
    (C) Both (A) and (B)
    (D) None of the above

40. The aortic valve protects the orifice between the
    - (A) Left ventricle
    - (B) Aorta
    - (C) Both (A) and (B)
    - (D) None of the above

41. Bicuspid valve is also called
    - (A) Mitral valve
    - (B) Bilateral valve
    - (C) Lateral valve
    - (D) Temporal valve

42. The right atrium receives deoxygenated blood from all part of the body except
    - (A) Kidney
    - (B) Brain
    - (C) Lungs
    - (D) Liver

43. Right atrium receive blood through
    - (A) Superior vena cava
    - (B) Inferior vena cava
    - (C) Coronary sinus
    - (D) All of the above

44. Which vena cava is also known as anterior vena cava?
    - (A) Distal vena cava
    - (B) Superior vena cava
    - (C) Inferior vena cava
    - (D) Proximal vena cava

45. Superior vena cava returns the venous blood from
    - (A) Head
    - (B) Neck
    - (C) Arms
    - (D) All of the above

46. Which vena cava is also known as posterior vena cava?
    - (A) Inferior vena cava
    - (B) Superior vena cava
    - (C) Anterior vena cava
    - (D) Proximal vena cava

47. Inferior vena cava brings the blood from
    - (A) Legs
    - (B) Abdomen
    - (C) Both (A) and (B)
    - (D) None of the above

48. Which veins drains the blood from most of the vessels that supply to the heart
    - (A) Coronary sinus
    - (B) Nasal sinus
    - (C) Coronary fissures
    - (D) Temporal sinus

49. Which vein is the largest vein in human body?
    - (A) Superior vena cava
    - (B) Inferior vena cava
    - (C) Pulmonary vein
    - (D) Renal vein

50. Which of the following is not chamber of heart?
    - (A) Left ventricle
    - (B) Right atrium
    - (C) Left atrium
    - (D) Distal ventricle

Answer Key

Cardiovascular System (Part-02)

Question	Answer	Question	Answer
01	A = Endocardium	26	A = Left Atrium
02	B = Endocardium	27	B = Pulmonary Vein
03	C = Both A and B	28	A = Pulmonary Artery
04	D = All of the Above	29	D = Left Atrioventricular Orifice
05	A = Endothelium	30	B = Four
06	C = Subendocardial Layer	31	C = Both and B
07	C = Both A and B	32	B = Two
08	A = Subendothelial layer	33	C = Two
09	D = Four	34	A = AV Valves
10	A = Atrium	35	B = Tricuspid Valve
11	C = Ventricle	36	A = Mitral Valve
12	C = Both A and B	37	A = Chordate Tendinae
13	C = Both A and B	38	C = Both A and B
14	A = Interatrial Septum	39	C = Both A and B
15	C = Intraventricular Septum	40	C = Both A and B
16	B = Auricle	41	A = Mitral Valve
17	A = Sulci	42	C = Lungs
18	C = Two	43	D = All of the Above
19	B = Two	44	B = Superior Vena Cava
20	B = Right Atrium	45	D = All of the Above
21	C = Both A and B	46	A = Inferior Vena Cava
22	A = Right Atrioventricular Orifice	47	C = Both A and B
23	D = SA Node	48	A = Coronary Sinus
24	B = Tricuspid Valve	49	B = Inferior Vena Cava
25	C = Bicuspid Valve	50	D = Distal Vernicle

Part-03

1. The interior surface of the left atrium can be divided into
   - (A) Inflow portion
   - (B) Outflow portion
   - (C) Both (A) and (B)
   - (D) None of the above

2. The inflow portion of right ventricle can be grouped into
   - (A) Ridges
   - (B) Bridges
   - (C) Pillars
   - (D) All of the above

3. The wall of inflow portion of left ventricle are lined by
   - (A) Trabeculae carneae
   - (B) Medullae cisternae
   - (C) Tubular cristae
   - (D) Medullae cristae

4. The outflow part of left ventricle is known as
   - (A) Aortic vestibule
   - (B) Aortic fissure
   - (C) Aortic cristae
   - (D) Aortic cisternae

5. The largest artery in the body is
   - (A) Aorta
   - (B) Pulmonary artery
   - (C) Renal artery
   - (D) Facial artery

6. Aorta receives the cardiac output from
   - (A) Right atrium
   - (B) Pulmonary artery
   - (C) Left ventricle
   - (D) Right ventricle

7. Which artery of heart supplies oxygenated blood to the body
   - (A) Pulmonary artery
   - (B) Aorta
   - (C) Renal artery
   - (D) Gastric artery

8. Which of the following is section of aorta?
   - (A) Ascending artery
   - (B) Aortic arch
   - (C) Thoracic artery
   - (D) All of the above

9. The length of ascending aorta is
   - (A) 10 inches
   - (B) 20 inches
   - (C) 2 inches
   - (D) 12 inches

10. The ascending aorta arises from the
    - (A) Aortic orifice
    - (B) Ventricle orifice
    - (C) Atrium orifice
    - (D) Gastric orifice

11. The aortic arch ends at the level of
    - (A) C9 vertebrae
    - (B) T4 vertebrae
    - (C) S10 vertebrae
    - (D) L12 vertebrae

12. The aortic arch is still connected to the pulmonary trunk by the
    - (A) Ligamentum arteriosum
    - (B) Tendon arteriosum
    - (C) Cartilage arteriosum
    - (D) Collagen arteriosum

13. The major branches arising from the aortic arch are
    - (A) Brachiocephalic trunk
    - (B) Left common carotid artery
    - (C) Left subclavian artery
    - (D) All of the above

14. The first and largest branch of aortic arch
    - (A) Brachiocephalic trunk
    - (B) Branchirenal trunk
    - (C) Brachialveolar trunk
    - (D) Branchigonadal trunk

15. The left common carotid artery supplies the left side of the
    - (A) Neck
    - (B) Head
    - (C) Both (A) and (B)
    - (D) None of the above

16. Which aortic arch supplies the left upper limb
    - (A) Left subrenal artery
    - (B) Right subadrenal artery
    - (C) Left subclavian artery
    - (D) Right suprarenal artery

17. The branches of thoracic aorta are
    - (A) Bronchial arteries
    - (B) Mediastinal arteries
    - (C) Oesophageal arteries
    - (D) All of the above

18. The mediastinal is small arteries that supply the
    - (A) Lymph glands
    - (B) Loose areolar tissue
    - (C) Both (A) and (B)
    - (D) None of the above

19. The branch of abdominal aorta is
    - (A) Inferior phrenic arteries
    - (B) Renal arteries
    - (C) Gonadal arteries
    - (D) All of the above

20. The median sacral artery supplies the
    - (A) Coccyx
    - (B) Lumbar vertebrae
    - (C) Sacrum
    - (D) All of the above

21. Which arteries supply the kidney
    - (A) Renal arteries
    - (B) Gonadal arteries
    - (C) Lumbar arteries
    - (D) Inferior phrenic arteries

22. Coeliac artery supplies the
    (A) Liver
    (B) Stomach
    (C) Spleen
    (D) All of the above

23. Middle suprarenal arteries supply the
    (A) Pineal gland
    (B) Thyroid gland
    (C) Adrenal gland
    (D) Thymus gland

24. The branches of subclavian artery supplying the head and neck area are
    (A) Vertebral arteries
    (B) Thyrocervical arteries
    (C) Costocervical arteries
    (D) All of the above

25. Which arteries supplies the parathyroid gland, larynx, trachea, oesophagus and pharynx
    (A) Thyrocervical arteries
    (B) Renal arteries
    (C) Gonadal arteries
    (D) Suprarenal arteries

26. The branch of external carotid artery is
    (A) Lingual artery
    (B) Facial artery
    (C) Occipital artery
    (D) All of the above

27. Facial artery supplies the
    (A) Lips
    (B) Nose
    (C) Palate
    (D) All of the above

28. Which artery passes behind the ear
    (A) Gonadal artery
    (B) Occipital artery
    (C) Maxillary artery
    (D) Renal artery

29. Maxillary artery supplies the
    (A) Teeth
    (B) Gums
    (C) Cheeks
    (D) All of the above

30. The branches of internal carotid artery
    (A) Ophthalmic artery
    (B) Choroidal artery
    (C) Anterior cerebral artery
    (D) All of the above

31. The largest branch of internal carotid artery is
    (A) Occipital artery
    (B) Facial artery
    (C) Middle cerebral artery
    (D) Lingual artery

32. The smallest terminal branch of internal carotid artery is
    (A) Facial artery
    (B) Anterior cerebral artery
    (C) Renal artery
    (D) Facial artery

33. Which of the following is arteries of foramen?
    (A) Radial artery
    (B) Ulnar artery
    (C) Both (A) and (B)
    (D) None of the above
34. Which artery run from the elbow to the wrist
    (A) Ulnar artery
    (B) Renal artery
    (C) Facial artery
    (D) Lingual artery
35. Which of the following is arch of palmar arches?
    (A) Superficial palmar arch
    (B) Deep palmar arch
    (C) Both (A) and (B)
    (D) None of the above
36. The anterior abdominal wall is primarily supplied by branches of
    (A) Internal thoracic artery
    (B) External iliac arteries
    (C) Both (A) and (B)
    (D) None of the above
37. Which of the following is not a branch of abdominal viscera?
    (A) Celiac artery
    (B) Facial artery
    (C) Renal arteries
    (D) Suprarenal arteries
38. The arteries in popliteal fossa and leg are
    (A) Popliteal artery
    (B) Anterior tibial artery
    (C) Posterior tibial artery
    (D) All of the above
39. The venous blood drained from the head and neck area reaches the superior vena cava through the veins are
    (A) External jugular vein
    (B) Internal jugular vein
    (C) Both (A) and (B)
    (D) None of the above
40. Which vein is formed in the neck at the level of angle of jaw by the union of superficial veins of the scalp?
    (A) External jugular vein
    (B) Gonadal vein
    (C) Renal vein
    (D) Tibial vein
41. The tributaries of internal jugular vein are
    (A) Facial vein
    (B) Intracranial venous sinuses
    (C) Superior sagittal sinus
    (D) All of the above
42. The main superficial vein is
    (A) Cephalic vein
    (B) Basilic vein
    (C) Medial vein
    (D) All of the above

43. Which vein runs upwards from the hand to shoulder in the lateral side of the arm
    (A) Cephalic vein
    (B) Renal vein
    (C) Thoracic vein
    (D) Gonadal vein

44. Deep vein of upper limb is present in
    (A) Hands
    (B) Forearm
    (C) Upper arm
    (D) All of the above

45. Which vein is formed by the union of ulnar and redial veins just above the elbow
    (A) Renal veins
    (B) Brachial veins
    (C) Gonadal veins
    (D) Tibial veins

46. The vein of the two sides join to form the superior vena cava which opens in the right atrium of the heart
    (A) Brachiocephalic veins
    (B) Gonadal veins
    (C) Renal veins
    (D) Tibial vein

47. The veins draining blood from the thorax include
    (A) Internal thoracic vein
    (B) Intercoastal veins
    (C) Lumbar veins
    (D) All of the above

48. Most of the blood from the right side of thoracic cavity and abdominal wall is drained by
    (A) Renal veins
    (B) Azygos veins
    (C) Suprarenal veins
    (D) Facial veins

49. The tributaries of azygos vein include
    (A) Posterior intercoastal veins
    (B) Ascending lumbar veins
    (C) Both (A) and (B)
    (D) None of the above

50. Most of the blood from the left side of thoracic cavity and abdominal wall is drained by
    (A) Hemiazygos vein
    (B) Renal vein
    (C) Lingual vein
    (D) Occipital vein

Answer Key

Cardiovascular System (Part-03)

Question	Answer	Question	Answer
01	C = Both A and B	26	D = All of the Above
02	D = All of the Above	27	D = All of the Above
03	A = Trabeculae Carneae	28	B = Occipital Artery
04	A = Aortic Vestibule	29	D = All of the Above
05	A = Aorta	30	D = All of the Above
06	C = Left Ventricle	31	C = Middle Cerebral Artery
07	B = Aorta	32	B = Anterior Cerebral Artery
08	D = All of the Above	33	C = Both A and B
09	C = 2 inch	34	A = Ulnar Artery
10	A = Aortic Orifice	35	C = Both A and B
11	B = T_4 Vertebrae	36	C = Both A and B
12	A = Ligamentum Arteriosum	37	B = Facial Artery
13	D = All of the Above	38	D = All of the Above
14	A = Brachiocephalic Trunk	39	C = Both A and B
15	C = Both A and B	40	A = External Jugular Vein
16	C = Left Subclavian Artery	41	D = All of the Above
17	D = All of the Above	42	D = All of the Above
18	C = Both A and B	43	A = Cephalic Vein
19	D = All of the Above	44	D = All of the Above
20	D = All of the Above	45	B = Brachial Veins
21	A = Renal Arteries	46	A = Brachiocephalic Veins
22	D = All of the Above	47	D = All of the Above
23	C = Adrenal Gland	48	B = Azygos Veins
24	D = All of the Above	49	C = Both A and B
25	A = Thyrocervical Arteries	50	A = Hemiazygos Vein

Part-04

1. Which veins opens into the inferior vena cava?
   (A) Renal vein
   (B) Lumbar vein
   (C) Phrenic vein
   (D) All of the above

2. The inferior vena cava is the major venous trunk collecting the deoxygenated blood from
   (A) Abdominal viscera
   (B) Pelvic viscera
   (C) Both (A) and (B)
   (D) None of the above

3. In portal circulation the portal vein passes to the
   (A) Liver
   (B) Kidney
   (C) Lungs
   (D) Brain

4. The tributaries of portal vein include
   (A) Superior mesenteric vein
   (B) Splenic vein
   (C) Gastric vein
   (D) All of the above

5. Superior mesenteric vein drains blood from
   (A) Small intestine
   (B) Ascending colon
   (C) Transverse colon
   (D) All of the above

6. Splenic vein drains blood from
   (A) Spleen
   (B) Pancreas
   (C) Part of stomach
   (D) All of the above

7. Which vein drains blood from the descending colon, sigmoid colon and rectum
   (A) Inferior mesenteric vein
   (B) Facial vein
   (C) Tibial vein
   (D) Occipital vein

8. The gastric vein drain blood from
   (A) Stomach
   (B) Distal end of oesophagus
   (C) Both (A) and (B)
   (D) None of the above

9. The vein drain blood from gallbladder and join the portal vein
   (A) Facial vein
   (B) Occipital vein
   (C) Cystic vein
   (D) Tibial vein

10. The vein draining blood from different structures of the lower limbs are arranged in groups
    (A) Superficial veins of lower limb
    (B) Deep veins of the lower limb
    (C) Both (A) and (B)
    (D) None of the above

11. The superficial veins of lower vein drain into
    (A) Small saphenous vein
    (B) Great saphenous vein
    (C) Both (A) and (B)
    (D) None of the above

12. Deep veins of the lower limb include
    (A) Anterior and posterior tibial veins
    (B) Popliteal vein
    (C) Femoral vein
    (D) All of the above

13. The blood is supplied to the heart by
    (A) Coronary arteries
    (B) Pulmonary arteries
    (C) Renal arteries
    (D) Temporal arteries

14. How many coronary arteries are there?
    (A) Two
    (B) Ten
    (C) Six
    (D) Eight

15. The coronary arteries are divided into
    (A) Right coronary artery
    (B) Left coronary artery
    (C) Both (A) and (B)
    (D) None of the above

16. Right coronary artery supplies blood to the
    (A) Right ventricle
    (B) Right atrium
    (C) Posterior part of left ventricle
    (D) All of the above

17. Left coronary artery supplies blood to the
    (A) Anterior part of left ventricle
    (B) Left atrium
    (C) Anterior part of the interventricular septum
    (D) All of the above

18. How long the coronary sinus
    (A) 10 cm
    (B) 2 cm
    (C) 20 cm
    (D) 12 cm

19. Coronary sinus drains most of the venous blood from the
    (A) Endometrium
    (B) Myometrium
    (C) Myocardium
    (D) Perimetrium

20. The tributaries of coronary sinus are
    (A) Great cardiac vein
    (B) Small cardiac vein
    (C) Oblique vein of left ventricle
    (D) All of the above

21. Anterior cardiac vein draining venous blood mainly from
    (A) Left atrium
    (B) Pulmonary vein
    (C) Right ventricle
    (D) Pulmonary artery

22. The vessels which carry the blood away from the heart are
    (A) Arteries
    (B) Arterioles
    (C) Both (A) and (B)
    (D) None of the above

23. The layer of blood vessels is
    (A) Tunica interna
    (B) Tunica media
    (C) Tunica externa
    (D) All of the above

24. The innermost layer of blood vessel is
    (A) Tunica interna
    (B) Tunica externa
    (C) Tunica media
    (D) Tunica medulla

25. Tunica interna composed of
    (A) Endothelium
    (B) Basement membrane
    (C) Elastic layer
    (D) All of the above

26. The endothelium layer of blood vessel is composed of
    (A) Cuboidal epithelium
    (B) Squamous epithelium
    (C) Columnar epithelium
    (D) Loose connective tissue

27. The middle layer of blood vessel is
    (A) Tunica externa
    (B) Tunica interna
    (C) Tunica media
    (D) Tunica medullar

28. Tunica media is composed of
    (A) Smooth muscles
    (B) Elastic fibres
    (C) Both (A) and (B)
    (D) None of the above

29. The outer covering of blood vessels is
    (A) Tunica externa
    (B) Tunica medullar
    (C) Tunica interna
    (D) Tunica media

30. Tunica externa consists of
    (A) Squamous epithelium
    (B) Loose connective tissue
    (C) Cuboidal epithelium
    (D) Columnar epithelium

31. Tunica interna is also called
   (A) Tunica intima
   (B) Tunica externa
   (C) Tunica media
   (D) Tunica adventitia

32. Tunica externa is also called
   (A) Tunica intima
   (B) Tunica media
   (C) Tunica adventitia
   (D) Tunica interna

33. Types of arteries are
   (A) Elastic arteries
   (B) Muscular arteries
   (C) Small arteries
   (D) All of the above

34. Example of elastic arteries
   (A) Aorta
   (B) Pulmonary trunk
   (C) Subclavian artery
   (D) All of the above

35. Largest diameter arteries are
   (A) Elastic arteries
   (B) Small arteries
   (C) Continuous capillaries
   (D) Discontinuous capillaries

36. Example of muscular arteries
   (A) Brachial artery
   (B) Femoral artery
   (C) Both (A) and (B)
   (D) None of the above

37. Diameter of small arteries
   (A) 15 – 300 micrometres
   (B) 600 – 700 micrometres
   (C) 900 – 1000 micrometre
   (D) 1200 – 1500 micrometre

38. Functional unit of cardiovascular system
   (A) Arteries
   (B) Veins
   (C) Capillaries
   (D) None of the above

39. Size of capillaries is
   (A) 8 – 10 micrometres
   (B) 50 – 60 micrometres
   (C) 100 – 200 micrometres
   (D) 300 – 400 micrometres

40. Capillaries exist in clusters called
   (A) Capillary bands
   (B) Capillary beds
   (C) Capillary roots
   (D) Capillary sacs

41. Each capillary bed is supplied by
   (A) Orthoarteriole
   (B) Par arteriole
   (C) Metarteriole
   (D) Periarteriole

42. Types of capillaries are
    (A) Continuous capillaries
    (B) Fenestrated capillaries
    (C) Discontinuous capillaries
    (D) All of the above

43. The most abundant capillaries are
    (A) Continuous capillaries
    (B) Fenestrated capillaries
    (C) Discontinuous capillaries
    (D) Fascicles capillaries

44. The continuous capillaries found in
    (A) Brain
    (B) Muscle tissue
    (C) Skin
    (D) All of the above

45. The size of small pores of fenestrated capillaries
    (A) 200 – 300 nm
    (B) 70 – 100 nm
    (C) 500 – 600 nm
    (D) 800 – 900 nm

46. The fenestrated capillaries found in
    (A) Kidneys
    (B) Intestine
    (C) Endocrine glands
    (D) All of the above

47. The discontinuous capillaries are found in
    (A) Spleen
    (B) Liver
    (C) Bone marrow
    (D) All of the above

48. Blood vessels help in transportation of
    (A) Nutrition
    (B) Water mineral
    (C) Hormone
    (D) All of the above

49. In portal circulation which vein passes to the liver via the portal vein
    (A) Splenic vein
    (B) Mesenteric vein
    (C) Gastric vein
    (D) All of the above

50. How long the portal vein
    (A) 20 cm
    (B) 30 cm
    (C) 8 cm
    (D) 60 cm

Answer Key

Cardiovascular System (Part-04)

Question	Answer	Question	Answer
01	D = All of the Above	26	B = Squamous Epithelium
02	C = Both A and B	27	C = Tunica Media
03	A = Liver	28	C = Both A and B
04	D = All of the Above	29	A = Tunica Externa
05	D = All of the Above	30	B = Loose Connective Tissue
06	D = All of the Above	31	A = Tunica Intima
07	A = Inferior Mesenteric Vein	32	C = Tunica Adventitia
08	C = Both A and B	33	D = All of the Above
09	C = Cystic Vein	34	D = All of the Above
10	C = Both A and B	35	A = Elastic Arteries
11	C = Both A and b	36	C = Both A and B
12	D = All of the Above	37	A = 15-300 mm
13	A = Coronary Arteries	38	C = Capillaries
14	A = Two	39	A = 08-10 mm
15	C = Both A and B	40	B = Capillary Beds
16	D = All of the Above	41	C = Metarterioles
17	D = All of the Above	42	D = All of the Above
18	B = 2 cm	43	A = Continuous Capillaries
19	C = Myocardium	44	D = All of the Above
20	D = All of the Above	45	B = 70-100 nm
21	C = Right ventricle	46	D = All of the Above
22	C = Both A and B	47	D = All of the Above
23	D = All of the Above	48	D = All of the Above
24	A = Tunica Interna	49	D = All of the Above
25	D = All of the Above	50	C = 08 cm

Part-05

1. In portal circulation, venous blood first travel to the from the capillary beds of the abdominal part of the
   - (A) Digestive system
   - (B) Spleen
   - (C) Pancreas
   - (D) All of the above

2. The circulation of blood from the right ventricle of heart to the lungs and returning back of blood to the left atrium of the heart called
   - (A) Renal circulation
   - (B) Gastric circulation
   - (C) Pulmonary circulation
   - (D) Splenic circulation

3. The valve of heart that lies between the right ventricle and the pulmonary artery
   - (A) Renal valve
   - (B) Pulmonic valve
   - (C) Gastric valve
   - (D) Pancreatic valve

4. The temporary structure that provides an interface between mother and fetus
   - (A) Placenta
   - (B) Fascicles
   - (C) Globules
   - (D) Channels

5. The mature placenta is pancake – shaped and weight is about
   - (A) 1500 mg
   - (B) 500 mg
   - (C) 2000 mg
   - (D) 3000 mg

6. The diameter of mature placenta is
   - (A) 40 cm
   - (B) 60 cm
   - (C) 20 cm
   - (D) 70 cm

7. Branches of the uterine artery bring maternal blood about
   - (A) 500 mL/min
   - (B) 1000 mL/min
   - (C) 2000 mL/min
   - (D) 1500 mL/min

8. Branches of the uterine artery bring maternal blood into chambers in the placenta called
   - (A) Intravenous spaces
   - (B) Intramuscular spaces
   - (C) Intervillous spaces
   - (D) Interstitial spaces

9. The placenta attached to the fetus by a
   - (A) Umbilical cord
   - (B) Spinal cord
   - (C) Fascicle cord
   - (D) Tubular cord

10. How long the umbilical cord
   - (A) 100 cm
   - (B) 5 cm
   - (C) 50 cm
   - (D) 10 cm

11. How many umbilical arteries contain in umbilical cord?
   - (A) Four
   - (B) Two
   - (C) Six
   - (D) Seven

12. The cord enters the fetus at a spot on the abdomen called the
   - (A) Umbilicus
   - (B) Fascicle
   - (C) Cisternae
   - (D) Crista

13. Any agent that causes an abnormality in fetus is called
   - (A) Teratogen
   - (B) Carcinogen
   - (C) Pathogen
   - (D) Histogen

14. The teratogens include
   - (A) Alcohol
   - (B) Tobacco
   - (C) Some drugs
   - (D) All of the above

15. Which of the following is teratogenic drug?
   - (A) Benazepril
   - (B) Captopril
   - (C) Ramipril
   - (D) All of the above

16. The unique modification in the Fetal circulation includes special structure like
   - (A) Placenta
   - (B) Umbilical arteries
   - (C) Umbilical vein
   - (D) All of the above

17. Fetal blood is oxygenated by
   - (A) Fetal lungs
   - (B) Fetal liver
   - (C) Placenta
   - (D) Inferior vena cava

18. The placental function includes
   - (A) Exchange of substances
   - (B) Protection of the fetus
   - (C) Maintenance of pregnancy
   - (D) All of the above

19. The deoxygenated blood in fetus returns to the placenta via
   - (A) Renal veins
   - (B) Umbilical arteries
   - (C) Uterine arteries
   - (D) Gastric veins

20. Which of the following returns the oxygenated blood back to the fetus?
    (A) Umbilical vein
    (B) Umbilical arteries
    (C) Uterine arteries
    (D) Renal arteries

21. The branch of umbilical vein that drains most of the oxygenated blood into the inferior vena cava
    (A) Ductus arteriosus
    (B) Ductus venosus
    (C) Fascicle venous
    (D) Fascicle arteries

22. The small opening present in the septum between the right and left atria
    (A) Foramen ovale
    (B) Foramen magnum
    (C) Vertebral foramen
    (D) Foramen rotundum

23. The small vessel that connects the pulmonary artery with the aorta
    (A) Tibial artery
    (B) Ductus arteriosus
    (C) Renal artery
    (D) Facial artery

24. Which hormone secreted in early pregnancy?
    (A) HCG
    (B) Prolactin
    (C) Oxytocin
    (D) Growth hormone

25. Which organ possess the property of auto rhythmicity?
    (A) Liver
    (B) Kidney
    (C) Heart
    (D) Lungs

26. The source of electrical activity is a network of specialized cardiac muscle fibres called
    (A) Autorhythmic fibres
    (B) Collagen fibres
    (C) Elastic fibres
    (D) Projection fibres

27. How many percentages of cardiac muscle fibres become autorhythmic fibres during development of the embryo?
    (A) 10 %
    (B) 1 %
    (C) 30 %
    (D) 40 %

28. The intrinsic system is also called
    (A) Cardiac conduction system
    (B) Hepatic portal system
    (C) Reticuloendothelial system
    (D) Renin angiotensin aldosterone system

29. Functions of autorhythmic system
    (A) Initiate and conduct the impulse
    (B) Contraction of the heart
    (C) Both (A) and (B)
    (D) None of the above

30. Types of cells that control heartbeat
   (A) Conducting cells
   (B) Muscle cells
   (C) Both (A) and (B)
   (D) None of the above

31. Which cells carry the electric signals?
   (A) Muscle cells
   (B) Conducting cells
   (C) Mast cells
   (D) Bone cells

32. Cardiac conduction system contains specialized cells and nodes that control the heartbeat
   (A) Sinoatrial node
   (B) Atrioventricular node
   (C) Bundle of His
   (D) All of the above

33. The small mass of specialised cells that lies in the wall of the right atrium near the opening of the superior vena cava
   (A) Sinoatrial node
   (B) Bundle of His
   (C) Purkinje fibres
   (D) Collagen fibres

34. Which of the following is called pacemaker?
   (A) SA node
   (B) AV node
   (C) Purkinje fibres
   (D) Bundle of His

35. Which cells generates the electric impulses
   (A) AV node
   (B) SA node
   (C) SN node
   (D) SV node

36. SA node has dimensions up to
   (A) 25 mm
   (B) 100 mm
   (C) 120 mm
   (D) 200 mm

37. The SA node receives its blood supply from the sinoatrial nodal branch of
   (A) Renal artery
   (B) Coronary artery
   (C) Gastric artery
   (D) Tibial artery

38. The internodal conduction pathways are a part of the intra – atrial conduction network initially described by
   (A) Thomas N. James
   (B) Robert Koch
   (C) Alexander Fleming
   (D) Robert Hooke

39. The internodal conduction pathway is divided into
   (A) Anterior branches
   (B) Middle branches
   (C) Posterior branches
   (D) All of the above

40. The band of specialized muscle fibres that run from SA node to left atrium
   (A) Interatrial tract
   (B) Interventricular tract
   (C) Interstitial tract
   (D) Intracellular tract

41. The internodal conduction paths which connect SA node to AV node include

    (A) Anterior internodal pathway of Bachman

    (B) Middle internodal pathway of Wenckebach

    (C) Posterior internodal pathway of Thorel

    (D) All of the above

42. The rate of production of rhythmic impulses by SA node

    (A) 20 – 30 per minute   (B) 70 – 80 per minute

    (C) 30 – 40 per minute   (D) 50 – 55 per minute

43. The impulses from the SA node arrives at the AV node about

    (A) 0.1 sec   (B) 1 sec

    (C) 2 sec   (D) 0.9 sec

44. The small mass of neuromuscular tissue that is situated in the wall of the atrial septum near the atrioventricular valve

    (A) AN node   (B) AV node

    (C) SV node   (D) SN node

45. The impulse that was initiated by the SA node reaches the

    (A) AV node   (B) AN node

    (C) AT node   (D) SN node

46. The rate of production of rhythmic impulses by AV node is

    (A) 20 – 25 per min   (B) 10 – 15 per min

    (C) 40 – 60 per min   (D) 10 – 20 per min

47. The AV node receives its arterial blood supply from

    (A) Atrioventricular nodal artery   (B) Renal artery

    (C) Facial artery   (D) Anterior tibial artery

48. The atrioventricular node delays impulses for

    (A) 2 sec   (B) 0.1 sec

    (C) 0.9 sec   (D) 1 sec

49. The AV node stimulated by the excitation wave that travels through

    (A) Internodal tracts   (B) Atrial myocardium

    (C) Both (A) and (B)   (D) None of the above

50. What does systemic circulation provide tissues?

    (A) Nutrient   (B) Oxygen

    (C) Water   (D) All of the above

Answer Key

Cardiovascular System (Part-05)

Question	Answer	Question	Answer
01	D = All of the Above	26	A = Autorhythmic Fibres
02	C = Pulmonary Circulation	27	B = 1%
03	B = Pulmonic Valve	28	A = cardiac Conduction System
04	A = Placenta	29	C = Both A and B
05	B = 500 mg	30	C = Both A and B
06	C = 20 cm	31	B = Conducting Cells
07	A = 500ml/min	32	D = All of the Above
08	C = Intervillous Spaces	33	A = Sinoatrial Node
09	A = Umbilical Cord	34	A = SA Node
10	C = 50 cm	35	B = SA Node
11	B = Two	36	A = 25 mm
12	A = Umbilicus	37	B = Coronary Artery
13	A = Teratogen	38	A = Thomas N James
14	D = All of the Above	39	D = All of the Above
15	D = All of the Above	40	A = Intraarterial Tract
16	D = All of the above	41	D = All of the Above
17	C = Placenta	42	B = 70-80 per Minute
18	D = All of the Above	43	A = 0.1 sec
19	B = Umbilical Arteries	44	B = AV Node
20	A = Umbilical Vein	45	A = AV Node
21	B = Ductus Venosus	46	C = 40-60 per min
22	A = Foramen Ovale	47	A = Atrioventricular Nodal Artery
23	B = Ductus Arteriosus	48	B = 0.1 Sec
24	A = HCH	49	C = Both A and B
25	C = Heart	50	D = All of the Above

Part-06

1. From the AV node, the impulse enters the
   - (A) Atrioventricular bundle
   - (B) Intercoastal bundle
   - (C) Intervertebral bundle
   - (D) Interstitial bundle

2. The atrioventricular bundle is also called
   - (A) Bundle of His
   - (B) Fascicle bundle
   - (C) Bundle of bone
   - (D) Bundle of lamina

3. The mass of specialized fibres that originate from the AV node
   - (A) AN bundle
   - (B) AV bundle
   - (C) AE bundle
   - (D) Lamina bundle

4. The only site where impulses can be conducted from atria to the ventricle
   - (A) AV bundle
   - (B) Lamina bundle
   - (C) Bone bundle
   - (D) SV bundle

5. The AV bundle branches and continues down towards both side of the eptum as
   - (A) Right bundle branches
   - (B) Left bundle branches
   - (C) Both (A) and (B)
   - (D) None of the above

6. The right and left bundle branches further break up into fine fibres called
   - (A) Myosin fibres
   - (B) Purkinje fibres
   - (C) Collagen fibres
   - (D) Tendon fibres

7. Which of the following spread out deep to the endocardium and reach all parts of the ventricles, including the bas of papillary muscles?
   - (A) Collagen fibres
   - (B) Sharpey's fibres
   - (C) Purkinje fibres
   - (D) Myosin fibres

8. Both SA node and AV node are richly supplied by
   - (A) Sympathetic nervous system
   - (B) Parasympathetic nervous system
   - (C) Both (A) and (B)
   - (D) None of the above

9. Parasympathetic fibres of heart come from
   (A) Vagus nerve
   (B) Olfactory nerve
   (C) Auditory nerve
   (D) Optic nerve

10. SA node is supplied by
   (A) Auditory nerve
   (B) Right vagus nerve
   (C) Optic nerve
   (D) Accessory nerve

11. AV node is supplied by
   (A) Accessory nerve
   (B) Auditory nerve
   (C) Optic neve
   (D) Left vagus nerve

12. The main factors affecting heart rate
   (A) Autonomic activity
   (B) Circulating hormone
   (C) Activity and exercise
   (D) All of the above

13. The main forces drive ions across cell membranes
   (A) Chemical potential
   (B) Electrical potential
   (C) Both (A) and (B)
   (D) None of the above

14. The electrical activity that takes place in the cardiac muscle is called
   (A) Action potential
   (B) Action kinetics
   (C) Action mechanism
   (D) Action direction

15. The resting potential in a cardiomyocyte is
   (A) -30 mV
   (B) -10 mV
   (C) $+10$ mV
   (D) -90 mV

16. In which phase both voltage – gated sodium and voltage – gated potassium ions channels are closed
   (A) Depolarization
   (B) Repolarization
   (C) Hyperpolarization
   (D) Resting potential

17. Duration of action potential in cardiac cycle is
   (A) $1.23 - 1.30$ sec
   (B) $0.25 - 0.35$ sec
   (C) $1.30 - 1.33$ sec
   (D) $0.91 - 0.98$ sec

18. The phases of action potential in a single cardiac muscle fibre
   (A) Depolarization
   (B) Plateau phase
   (C) Repolarization
   (D) All of the above

19. The depolarization phase is very rapid and lasts for about
   (A) 2 Millisecond
   (B) 10 Millisecond
   (C) 30 Millisecond
   (D) 40 Millisecond

20. The depolarization occurs due to rapid opening of voltage gated

    (A) Calcium channel
    (B) Potassium channel
    (C) Sodium channel
    (D) Chloride channel

21. Which phase occurs due to opening of voltage – gated slow calcium channel

    (A) Plateau phase
    (B) Depolarization
    (C) Resting potential
    (D) Repolarization phase

22. Plateau phase lasts for about

    (A) 1 sec
    (B) 0.25 sec
    (C) 0.78 sec
    (D) 0.98 sec

23. Repolarization is slow process and lasts for about

    (A) 0.05 – 0.08 sec
    (B) 1 – 2 sec
    (C) 2- 3 sec
    (D) 0.9 – 0.99 sec

24. The phase starts at the end of plateau phase when the voltage – gated potassium channels open

    (A) Depolarization
    (B) Hypo polarization
    (C) Repolarization
    (D) Resting potential

25. The duration of action potential in heart

    (A) 200 Millisecond
    (B) 500 Millisecond
    (C) 800 Millisecond
    (D) 900 Millisecond

26. The properties of cardiac muscle

    (A) Excitability
    (B) Contractility
    (C) Conductivity
    (D) All of the above

27. The baroreceptors and mechanoreceptors located in

    (A) Carotid sinus
    (B) Aortic arch
    (C) Both (A) and (B)
    (D) None of the above

28. If an increase in arterial pressure is detected the

    (A) Parasympathetic nervous system
    (B) Sympathetic nervous system
    (C) Both (A) and (B)
    (D) None of the above

29. If a decrease in arterial pressure is detected the
   (A) Parasympathetic nervous system
   (B) Sympathetic nervous system
   (C) Both (A) and (B)
   (D) None of the above

30. The succession of all the coordinated events that take place during every heart beat is called
   (A) Renal cycle
   (B) Cardiac cycle
   (C) Gastric cycle
   (D) Splenic cycle

31. Stages of cardiac cycle is
   (A) Atrial systole
   (B) Ventricular systole
   (C) Relaxation period
   (D) All of the above

32. The period of contraction is called
   (A) Systole
   (B) Diastole
   (C) Dialysis
   (D) Reduced

33. The period of relaxation is called
   (A) Systole
   (B) Diastole
   (C) Dialysis
   (D) Dilute

34. The normal heart rate is
   (A) 100 times/min
   (B) 30 times/min
   (C) 72 times/min
   (D) 45 times/min

35. The duration of each cardiac cycle is about
   (A) 0.8 sec
   (B) 0.1 sec
   (C) 1.2 sec
   (D) 1.9 sec

36. The cardiac cycle is essentially split into
   (A) Systole
   (B) Diastole
   (C) Both (A) and (B)
   (D) None of the above

37. The duration of systole is
   (A) 0.97 sec
   (B) 0.27 sec
   (C) 0.87 sec
   (D) 0.77 sec

38. The duration of diastole is
   (A) 0.53 sec
   (B) 0.10 sec
   (C) 0.99 sec
   (D) 1.5 sec

39. The atrial systole, that is contraction of the atria, lasts for about
   (A) 0.9 sec
   (B) 0.1 sec
   (C) 0.8 sec
   (D) 0.79 sec

40. Which phase is also called the last rapid filling phase?
    (A) Atrial systole
    (B) Ventricular systole
    (C) Atrial diastole
    (D) Ventricular diastole

41. The atrial systole pushes blood into the ventricle about
    (A) 5 mL
    (B) 100 mL
    (C) 52 mL
    (D) 150 mL

42. The stage of ventricular systole is
    (A) Isometric contraction
    (B) Ejection period
    (C) Both (A) and (B)
    (D) None of the above

43. The isometric contraction phase lasts for
    (A) 0.05 sec
    (B) 0.5 sec
    (C) 0.4 sec
    (D) 0.6 sec

44. The ejection period lasts for about
    (A) 0.99 sec
    (B) 0.25 sec
    (C) 0.85 sec
    (D) 0.92 sec

45. The left ventricle eject blood into aorta about
    (A) 70 mL
    (B) 150 mL
    (C) 190 mL
    (D) 200 mL

46. The volume of blood remaining in each ventricle at the end of ventricular systole about
    (A) 200mL
    (B) 180 mL
    (C) 60 mL
    (D) 150 mL

47. In which phase both ventricles contract, blood is forced to the lung via the pulmonary trunk and the rest of the body via aorta
    (A) Ventricular systole
    (B) Ventricular diastole
    (C) Atrial systole
    (D) Atrial diastole

48. During atrial systole the pressure in the aorta is about
    (A) 180 mm Hg
    (B) 120 mm Hg
    (C) 80 mm Hg
    (D) 160 mm Hg

49. A cardiac output pumps blood every minute about
    (A) 10 – 11 litres
    (B) 5 – 6 litres
    (C) 1 – 2 litres
    (D) 11 – 12 litres

50. Factors affecting cardiac output
    (A) Blood volume reflexes
    (B) Autonomic innervation
    (C) Hormones
    (D) All of the above

Answer Key

Cardiovascular System (Part-06)

Question	Answer	Question	Answer
01	A = Atrioventricular Bundle	26	D = All of the Above
02	A = Bundle of His	27	C = Both (A) and (B)
03	B = AV Bundle	28	A = Parasympathetic Nervous System
04	A = AV Bundle	29	B = Sympathetic Nervous System
05	C = Both (A) and (B)	30	B = Cardiac Cycle
06	B = Purkinje Fibres	31	D = All of the Above
07	C = Purkinje Fibres	32	A = Systole
08	C = Both (A) and (B)	33	B = Diastole
09	A = Vagus Nerve	34	C = 72 times/min
10	B = Right Vagus Nerve	35	A = 0.8 sec
11	D = Left Vagus Nerve	36	C = Both (A) and (B)
12	D = All of the Above	37	B = 0.27 sec
13	C = Both (A) and (B)	38	A = 0.53 sec
14	A = Action Potential	39	B = 0.1 sec
15	D = - 90 mV	40	A = Atrial systole
16	D = Resting Potential	41	C = 52 mL
17	B = 0.25 – 0.35 sec	42	C = Both (A) and (B)
18	D = All of the Above	43	A = 0.05 sec
19	A = 2 Milliseconds	44	B = 0.25 sec
20	C = Sodium Channel	45	A = 70 mL
21	A = Plateau Phase	46	C = 60 mL
22	B = 0.25 sec	47	A = Ventricular Systole
23	A = 0.05 – 0.08 sec	48	C = 80 mm Hg
24	C = Repolarization	49	B = 5 – 6 litres
25	A = 200 Milliseconds	50	D = All of the Above

Part-07

1. In which phase the ventricles contract and emptying, pulmonary artery and aortic valve close
   - (A) Ventricular ejections
   - (B) Isovolumic relaxation
   - (C) Atrial systole
   - (D) Rapid filling phase

2. The isometric contraction and ejection phase together form the
   - (A) Atrial systole
   - (B) Arterial diastole
   - (C) Ventricular systole
   - (D) Relaxation period

3. The sum of duration of isometric contraction and ejection phase is called
   - (A) Atrial systole
   - (B) Ventricular systole
   - (C) Relaxation period
   - (D) Ventricular diastole

4. When both atria and ventricular are relaxed is called
   - (A) Relaxation period
   - (B) Ventricular systole
   - (C) Atrial systole
   - (D) Ejection period

5. Ventricular period is lasts for
   - (A) 0.04 sec
   - (B) 0.4 sec
   - (C) 0.5 sec
   - (D) 0.09 sec

6. The period of isovolumetric relaxation is lasts for
   - (A) 0.01 sec
   - (B) 0.02 sec
   - (C) 0.08 sec
   - (D) 0.8 sec

7. Closure of semilunar valves prevents the movement of blood back into the ventricles and produces the
   - (A) First heart sound
   - (B) Second heart sound
   - (C) Third heart sound
   - (D) Fourth heart sound

8. The ventricle volume remains constant, this phase is called
   - (A) Isometric relaxation phase
   - (B) Monometric relaxation phase
   - (C) Ventricular ejection
   - (D) Isovolumetric contraction

9. When AV valves are opened, there is a sudden rush of blood into the ventricles and major part (70%) of ventricular filling occurs
   - (A) Rapid filling phase
   - (B) Slow filling phase
   - (C) Instant filling phase
   - (D) Down filling phase

10. Rapid filling phase lasts for
    - (A) 0.91 sec
    - (B) 0.11 sec
    - (C) 0.81 sec
    - (D) 0.88 sec

11. After sudden rush of blood, the filling of ventricles becomes slow, this phase is called
    - (A) Down filling phase
    - (B) Slow filling phase
    - (C) Instant filling phase
    - (D) Rapid filling phase

12. Slow filling phase is lasts for
    - (A) 0.99 sec
    - (B) 0.92 sec
    - (C) 0.19 sec
    - (D) 0.77 sec

13. Which of the following include in relaxation period?
    - (A) Ejection period
    - (B) Isovolumetric contraction
    - (C) Ventricular diastole
    - (D) Atrial systole

14. The process of listening to sound of heart within the body is called
    - (A) Articulation
    - (B) Auscultation
    - (C) Orientation
    - (D) Ossification

15. The sound of heart is usually listened by
    - (A) Endoscope
    - (B) Microscope
    - (C) Stethoscope
    - (D) Telescope

16. The first sound is fairly loud and is due to the closure of the atrioventricular valves are
    - (A) Lub
    - (B) Tub
    - (C) Dup
    - (D) Tup

17. The second sound is softer and is due to the closure of the aortic and pulmonary valves are
    - (A) Tub
    - (B) Tup
    - (C) Dup
    - (D) Lup

18. Which sound is generated by vibrations created by the closing of both AV valves?
    - (A) First heart sound
    - (B) Second heart sound
    - (C) Third heart sound
    - (D) Fourth heart sound

19. Which sound is produced by aortic and pulmonary valves close and cause vibrations?

    (A) Third heart sound
    (B) First heart sound
    (C) Second heart sound
    (D) Fourth heart sound

20. Which sound is normally not loud enough to be heard and can be heard using a microphone?

    (A) Fifth heart sound
    (B) Second heart sound
    (C) First heart sound
    (D) Third heart sound

21. Which sound is inaudible and can only by recorded graphically using a phonocardiogram?

    (A) Fourth heart sound
    (B) Second heart sound
    (C) First heart sound
    (D) Fifth heart sound

22. In which phase of cardiac cycle, the first heart sound heard

    (A) Beginning of ventricular diastole

    (B) Beginning of ventricular systole

    (C) Rapid ventricular filling

    (D) Trial contraction

23. In which phase of cardiac cycle, the second heart sound heard

    (A) Trial contraction

    (B) Rapid ventricular filling

    (C) Beginning of ventricular diastole

    (D) Beginning of ventricular systole

24. Which sound generate when rushing of blood into ventricles

    (A) Third heart sound
    (B) Second heart sound
    (C) First heart sound
    (D) Fifth heart sound

25. In which phase of cardiac cycle the third heart sound heard

    (A) Atrial contraction

    (B) Rapid ventricular filling

    (C) Beginning of ventricular diastole

    (D) Beginning of ventricular systole

26. In which phase of cardiac cycle, the fourth heart sound heard

    (A) Rapid ventricular filling

    (B) Atrial contraction

    (C) Beginning of ventricular systole

    (D) Beginning of ventricular diastole

27. Which sound generates by blood turbulence and contraction of atrial muscle
    - (A) Third heart sound
    - (B) Fifth heart sound
    - (C) Second heart sound
    - (D) Fourth heart sound

28. The characteristics of third heart sound is
    - (A) Heard by microscope
    - (B) Heard by microphone
    - (C) Resembles the LUBB
    - (D) Louder and longer

29. The characteristics of fourth heart sound is
    - (A) Recorded by phonocardiogram
    - (B) Heard by microphone
    - (C) Shorter and softer
    - (D) Louder and longer

30. The recording of the electrical activities of heart
    - (A) Microscope
    - (B) Electrocardiogram
    - (C) Radiographic
    - (D) Sonographic

31. The instrument which is used to record the electrical activities of the heart is called
    - (A) Electrocardiograph
    - (B) Thermometer
    - (C) Radiograph
    - (D) Hysteroscope

32. Electrocardiography technique is discovered by
    - (A) Zacharias Janssen
    - (B) Thomas Edison
    - (C) Galileo Galilei
    - (D) Willem Einthoven

33. Who is the father of ECG?
    - (A) Willem Einthoven
    - (B) Thomas Edison
    - (C) Zacharias Janssen
    - (D) Galileo Galilei

34. The markings on the paper of ECG are called
    - (A) ECG band
    - (B) ECG grid
    - (C) ECG bold
    - (D) ECG view

35. Which represent the impulse from the SA node sweeping over the atria (atrial depolarization)
    - (A) C wave
    - (B) B wave
    - (C) P wave
    - (D) D wave

36. Which of the following is the first wave of ECG and is small upward deflection on the ECG?
    - (A) B wave
    - (B) P wave
    - (C) D wave
    - (D) F wave

37. Which of the following is not a wave of ECG tracing?

    (A) A wave
    (B) P wave
    (C) Q wave
    (D) R wave

38. Which of the following obtain due to depolarization of the ventricles?

    (A) ABC complex
    (B) XYZ complex
    (C) QRS complex
    (D) UVW complex

39. Which wave arises when the impulse from the SA node spreads throughout both the atria

    (A) Q wave
    (B) S wave
    (C) P wave
    (D) R wave

40. Which wave is arising due to the depolarization of the basal portion of the interventricular septum?

    (A) P wave
    (B) Q wave
    (C) T wave
    (D) B wave

41. Which wave arises due to the depolarization of apical portion of the interventricular septum and ventricular muscle

    (A) R wave
    (B) P wave
    (C) Q wave
    (D) D wave

42. Which wave arises due to the depolarization of the basal portion of ventricular muscle

    (A) D wave
    (B) S wave
    (C) B wave
    (D) P wave

43. Blood pressure is directly proportional to the

    (A) Cardiac output
    (B) Cardiac input
    (C) Sugar levels
    (D) Salts levels

44. Cardiac output can be calculated by

    (A) Cardiac output = stroke volume − heart rate
    (B) Cardiac output = stroke volume + heart rate
    (C) Cardiac output = stroke volume × heart rate
    (D) Cardiac output = stroke volume ÷ heart rate

45. As increase in blood volume the cardiac volume will be

    (A) Decrease
    (B) Increase
    (C) No change
    (D) Constant

46. The increase in stroke volume then cardiac volume will be
    (A) Increase
    (B) Decrease
    (C) No change
    (D) Constant

47. Cardiac output can be determined by
    (A) Stroke volume
    (B) Glucose level
    (C) Bilirubin level
    (D) Tidal volume

48. The amount of blood pumped out by each ventricle during each beat is called
    (A) Stroke volume
    (B) Tidal volume
    (C) Reverse volume
    (D) Residual volume

49. The opposition or resistance to the blood flow due to friction between blood and walls of the blood vessels is called
    (A) Central resistance
    (B) Peripheral resistance
    (C) Temporary resistance
    (D) Permanent resistance

50. The blood pressure is directly proportional to the
    (A) Peripheral resistance
    (B) Central resistance
    (C) Occipital resistance
    (D) Temporary resistance

Answer Key

Cardiovascular System (Part-07)

Question	Answer	Question	Answer
01	A = Ventricular ejections	26	B = Atrial contraction
02	C = Ventricular systole	27	D = Fourth heart sound
03	B = Ventricular systole	28	B = Heard by microphone
04	A = Relaxation period	29	A = Recorded by phonocardiogram
05	A = 0.04 sec	30	B = Electrocardiogram
06	C = 0.08 sec	31	A = Electrocardiograph
07	B = Second heart sound	32	D = Willem Einthoven
08	A = isometric relaxation phase	33	A = Willem Einthoven
09	A = Rapid filling phase	34	B = ECG grid
10	B = 0.11 sec	35	C = P wave
11	B = Slow filling phase	36	B = P wave
12	C = 0.19 sec	37	A = A wave
13	C = Ventricular diastole	38	C = QRS wave
14	B = Auscultation	39	C = P wave
15	C = stethoscope	40	B = Q wave
16	A = Lub	41	A = R wave
17	C = Dup	42	B = S wave
18	A = First heart sound	43	A = Cardiac output
19	C = Second heart sound	44	C = Cardiac output = stroke volume × heart rate
20	D = Third heart sound	45	B = Increase
21	A = Fourth heart sound	46	A = Increase
22	B = Beginning of ventricular systole	47	A = Stroke volume
23	C =Beginning of ventricular diastole	48	A = Stroke volume
24	A = Third heart sound	49	B = Peripheral resistance
25	B = Rapid ventricular filling	50	A = Peripheral resistance

Part-08

1. The smaller the diameter of the blood vessels, the resistance will be
   (A) Greater
   (B) Lesser
   (C) No change
   (D) Constant

2. The vasoconstriction constricts the arterioles and the resistance is
   (A) Decreases
   (B) Increases
   (C) Constant
   (D) No change

3. The diameter of blood vessels is inversely proportional to the
   (A) Glucose levels
   (B) Urea levels
   (C) Blood pressure
   (D) Creatinine levels

4. The viscosity of blood depends on the ratio of
   (A) RBCs to plasma
   (B) WBCs to plasma
   (C) Platelets to hormones
   (D) Platelets to electrolytes

5. Increased the viscosity of blood the resistance will be
   (A) Decrease
   (B) No change
   (C) Constant
   (D) Increase

6. The resistance increased, the blood pressure will be
   (A) Decrease
   (B) Increase
   (C) Constant
   (D) No change

7. Blood pressure is directly proportional to the
   (A) Viscosity of blood
   (B) Diameter of blood vessels
   (C) Elasticity of blood vessels
   (D) None of the above

8. In anaemia decreased the viscosity of blood, the resistance will be
   (A) Increased
   (B) Decreased
   (C) No change
   (D) Constant

9. The volume of blood flowing back to the heart through veins and the pressure generated by the contraction of the left ventricle of the heart is responsible for the
   (A) Venous return
   (B) Venous instant
   (C) Atrial pressure
   (D) Blood pressure

10. Blood pressure is directly proportional to the
    (A) Venous instant
    (B) Atrial back
    (C) Venous return
    (D) Elasticity of blood vessels

11. The blood pressure is inversely proportional to the
    (A) Venous return
    (B) Elasticity of blood vessels
    (C) Viscosity of blood
    (D) Peripheral resistance

12. The nervous mechanism for BP regulation is also called
    (A) Long – term BP regulation
    (B) Renal mechanism
    (C) Short – term BP regulation
    (D) Hormonal regulation

13. The long – term BP regulation is also called
    (A) Nervous regulation
    (B) Renal regulation
    (C) Hormonal regulation
    (D) Gastric regulation

14. The nervous system regulates BP through
    (A) RAAS system
    (B) Angiotensin II
    (C) Aldosterone
    (D) Vasomotor system

15. Which of the following is not a part of vasomotor system?
    (A) Vasodilator fibres
    (B) Vasoconstrictor fibres
    (C) Bronchoconstrictor fibres
    (D) Vasomotor centre

16. Vasomotor centre is also called
    (A) Cardiovascular centre
    (B) Gastrointestinal centre
    (C) Respiratory centre
    (D) Urinary centre

17. Vasomotor centre is present in
    (A) Medulla oblongata
    (B) Pons of the brain stem
    (C) Both (A) and (B)
    (D) None of the above

18. The cardiovascular centre is a collection of interconnected neurones that help to regulate
    (A) Glucose level
    (B) Blood pressure
    (C) Urea level
    (D) Bile level

19. The vasomotor centre controls the diameter of blood vessels by causing
    (A) Nasodilation
    (B) Bronchodilation
    (C) Vasoconstriction
    (D) Bronchodilation

20. The vasoconstrictor centre sends impulses to blood vessels through sympathetic vasoconstrictor fibres, which stimulated cause constriction of blood vessels and blood pressure will be
    (A) Decreases
    (B) Increases
    (C) No change
    (D) Constant

21. The vasodilator centre supresses the vasoconstrictor centre and causes vasodilation, which leads to blood pressure

    (A) Decreases   (B) No change

    (C) Constant   (D) Increase

22. The impulses from the vasodilator centre are passed through the

    (A) Auditory nerve   (B) Optic nerve

    (C) Vagus nerve   (D) Olfactory nerve

23. The sympathetic nerve fibres of ANS cause vasoconstriction by the release of neurotransmitter

    (A) Adrenaline   (B) Serotonin

    (C) GABA   (D) Melanin

24. The parasympathetic nerve fibres ANS and cause vasodilation by the release of neurotransmitter

    (A) GABA   (B) Melanin

    (C) Acetylcholine   (D) Serotonin

25. The receptors that produce response to change in BP is

    (A) Baroreceptors   (B) Proprioceptors

    (C) Nociceptor   (D) Cutaneous receptor

26. Baroreceptors are situated in the

    (A) Arch of ilium   (B) Arch of aorta

    (C) Arch of carpal   (D) Arch of sternal

27. A rise in BP in the aorta and carotid sinus stimulates

    (A) Nociceptor   (B) Proprioceptors

    (C) Baroreceptors   (D) Cutaneous receptor

28. The baroreceptors send the impulses to

    (A) Nasomotor centre   (B) Vasomotor centre

    (C) Gastrointestinal centre   (D) Respiratory centre

29. Which receptors produce response to changes in the chemical constituents of blood

    (A) Nociceptor   (B) Thermoreceptors

    (C) Chemoreceptors   (D) Proprioceptors

30. Which detect changes in the blood levels of oxygen, carbon dioxide and hydrogen ions

    (A) Baroreceptors   (B) Chemoreceptors

    (C) Cutaneous receptor   (D) Thermoreceptors

31. The vasomotor centre is also controlled by impulses from higher centres in the brain are
    (A) Cerebral cortex
    (B) Hypothalamus
    (C) Both (A) and (B)
    (D) None of the above

32. During emotional stress the cerebral cortex sends impulses to the vasomotor centre which activates and the stimulates the
    (A) Vasoconstrictor fibres
    (B) Vasodilator fibres
    (C) Bronchodilator fibres
    (D) Bronchoconstrictor fibres

33. Stimulation of the anterior hypothalamus causes
    (A) Vasodilation
    (B) Vasoconstriction
    (C) Bronchodilation
    (D) Bronchoconstriction

34. Stimulation of posterior hypothalamus causes
    (A) Bronchodilation
    (B) Vasoconstriction
    (C) Bronchoconstriction
    (D) Vasodilation

35. Which of the following play an important role in the long – term regulation of blood pressure?
    (A) Stomach
    (B) Pancreas
    (C) Kidney
    (D) Intestine

36. The kidneys regulate BP in the way of
    (A) RAAP
    (B) RAAS
    (C) SAAR
    (D) RAAD

37. The renin is release by juxtaglomerular cells of the
    (A) Kidney
    (B) Liver
    (C) Lungs
    (D) Brain

38. The renin converts Angiotensinogen into
    (A) Angiotensin V
    (B) Angiotensin IV
    (C) Angiotensin III
    (D) Angiotensin I

39. Angiotensinogen is release from
    (A) Lungs
    (B) Liver
    (C) Stomach
    (D) Pancreas

40. Angiotensin I is converted into
    (A) Angiotensin II
    (B) Angiotensin III
    (C) Angiotensin IV
    (D) Angiotensin V

41. Angiotensin I is converted into Angiotensin II by an enzyme
    (A) Pyruvate kinase
    (B) Hexokinase
    (C) Angiotensin – converting enzyme
    (D) Triosephosphate isomerase

42. Angiotensin – converting enzyme released from
    (A) Stomach
    (B) Pancreas
    (C) Lungs
    (D) Brain

43. Angiotensin II stimulates the release of
    (A) Aldosterone
    (B) Serotonin
    (C) Melatonin
    (D) Thyroxin

44. Angiotensin II causes
    (A) Vasodilation
    (B) Vasoconstriction
    (C) Bronchodilation
    (D) Bronchoconstriction

45. As the blood pressure decrease the hormone release are
    (A) Oxytocin
    (B) Growth hormone
    (C) Antidiuretic hormone
    (D) Prolactin

46. Antidiuretic hormones release from
    (A) Thyroid gland
    (B) Anterior pituitary
    (C) Posterior pituitary
    (D) Pineal gland

47. Antidiuretic hormone is also called
    (A) Vasopressin
    (B) Oxytocin
    (C) Thyroxine
    (D) Melatonin

48. Which of the following is example of local vasoconstrictor?
    (A) Melanin
    (B) Acetylcholine
    (C) Endothelin's
    (D) Endothelium – derived relaxing factor

49. Angiotensin II also cause
    (A) Water retention
    (B) Calcium retention
    (C) Hormone retention
    (D) Iron retention

50. ANP stands for
    (A) Anterior normal peptide
    (B) Atrial natriuretic peptide
    (C) Automatic normal protein
    (D) Automatic natriuretic plasma

Answer Key

Cardiovascular System (Part-08)

Question	Answer	Question	Answer
01	A = Greater	26	B = Arch of aorta
02	B = Increase	27	C = Baroreceptors
03	C = Blood pressure	28	B = Vasomotor centre
04	A = RBCs to plasma	29	C = Chemoreceptors
05	D = Increase	30	B = Chemoreceptors
06	B = Increase	31	C = Both (A) and (B)
07	A = Viscosity of blood	32	A = Vasoconstrictor fibres
08	B = Decreased	33	B = Vasoconstriction
09	A = Venous return	34	D = Vasodilation
10	C = Venous return	35	C = Kidney
11	B = Elasticity of blood vessels	36	B = RAAS
12	C = Short – term BP regulation	37	A = Kidney
13	B = Renal regulation	38	D = angiotensin I
14	D = Vasomotor system	39	B = Liver
15	C = Bronchoconstrictor fibres	40	A = Angiotensin I
16	A = Cardiovascular centre	41	C = Angiotensin – Converting Enzyme
17	C = Both (A) and (B)	42	C = Lungs
18	B = Blood pressure	43	A = Aldosterone
19	C = vasoconstriction	44	B = Vasoconstriction
20	B = Increase	45	C = Antidiuretic hormone
21	A = Decrease	46	C = Posterior pituitary
22	C = Vagus nerve	47	A = Vasopressin
23	A = Adrenaline	48	C = Endothelin's
24	C = Acetylcholine	49	A = Water retention
25	A = Baroreceptors	50	B = Atrial natriuretic peptide

Part-09

1. The maximum amount of blood that can be pumped out of the heart above the normal value
   - (A) Cardiac reverse
   - (B) Cardiac instant
   - (C) Cardiac reset
   - (D) Cardiac refresh

2. The cardiac output would be
   - (A) 15 L/min
   - (B) 5 L/min
   - (C) 20 L/min
   - (D) 25 /min

3. Which of the following receives maximum amount of blood pumped by the heart?
   - (A) Stomach
   - (B) Kidney
   - (C) Liver
   - (D) Intestine

4. The liver receives amount of blood pumped by the heart is
   - (A) 90 %
   - (B) 30 %
   - (C) 60 %
   - (D) 70 %

5. The heart which pumps blood to all organs receives the amount of blood
   - (A) 40 %
   - (B) 30 %
   - (C) 5 %
   - (D) 45 %

6. The value of cardiac reverse in average person at rest is
   - (A) 10 – 12 times
   - (B) 20 – 25 times
   - (C) 30 – 40 times
   - (D) 4 – 5 times

7. The physiological variations in cardiac output is
   - (A) Age
   - (B) Emotional conditions
   - (C) Exercise
   - (D) All of the above

8. Cardiac output is increased at high altitude because of decreased
   - (A) Nitrogen
   - (B) Carbon dioxide
   - (C) Oxygen
   - (D) Carbon monoxide

9. Which of the following increases the cardiac output?
   - (A) Melanin
   - (B) Melatonin
   - (C) Adrenaline
   - (D) Histamine

10. During the later months of pregnancy, the cardiac output increases by
    (A) 45 – 50 %
    (B) 60 – 65 %
    (C) 70 – 80 %
    (D) 80 – 90 %

11. The pathological variations which increased cardiac output
    (A) Fever
    (B) Anaemia
    (C) Hyperthyroidism
    (D) All of the above

12. Which condition decreased the cardiac output
    (A) Fever
    (B) Hypothyroidism
    (C) Anaemia
    (D) Hyperthyroidism

13. Which factors regulate stroke volume
    (A) Preload
    (B) Force of contraction
    (C) Afterload
    (D) All of the above

14. The filling pressure of the heart at the end of diastole is called
    (A) Reload
    (B) Post load
    (C) Preload
    (D) Afterload

15. The greater the preload, the volume of blood in the heart at the end of diastole will be
    (A) Greater
    (B) Lesser
    (C) No change
    (D) Constant

16. Which of the following depends on the amount of blood returning to the heart through the superior and inferior vena cava?
    (A) Reload
    (B) Preload
    (C) Post load
    (D) Before load

17. The difference between end diastolic volume (EDV) and end systolic volume (ESV) is called
    (A) Stroke volume
    (B) Standard volume
    (C) Standard rate
    (D) Strong volume

18. The pressure against which the heart must work to eject blood during systole is called
    (A) Preload
    (B) Post load
    (C) Afterload
    (D) Reload

19. The lower the afterload, the blood eject with contraction of the heart will be
    (A) More
    (B) Less
    (C) Constant
    (D) No change

20. The formula of stroke volume is
   (A) End diastolic volume + end systolic volume
   (B) End diastolic volume − end systolic volume
   (C) End diastolic volume × end systolic volume
   (D) End diastolic volume ÷ end systolic volume

21. The increased the end diastolic volume, increases stretch on the heart so, the force of contraction will be
   (A) Increases
   (B) Decreases
   (C) No change
   (D) Constant

22. The substances that increase the force of contraction are called
   (A) Negative inotropic agents
   (B) Positive inotropic agents
   (C) Neutral inotropic agents
   (D) Negative oligotrophic agents

23. The substances that decrease the force of contraction are called
   (A) Neutral inotropic agents
   (B) Negative inotropic agents
   (C) Positive inotropic agents
   (D) Positive oligotrophic agents

24. The condition in which plaque builds up inside the coronary artery
   (A) Atherosclerosis
   (B) Angina
   (C) Shock
   (D) Lymphoma

25. Plaque is made up of
   (A) Fats
   (B) Cholesterol
   (C) Calcium
   (D) All of the above

26. Which cause the narrows the arteries and reduction in blood flow to heart muscle
   (A) Water
   (B) Plasma
   (C) Plaque
   (D) WBCs

27. Hypovolaemic shock occurs when blood volume is reduced by
   (A) 50 – 60 %
   (B) 15 – 25 %
   (C) 70 – 80 %
   (D) 50 – 55 %

28. Which shock occurs in acute heart disease when damaged heart muscle cannot maintain an adequate cardiac output
   (A) Cardiogenic shock
   (B) Neurogenic shock
   (C) Septic shock
   (D) Anaphylactic shock

29. Which shock occurs due to active infection in the bloodstream

    (A) Neurogenic shock
    (B) Cardiogenic shock
    (C) Septic shock
    (D) Anaphylactic shock

30. Which shock occurs due to sudden acute pain, severe emotional experience, spinal anaesthesia and spinal cord damage

    (A) Septic shock
    (B) Anaphylactic shock
    (C) Cardiogenic shock
    (D) Neurogenic shock

31. Which shock occurs due to severe allergic response than may be triggered in sensitive individual by some substances

    (A) Septic shock
    (B) Neurogenic shock
    (C) Cardiogenic shock
    (D) Anaphylactic shock

32. The formation of blood clot inside the blood vessel, interrupting blood supply to the tissue is called

    (A) Thrombosis
    (B) Angina
    (C) Diphtheria
    (D) Emphysema

33. The blocking of a blood vessel by any mass of material travelling in the blood

    (A) Bronchiectasis
    (B) Embolism
    (C) Emphysema
    (D) Diphtheria

34. The chest pain or discomfort when there is not enough blood flow to heart muscle is called

    (A) Emphysema
    (B) Sinusitis
    (C) Angina
    (D) Diphtheria

35. The abnormal heart sound produced because of changed pattern of blood flow or turbulent blood flow is called

    (A) Dyspnoea
    (B) Cardiac murmurs
    (C) Angina
    (D) Bronchitis

36. The inflammation of pericardium is called

    (A) Lymphangitis
    (B) Tonsilitis
    (C) Bronchitis
    (D) Pericarditis

37. Cardiac murmurs caused by

    (A) Heart attack
    (B) High blood pressure
    (C) Rhematic fever
    (D) All of the above

38. The inability of the heart to supply sufficient blood flow to body is called

    (A) Congestive heart failure
    (B) Bronchiectasis
    (C) Asbestosis
    (D) Cystic fibrosis

39. The medical procedure done to open blocked or narrowed coronary arteries is called

(A) Laparoscopy

(B) Angioplasty

(C) Hysteroscopy

(D) Myomectomy

40. The inflammation of myocardium is called

(A) Bronchitis

(B) Bronchiectasis

(C) Myocarditis

(D) Tonsilitis

41. The inflammation of inside lining of the heart chambers and heart valves is called

(A) Endocarditis

(B) Tonsilitis

(C) Bronchitis

(D) Diphtheria

42. Which of the following occur due to change the rhythm or heart rate?

(A) Diphtheria

(B) Cardiac arrhythmia

(C) Angina

(D) Embolism

43. Which of the following refers to slow heart rate (below 60 beats/min)

(A) Bradycardia

(B) Tachycardia

(C) Endocarditis

(D) Myocarditis

44. Which of the following refers to rapid heart rate (above 100 beats/min)

(A) Endocarditis

(B) Myocarditis

(C) Tachycardia

(D) Bradycardia

45. The myocardium may infarct when a branch of a coronary artery is blocked, usually by an atheromatous plaque complicated by thrombosis

(A) Myocardial infraction

(B) Angina

(C) Emphysema

(D) Bronchiectasis

46. Which of the following occurs when the normal impulse transmission is blocked or impaired?

(A) Emphysema

(B) Heart block

(C) Shock

(D) Thrombosis

47. Which of the following is commonly called hole in the heart?

(A) Septal defect

(B) Shock

(C) Angina

(D) Myocardial infraction

48. Which of the following occurs due to narrowing of a valve opening, impeding blood flow through the valve?

(A) Embolism

(B) Stenosis

(C) Emphysema

(D) Diphtheria

49. Which of the following refers to high blood pressure?
    (A) Hyperthyroidism
    (B) Hypotension
    (C) Hypertension
    (D) Hypothyroidism

50. Which of the following refers to low blood pressure?
    (A) Hypotension
    (B) Hyperthyroidism
    (C) Hypothyroidism
    (D) Hypertension

Answer Key

Cardiovascular System (Part-09)

Question	Answer	Question	Answer
01	A = Cardiac reserve	26	C = Plaque
02	B = 5 L/min	27	B = 15 – 25%
03	C = Liver	28	A = Cardiogenic shock
04	B = 30%	29	C = Septic shock
05	C = 5%	30	D = Neurogenic shock
06	D = 4 – 5 times	31	D = Anaphylactic shock
07	D = All of the above	32	A = Thrombosis
08	C = Oxygen	33	B = Embolism
09	C = Adrenaline	34	C = Angina
10	A = 45 – 50%	35	B = Cardiac murmurs
11	D = All of the above	36	D = Pericarditis
12	B = Hypothyroidism	37	D = All of the above
13	D = All of the above	38	A = Congestive heart failure
14	C = Preload	39	B = Angioplasty
15	A = Greater	40	C = Myocarditis
16	B = Preload	41	A = Endocarditis
17	A = Stroke volume	42	B = Cardiac arrhythmia
18	C = Afterload	43	A = Bradycardia
19	A = More	44	C = Tachycardia
20	B = End diastolic volume – end systolic volume	45	A = Myocardial infraction
21	A = Increases	46	B = Heart block
22	B = Positive inotropic agents	47	A = Septal defect
23	B = Negative inotropic agents	48	B = Stenosis
24	A = Atherosclerosis	49	C = Hypertension
25	D = All of the above	50	A = Hypotension

Unit - VIII

Digestive System

Part-01

1. Which system breaks down the food into smaller molecules
   - (A) Respiratory system
   - (B) Digestive system
   - (C) Urinary system
   - (D) Nervous system

2. Digestive system starts from
   - (A) Mouth
   - (B) Nose
   - (C) Iris
   - (D) Stomach

3. Which system describe the alimentary canal, its accessory organs and variety of process for food absorption
   - (A) Respiratory system
   - (B) Urinary system
   - (C) Digestive system
   - (D) Cardiovascular system

4. The consumption of food materials is called
   - (A) Mixing
   - (B) Digestion
   - (C) Ingestion
   - (D) Absorption

5. The movement of food contents is called
   - (A) Absorption
   - (B) Propulsion
   - (C) Digestion
   - (D) Elimination

6. The churning of food is called
   - (A) Ingestion
   - (B) Absorption
   - (C) Digestion
   - (D) Mixing

7. The mechanical and chemical breakdown of food is called
   - (A) Digestion
   - (B) Propulsion
   - (C) Ingestion
   - (D) Elimination

8. The removal of unwanted substance from the body is called
   - (A) Ingestion
   - (B) Elimination
   - (C) Propulsion
   - (D) Mixing

429

9. The process by which the products of digestion pass into blood and lymph is called

   (A) Elimination
   (B) Ingestion
   (C) Absorption
   (D) Propulsion

10. Alimentary canal is also called

   (A) Gastrointestinal tract
   (B) Urinary tract
   (C) Respiratory tract
   (D) Nervous tract

11. The length of alimentary canal is about

   (A) 30 metres
   (B) 10 metres
   (C) 50 metres
   (D) 25 metres

12. The alimentary canal terminates at

   (A) Oesophagus
   (B) Mouth
   (C) Anus
   (D) Bladder

13. The parts of alimentary canal include

   (A) Mouth
   (B) Pharynx
   (C) Stomach
   (D) All of the above

14. Which of the following is not part of alimentary canal?

   (A) Oesophagus
   (B) Large intestine
   (C) Kidney
   (D) Stomach

15. Which of the following is accessory organ of digestive system?

   (A) Kidney
   (B) Lungs
   (C) Liver
   (D) Urethra

16. How many pairs of salivary glands are there?

   (A) Four
   (B) Three
   (C) Five
   (D) Six

17. The layer of GI tract includes

   (A) Mucosa
   (B) Submucosa
   (C) Muscularis
   (D) All of the above

18. The outermost layer of alimentary canal is

   (A) Serosa
   (B) Submucosa
   (C) Mucosa
   (D) Muscularis

19. The innermost layer of alimentary canal is

   (A) Serosa
   (B) Mucosa
   (C) Muscularis
   (D) Submucosa

20. The largest serous membrane of the body
    (A) Myocardium
    (B) Pleura
    (C) Peritoneum
    (D) Pericardium

21. The single membrane, forming a closed sac and containing a small amount of serous fluid, within the abdominal cavity
    (A) Peritoneum
    (B) Pleura
    (C) Myocardium
    (D) Pericardium

22. Which portion lines the abdominal and pelvic cavities
    (A) Fissure peritoneum
    (B) Parietal peritoneum
    (C) Ventral peritoneum
    (D) Distal peritoneum

23. Which of the following covers the external surfaces of most abdominal organs?
    (A) Visceral peritoneum
    (B) Proximal peritoneum
    (C) Distal peritoneum
    (D) Ventral peritoneum

24. The mucosal layer that has direct access to the contents in the lumen of the GI tract
    (A) Connective layer
    (B) Epithelial layer
    (C) Nervous layer
    (D) Cardiac tissue layer

25. Types of epithelia in the mucosa of digestive system
    (A) Simple columnar epithelium
    (B) Squamous epithelium
    (C) Both (A) and (B)
    (D) None of the above

26. The squamous epithelium presents in
    (A) Mouth
    (B) Stomach
    (C) Small intestine
    (D) Large intestine

27. The simple columnar epithelium presents in
    (A) Mouth
    (B) Pharynx
    (C) Stomach
    (D) Oesophagus

28. Which of the following connects the epithelium to muscularis mucosa?
    (A) Lamina propria
    (B) Submucosa
    (C) Lamina cheeks
    (D) Lamina cortical

29. Lamina propria is composed of
    (A) Squamous epithelium
    (B) Simple columnar epithelium
    (C) Loose connective tissue
    (D) Stratified cuboidal epithelium

30. The thin layer present outside the lamina propria that permits enfolding of the mucosa membrane of the stomach and small intestine

    (A) Muscularis mucosa
    (B) Cutaneous mucosa
    (C) Nasal mucosa
    (D) Oral mucosa

31. The layer present between the mucosa and the muscularis called

    (A) Submucosa
    (B) Central mucosa
    (C) Lateral mucosa
    (D) Ventral mucosa

32. Which of the following formed by a thick layer of smooth muscle fibres surrounding the submucosa

    (A) Muscle coat
    (B) Muscle band
    (C) Muscle sac
    (D) Muscle cone

33. Which layer binds submucosa and serosa

    (A) Dermis
    (B) Subcutaneous
    (C) Muscularis
    (D) Synovial

34. Muscularis is composed of

    (A) Skeletal muscle
    (B) Smooth muscle
    (C) Both (A) and (B)
    (D) None of the above

35. The inner layer of smooth muscle of muscularis is

    (A) Rectangular smooth muscle fibres
    (B) Circular smooth muscle fibres
    (C) Longitudinal smooth muscle fibres
    (D) Triangular smooth muscle fibres

36. The outer layer of smooth muscle of muscularis is

    (A) Longitudinal smooth muscle fibres
    (B) Triangular smooth muscle fibres
    (C) Circular smooth muscle fibres
    (D) Rectangular smooth muscle fibres

37. Circular smooth muscle fibres and longitudinal smooth muscle fibres of muscularis are found in

    (A) Mouth
    (B) Stomach
    (C) Pharynx
    (D) Anal sphincter

38. Skeletal muscle of muscularis is present in

    (A) Small intestine
    (B) Large intestine
    (C) Mouth
    (D) Stomach

39. Simple columnar epithelium of epithelial layer of mucosa are present in

    (A) Mouth   (B) Pharynx

    (C) Oesophagus   (D) Stomach

40. Which layer of smooth muscle are used for peristalsis?

    (A) Muscularis propria   (B) Perimysium

    (C) Endomysium   (D) Epimysium

41. Which fold of peritoneum attaches the transverse colon to the posterior abdominal wall

    (A) Splenorenal ligament   (B) Transverse mesocolon

    (C) Sigmoid mesocolon   (D) Gastroparetic ligament

42. Which fold of peritoneum connects spleen to the left kidney

    (A) Gastrosplenic ligament   (B) Gastrophrenic ligament

    (C) Splenorenal ligament   (D) Transverse mesocolon

43. Which of the following refers the space between the visceral and parietal layers of peritoneum?

    (A) Peritoneal cavity   (B) Vertebral cavity

    (C) Cranial cavity   (D) Pericardial cavity

44. Which refers to the main part of peritoneal cavity, which extends from the roof of abdominal cavity to its floor

    (A) Shorter sac   (B) Greater sac

    (C) Lesser sac   (D) Shorter sac

45. The GI tract possess an integral nervous system called

    (A) Bilateral nervous system   (B) Enteric nervous system

    (C) Lateral nervous system   (D) Distal nervous system

46. Which of the following located between the longitudinal and circular layers of muscle in the tunica muscularis?

    (A) Myenteric plexus   (B) Lateral plexus

    (C) Vertical plexus   (D) Distal plexus

47. Which neurons receive information from sensory receptors in the mucosa and muscle

    (A) Motor neuron   (B) Efferent neuron

    (C) Sensory neuron   (D) Intraneuron

48. How many neurons contain in enteric nervous system?

    (A) 1000 – 2000 millions   (B) 100 – 500 million

    (C) 10 – 30 million   (D) 1500 – 1800 millions

49. Meissner's plexus is also called

   (A) Sublateral plexus

   (B) Myenteric plexus

   (C) Subdistal plexus

   (D) Submucosal plexus

50. Auerbach's plexus is also called

   (A) Myenteric plexus

   (B) Submucosal plexus

   (C) Subdistal plexus

   (D) Sublateral plexus

Answer Key

Digestive System (Part-01)

Question	Answer	Question	Answer
01	B = Digestive system	26	A = Mouth
02	A = Mouth	27	C = Stomach
03	C = Digestive system	28	A = Lamina propria
04	C = Ingestion	29	C = Loose connective tissue
05	B = Propulsion	30	A = Muscularis mucosa
06	D = Mixing	31	A = Submucosa
07	A = Digestion	32	A = Muscle coat
08	B = Elimination	33	C = Muscularis
09	C = Absorption	34	C = Both (A) and (B)
10	A = Gastrointestinal tract	35	B = Circular smooth muscle fibres
11	B = 10 metres	36	A = Longitudinal smooth muscle fibres
12	C = Anus	37	B = Stomach
13	D = All of the above	38	C = Mouth
14	C = Kidney	39	D = stomach
15	C = Liver	40	A = Muscularis propria
16	B = Three	41	B = Transverse mesocolon
17	D = All of the above	42	C = Splenorenal ligament
18	A = Serosa	43	A = Peritoneal cavity
19	B = Mucosa	44	B = Greater sac
20	C = Peritoneum	45	B = Enteric nervous system
21	A = Peritoneum	46	A = Myenteric plexus
22	B = Parietal peritoneum	47	C = sensory neuron
23	A = visceral peritoneum	48	B = 100 – 500 million
24	B = Epithelial layer	49	D = Submucosal plexus
25	C = Both (A) and (B)	50	A = Myenteric plexus

Part-02

1. The blood vessels in the digestive system form an extensive system called
   - (A) Splanchnic circulation
   - (B) Renal circulation
   - (C) Hepatic circulation
   - (D) Pulmonary circulation
2. Coeliac trunk supplied blood to the
   - (A) Rectum
   - (B) Sigmoid colon
   - (C) Oesophagus
   - (D) Descending colon
3. Coeliac trunk arises from the anterior aspect of the aorta, at the aortic hiatus of the diaphragm
   - (A) T12 level
   - (B) L1 level
   - (C) L3 level
   - (D) L9 level
4. Coeliac trunk runs forward for about
   - (A) 5 cm
   - (B) 1 cm
   - (C) 10 cm
   - (D) 19 cm
5. Coeliac trunk divided into major branches are
   - (A) Left gastric artery
   - (B) Common hepatic artery
   - (C) Splenic artery
   - (D) All of the above
6. Left gastric artery is distributed into
   - (A) Rectum
   - (B) Oesophagus
   - (C) Colon
   - (D) Appendix
7. Common hepatic artery distributed into
   - (A) Stomach
   - (B) Colon
   - (C) Appendix
   - (D) Ileum
8. Splenic artery distributed into
   - (A) Colon
   - (B) Appendix
   - (C) Spleen
   - (D) Rectum
9. Superior mesenteric artery arises anteriorly from the abdominal aorta at the level of the
   - (A) L1 vertebrae
   - (B) S1 vertebrae
   - (C) C10 vertebrae
   - (D) T10 vertebrae

10. Superior mesenteric artery supplies the
    (A) Oesophagus
    (B) Distal duodenum
    (C) Rectum
    (D) Colon

11. Superior pancreaticoduodenal artery supplies the
    (A) Inferior region of the head of the pancreas
    (B) Rectum
    (C) Appendix
    (D) Colon

12. The inferior mesenteric artery arises at
    (A) T12
    (B) T10
    (C) L3
    (D) C10

13. The branches of the inferior mesenteric artery supply the structure of the embryonic
    (A) Foregut
    (B) Hindgut
    (C) Midgut
    (D) Tipgut

14. The major branches of inferior mesenteric artery are
    (A) Left colic artery
    (B) Sigmoid artery
    (C) Superior rectal artery
    (D) All of the above

15. The inferior mesenteric artery supplies the
    (A) Rectum
    (B) Oesophagus
    (C) Liver
    (D) Stomach

16. The major vein of portal system is
    (A) Renal vein
    (B) Pulmonary vein
    (C) Portal vein
    (D) Tibial vein

17. Cystic veins drains
    (A) Gall bladder
    (B) Lungs
    (C) Stomach
    (D) Kidney

18. Which nerve supplies most of the alimentary canal and accessory organ
    (A) Olfactory nerve
    (B) Auditory nerve
    (C) Vagus nerve
    (D) Optic nerve

19. The effect of parasympathetic stimulation on the digestive system are
    (A) Increased muscular activity
    (B) Decrease muscular activity
    (C) Decrease glandular secretion
    (D) None of the above

20. The effects of sympathetic stimulation on the digestive system
    - (A) Increase glandular secretion
    - (B) Decrease glandular secretion
    - (C) Increase muscular secretion
    - (D) None of the above

21. The cheeks is formed by
    - (A) Buccinator muscle
    - (B) Obturators
    - (C) Sartorius
    - (D) Trapezius

22. Which of the following located anteriorly to the mouth?
    - (A) Tongue
    - (B) Cheeks
    - (C) Hard palate
    - (D) Lips

23. Which of the following form the opening of the oral cavity?
    - (A) Teeth
    - (B) Lips
    - (C) Tongue
    - (D) Oesophagus

24. Lips is made up of muscles called
    - (A) Orbicularis
    - (B) Deltoid
    - (C) Iliacus
    - (D) Psoas

25. The part of the mouth between the gums and the cheeks is the
    - (A) Lamina
    - (B) Medullar
    - (C) Vestibule
    - (D) Tubularae

26. Which of the following formed the roof of the mouth?
    - (A) Palate
    - (B) Cheeks
    - (C) Tongue
    - (D) Teeth

27. The anterior palate of the mouth is called
    - (A) Soft palate
    - (B) Hard palate
    - (C) Band palate
    - (D) Deep palate

28. The posterior palate of the mouth is called
    - (A) Deep palate
    - (B) Band palate
    - (C) Soft palate
    - (D) Hard palate

29. The muscular structure in the mouth covered by mucosa
    - (A) Teeth
    - (B) Tongue
    - (C) Hard palate
    - (D) Soft palate

30. Tongue is made up of
    (A) Stratified squamous epithelium cells
    (B) Simple cuboidal epithelium cells
    (C) Simple columnar epithelium cells
    (D) Simple squamous epithelium cells

31. The tongue contains muscle are
    (A) Extrinsic muscle
    (B) Intrinsic muscle
    (C) Both (A) and (B)
    (D) None of the above

32. Tongue is attached by its base
    (A) Hyoid bone
    (B) Temporal bone
    (C) Parietal bone
    (D) Lacrimal bone

33. The fold of mucous membrane found underneath the tongue
    (A) Soleus
    (B) Frenulum
    (C) Sortorius
    (D) Pectineus

34. The main arterial supply to the tongue
    (A) Renal artery
    (B) Hepatic artery
    (C) Lingual artery
    (D) Coronary artery

35. The nerve supply to the tongue which supplies the voluntary muscle
    (A) Optic nerve
    (B) Auditory nerve
    (C) Olfactory nerve
    (D) Hypoglossal nerve

36. The venous drainage by the tongue is
    (A) Hepatic vein
    (B) Lingual vein
    (C) Pulmonary vein
    (D) Renal vein

37. Which nerve responsible for taste in the tongue
    (A) Facial nerve
    (B) Auditory nerve
    (C) Optic nerve
    (D) Olfactory nerve

38. The more forward surface of the tongue is covered is numerous small bumps called
    (A) Papillae
    (B) Tubullae
    (C) Cuticle
    (D) Canals

39. The taste receptor are also known as
    (A) Optic cells
    (B) Cardiac cells
    (C) Gustatory cells
    (D) Olfactory cells

40. The tongue plays an important role in
    (A) Chewing
    (B) Swallowing
    (C) Speech
    (D) All of the above

41. The accessory digestive organs embedded in the sockets of the alveolar processes of the mandible and maxillae
    (A) Tongue
    (B) Teeth
    (C) Cheeks
    (D) Lips

42. The part of teeth that protrudes from the gum
    (A) Crown
    (B) Root
    (C) Neck
    (D) Band

43. The part of teeth that embedded in the bone
    (A) Band
    (B) Neck
    (C) Root
    (D) Crown

44. The part of teeth is slightly narrowed region where the crown merges with the root
    (A) Root
    (B) Neck
    (C) Crown
    (D) Band

45. Which of the following composed of calcified connective tissue that contains calcium
    (A) Dentine
    (B) Osteon
    (C) Callus
    (D) Tarsal

46. Which of the following form outermost hardest layer of teeth?
    (A) Osteon
    (B) Tarsal
    (C) Enamel
    (D) Callus

47. The root of the tooth covered by a substance and that attached the root of tooth to the socket
    (A) Tarsal
    (B) Osteon
    (C) Cementum
    (D) Pedicle

48. The space enclosed in dentine at the centre of the tooth is called
    (A) Pulp cavity
    (B) Pedicle cavity
    (C) Lacrimal cavity
    (D) Tarsal cavity

49. Most arterial blood supply to the teeth is by branches of the
    (A) Renal arteries
    (B) Pulmonary arteries
    (C) Maxillary arteries
    (D) Gastric arteries

50. The nerve supply to the upper teeth is by branches of the
    (A) Maxillary nerve
    (B) Optic nerve
    (C) Olfactory nerve
    (D) Auditory nerve

Answer Key

Digestive System (Part-02)

Question	Answer	Question	Answer
01	A = Splanchnic circulation	26	A = Palate
02	C = Oesophagus	27	B = Hard palate
03	A = T12 level	28	C = Soft palate
04	B = 1 cm	29	B = Tongue
05	D = All of the above	30	A = Stratified squamous epithelium cells
06	B = Oesophagus	31	C = Both (A) and (B)
07	A = Stomach	32	A = Hyoid bone
08	C = Spleen	33	B = Frenulum
09	A = L1 vertebrae	34	C = Lingual artery
10	B = Distal duodenum	35	D = Hypoglossal nerve
11	A = Inferior region of the head of the pancreas	36	B = Lingual vein
12	C = L3	37	A = Facial nerve
13	B = Hindgut	38	A = Papillae
14	D = All of the above	39	C = Gustatory cells
15	A = Rectum	40	D = All of the above
16	C = Portal vein	41	B = Teeth
17	A = Gall bladder	42	A = Crown
18	C = Vagus nerve	43	C = Root
19	A = Increased muscular activity	44	B = Neck
20	B = Decrease glandular secretion	45	A = Dentine
21	A = Buccinator muscle	46	C = Enamel
22	D = Lips	47	C = Cementum
23	B = Lips	48	A = Pulp cavity
24	A = Orbicularis	49	C = Maxillary arteries
25	C = Vestibule	50	A = Maxillary nerve

Part-03

1. The nerve supply to the lower teeth by branches of
   (A) Mandibular nerve
   (B) Vagus nerve
   (C) Olfactory nerve
   (D) Optic nerve

2. Maxillary nerve and mandibular nerve are both branches of
   (A) Optic nerve
   (B) Vagus nerve
   (C) Trigeminal nerve
   (D) Olfactory nerve

3. How many deciduous (milk) teeth are present in children
   (A) 28
   (B) 20
   (C) 32
   (D) 25

4. Total number of permanent teeth are
   (A) 20
   (B) 22
   (C) 32
   (D) 26

5. Which of the following is not a type of teeth?
   (A) Molars
   (B) Premolars
   (C) Canine
   (D) Pedicle

6. Total number of molars teeth are
   (A) 10
   (B) 8
   (C) 12
   (D) 16

7. The middlemost four teeth on the upper and lower jaws
   (A) Incisors
   (B) Canines
   (C) Premolars
   (D) Molars

8. Which gland release their secretions into duct that lead into the mouth
   (A) Pineal gland
   (B) Thyroid gland
   (C) Adrenal gland
   (D) Salivary gland

9. Which of the following is not a pair of salivary glands?
   (A) Parotid glands
   (B) Submandibular glands
   (C) Pedicle glands
   (D) Sublingual glands

10. Which salivary glands situated one on each side of the face, just below the external acoustic meatus
    (A) Pedicle glands
    (B) Parotid glands
    (C) Sublingual glands
    (D) Submandibular glands

11. Each parotid gland weighing is about
    (A) 90 – 100 gm
    (B) 50 – 60 gm
    (C) 20 – 30 gm
    (D) 70 – 80 gm

12. The largest salivary glands are
    (A) Pedicle glands
    (B) Sublingual glands
    (C) Submandibular glands
    (D) Parotid glands

13. Which salivary gland lie one on each side of the face under the angle of the jaw
    (A) Parotid glands
    (B) Sublingual glands
    (C) Submandibular glands
    (D) Pedicle glands

14. How many submandibular ducts open on the floor of the mouth?
    (A) Two
    (B) Four
    (C) Six
    (D) Five

15. Submandibular gland is supplied by the
    (A) Renal artery
    (B) Facial artery
    (C) Tibial artery
    (D) Hepatic artery

16. Which salivary gland lie under the mucous membrane of the floor of the mouth in front of the submandibular glands
    (A) Parotid glands
    (B) Sublingual glands
    (C) Pedicle gland
    (D) Sternal gland

17. The number of sublingual glands is
    (A) 40 – 60
    (B) 50 – 55
    (C) 8 – 20
    (D) 30 – 35

18. Salivary pH ranges from
    (A) 1.2 – 2.3
    (B) 2.2 – 2.9
    (C) 5.8 – 7.4
    (D) 3.3 – 3.8

19. Saliva contains the enzyme are
    (A) Amylase
    (B) Pepsin
    (C) Lactase
    (D) Lipase

20. The optimum pH for the action of salivary amylase is
    (A) 1.2
    (B) 2.3
    (C) 11.4
    (D) 6.8

21. How much saliva is produced daily?
    (A) 4.4 litres
    (B) 1.5 litres
    (C) 5.5 litres
    (D) 6.9 litres

22. Arterial supply to salivary glands is by various branches from the
    (A) External carotid arteries
    (B) Renal arteries
    (C) Coronary arteries
    (D) Tibial arteries

23. Composition of saliva
    (A) Water
    (B) Mineral salts
    (C) Mucous
    (D) All of the above

24. Functions of saliva
    (A) Taste
    (B) Lubrication of food
    (C) Non – specific defence
    (D) All of the above

25. Which phase of salivary secretion refers to secretion of saliva before entering the food into the mouth
    (A) Gastric phase
    (B) Intestinal phase
    (C) Cephalic phase
    (D) Oesophagus phase

26. After the process of chewing in mouth, the masticated food is propelled into the stomach through the process called
    (A) Deglutition
    (B) Agglutination
    (C) Ossification
    (D) Effusion

27. Which of the following is not a process of swallowing?
    (A) Voluntary stage
    (B) First involuntary stage
    (C) Second involuntary stage
    (D) Fifth involuntary stage

28. The first phase of swallowing is a voluntary phase are
    (A) Oral phase
    (B) Gastric phase
    (C) Pancreatic phase
    (D) Facial phase

29. The first involuntary stage is also called
    (A) Gastric stage
    (B) Pancreatic stage
    (C) Pharyngeal stage
    (D) Facial stage

30. The second involuntary stage is also called
    (A) Gastric stage
    (B) Oesophageal stage
    (C) Renal stage
    (D) Facial stage

31. The muscular tube that connects the oral and nasal cavity to the larynx and oesophagus
    (A) Pharynx
    (B) Epiglottis
    (C) Tongue
    (D) Teeth

32. The middle part of the pharynx is
    (A) Oropharynx
    (B) Nasopharynx
    (C) Cricoid cartilage
    (D) Laryngopharynx

33. The top part of pharynx is
    (A) Oropharynx
    (B) Nasopharynx
    (C) Orthopharynx
    (D) Laryngopharynx

34. The length of pharynx is about
    (A) 20 cm
    (B) 24 cm
    (C) 13 cm
    (D) 30 cm

35. The lowest part of pharynx is
    (A) Orthopharynx
    (B) Nasopharynx
    (C) Oropharynx
    (D) Laryngopharynx

36. The pharynx is continuous with the
    (A) Oesophagus
    (B) Stomach
    (C) Pancreas
    (D) Liver

37. The blood supply to the pharynx is by several branches of
    (A) Renal arteries
    (B) Facial arteries
    (C) Gastric arteries
    (D) Pulmonary arteries

38. Which of the following lies in the median plane in the thorax in front of the vertebral column and behind the trachea and the heart?
    (A) Stomach
    (B) Intestine
    (C) Pancreas
    (D) Oesophagus

39. Oesophagus begins in the neck at the level of
    (A) T12
    (B) C6
    (C) L12
    (D) S9

40. Oesophagus terminates by joining the cardiac orifice of the stomach at the level of
    (A) C3
    (B) C5
    (C) T11
    (D) L13

41. How long the oesophagus is
    (A) 25 cm
    (B) 40 cm
    (C) 50 cm
    (D) 35 cm

42. The diameter of oesophagus is
    (A) 10 cm
    (B) 12 cm
    (C) 2 cm
    (D) 8 cm

43. The arterial supplied to thoracic region of oesophagus by
    (A) Oesophageal arteries
    (B) Renal arteries
    (C) Gastric arteries
    (D) Pancreatic arteries

44. The arterial supplied to abdominal region of oesophagus by branches from
    (A) Renal arteries
    (B) Facial arteries
    (C) Inferior phrenic arteries
    (D) Temporal arteries

45. The mucous coat of oesophagus is formed by
    (A) Stratified squamous epithelium
    (B) Simple cardiac epithelium
    (C) Simple cuboidal epithelium
    (D) Simple columnar epithelium

46. Submucous coat of oesophagus is formed by
    (A) Adipose tissue
    (B) Cardiac tissue
    (C) Areolar tissue
    (D) Smooth muscle tissue

47. Lower oesophageal sphincter is
    (A) Renal sphincter
    (B) Cardiac sphincter
    (C) Facial sphincter
    (D) Pancreatic sphincter

48. Upper oesophageal sphincter is produced by
    (A) Cricopharyngeus muscle
    (B) Soleus muscle
    (C) Gracilis muscle
    (D) Sartorius muscle

49. The gastro – oesophageal junction is situated to the left of the
    (A) C1 vertebrae
    (B) L1 vertebrae
    (C) T11 vertebrae
    (D) S2 vertebrae

50. Which sphincter prevents the reflux of the gastric contents into the oesophagus
    (A) Cardiac sphincter
    (B) Cricopharyngeal sphincter
    (C) Renal sphincter
    (D) Pancreatic sphincter

Answer Key

Digestive System (Part-03)

Question	Answer	Question	Answer
01	A = Mandibular nerve	26	A = Deglutition
02	C = Trigeminal nerve	27	D = Fifth involuntary stage
03	B = 20	28	A = Oral phase
04	C = 32	29	C = Pharyngeal stage
05	D = Pedicle	30	B = Oesophageal stage
06	B = 8	31	A = Pharynx
07	A = Incisors	32	A = Oropharynx
08	D = Salivary gland	33	B = Nasopharynx
09	C = Pedicle gland	34	C = 13 cm
10	B = Parotid glands	35	D = Laryngopharynx
11	C = 20 – 30 gm	36	A = Oesophagus
12	D = Parotid glands	37	B = Facial arteries
13	C = Submandibular glands	38	D = Oesophagus
14	A = Two	39	B = C6
15	B = Facial artery	40	C = T11
16	B = Sublingual glands	41	A = 25 cm
17	C = 8 – 20	42	C = 2 cm
18	C = 5.8 – 7.4	43	A = Oesophageal arteries
19	A = Amylase	44	C = Inferior phrenic arteries
20	D = 6.8	45	A = Stratified squamous epithelium
21	B = 1.5 litres	46	C = Areolar tissue
22	A = External carotid arteries	47	C = Cardiac sphincter
23	D = All of the above	48	A = Cricopharyngeus muscle
24	D = All of the above	49	C = T11 vertebrae
25	C = Cephalic phase	50	A = Cardiac sphincter

Part-04

1. The J – shaped dilated portion of the alimentary canal situated in the epigastric, umbilical and left hypochondriac regions of the abdominal cavity
   (A) Stomach
   (B) Liver
   (C) Oesophagus
   (D) Pharynx

2. Which organ situated posterior to the stomach
   (A) Liver
   (B) Duodenum
   (C) Spleen
   (D) Small intestine

3. Which organ situated to the right of stomach
   (A) Spleen
   (B) Liver
   (C) Pancreas
   (D) Adrenal gland

4. Which organ situated superior to the stomach
   (A) Small intestine
   (B) Adrenal gland
   (C) Pancreas
   (D) Oesophagus

5. Which organ situated inferior to the stomach
   (A) Small intestine
   (B) Liver
   (C) Diaphragm
   (D) Oesophagus

6. Stomach is continuous with the oesophagus at the
   (A) Pyloric sphincter
   (B) Renal sphincter
   (C) Cardiac sphincter
   (D) Pancreatic sphincter

7. Stomach is continuous with duodenum at the
   (A) Renal sphincter
   (B) Pyloric sphincter
   (C) Cardiac sphincter
   (D) Pancreatic sphincter

8. The volume of stomach when it empty
   (A) 1000 mL
   (B) 50 mL
   (C) 700 mL
   (D) 1200 mL

9. The volume of stomach when it can expand to accommodate of solids and liquids under normal conditions
   (A) 4000 – 5000 mL
   (B) 5000 – 6000 mL
   (C) 1200 – 1500 mL
   (D) 100 – 120 mL

10. Which of the following is short, lies on the posterior surface of the stomach and is downward continuation of the posterior wall of the oesophagus?

    (A) Longer curvature   (B) Lesser curvature

    (C) Larger curvature   (D) Shorter curvature

11. The large convex border of the stomach is called

    (A) Greater curvature   (B) Small curvature

    (C) Shorter curvature   (D) Longer curvature

12. Which region of stomach surrounds the superior opening of the stomach at the T11 level

    (A) Cardia   (B) Fundus

    (C) Pylorus   (D) Body

13. Which region of stomach is rounded, often gas filled portion superior to and left of the cardia?

    (A) Body   (B) Pylorus

    (C) Fundus   (D) Cardia

14. The large central portion inferior to the fundus of the stomach

    (A) Cardia   (B) Body

    (C) Pylorus   (D) Fundus

15. The area of stomach connects the stomach to the duodenum

    (A) Cardia   (B) Fundus

    (C) Body   (D) Pylorus

16. The pylorus can be subdivided into

    (A) Pylorus antrum   (B) Pylorus canal

    (C) Both (A) and (B)   (D) None of the above

17. The outer layer of stomach is composed of

    (A) Longitudinal fibres   (B) Circular fibres

    (C) Rectangular fibres   (D) Oblique fibres

18. The middle layer of stomach is composed of

    (A) Oblique fibres   (B) Circular fibres

    (C) Rectangular fibres   (D) Longitudinal fibres

19. The outer layer of stomach is composed of

    (A) Rectangular fibres   (B) Circular fibres

    (C) Longitudinal fibres   (D) Oblique fibres

20. Mucosa of the stomach is present in the form of large folds called
    (A) Rugae
    (B) Cisternae
    (C) Cristae
    (D) Tubulae

21. The mucosa of the stomach contains cells are
    (A) Mast cells
    (B) Oligodendrocytes
    (C) Parietal cells
    (D) Stem cells

22. Arterial supply to the stomach is by
    (A) Facial artery
    (B) Renal artery
    (C) Left gastric artery
    (D) Pulmonary artery

23. The right and left gastric veins drain into the
    (A) Hepatic portal vein
    (B) Renal vein
    (C) Tibial vein
    (D) Facial vein

24. Which cells mainly secrete pepsinogen
    (A) Mast cells
    (B) Stem cells
    (C) Chief cells
    (D) Dendritic cells

25. Which cells secrets the hydrochloric acids
    (A) Parietal cells
    (B) Mast cells
    (C) Dendritic cells
    (D) Adipocyte

26. The pH of HCl acid in stomach is
    (A) 7.6
    (B) 1.5
    (C) 8.9
    (D) 12.6

27. Which glands are found in the mucosa of cardia just around the distal end of oesophagus?
    (A) Pyloric glands
    (B) Pineal glands
    (C) Adrenal glands
    (D) Cardiac tubular glands

28. Which glands are found in the antrum and pylorus region of the stomach?
    (A) Pyloric glands
    (B) Thymus glands
    (C) Adrenal glands
    (D) Pineal glands

29. Which cells is responsible for release of the hormone gastrin?
    (A) H cells
    (B) P cells
    (C) G cells
    (D) D cells

30. Which tissue consists in mucous coat which connecting the muscular and mucous coats of the stomach

   (A) Loose areolar connective tissue

   (B) Stratified squamous epithelium

   (C) Simple squamous epithelium

   (D) Simple cuboidal epithelium

31. Which plexus located between the layers of circular and longitudinal muscles of the stomach

   (A) Submucosal plexus

   (B) Meissner's plexus

   (C) Myenteric plexus

   (D) Pedicle plexus

32. Which plexus located in the submucosal layer of the stomach

   (A) Medullar plexus

   (B) Pedicle plexus

   (C) Meissner's plexus

   (D) Auerbach's plexus

33. Intrinsic factor secreted by

   (A) Parietal cells

   (B) Mast cells

   (C) Adipocyte

   (D) Stem cells

34. How much gastric juice secreted daily by stomach?

   (A) 8 litres

   (B) 2 litres

   (C) 5 litres

   (D) 7 litres

35. Enzymes present in gastric juice

   (A) Pepsin

   (B) Gastric lipase

   (C) Gastric amylase

   (D) All of the above

36. Gastric juice consists of

   (A) Water

   (B) Mineral salts

   (C) Hydrochloric acids

   (D) All of the above

37. Pepsin have evolved to act most effectively at a pH between

   (A) 1.5 to 3.5

   (B) 7.8 to 8.2

   (C) 8.9 to 9.3

   (D) 10.3 to 11.9

38. Pepsinogen is inactive precursor of

   (A) Gelatinase

   (B) Pepsin

   (C) Lactase

   (D) Maltase

39. Pepsin break protein into

   (A) Carbohydrates

   (B) Vitamins

   (C) Polypeptides

   (D) Fats

40. The stimulation increases the secretion of HCl by parietal cells and pepsin by chief cells

   (A) Olfactory stimulation

   (B) Vagal stimulation

   (C) Accessory stimulation

   (D) Auditory stimulation

41. Which of the following is not a phase of gastric secretion?

   (A) Cephalic phase

   (B) Gastric phase

   (C) Intestinal phase

   (D) Pedicle phase

42. In which phase the secretion of gastric juice occurs before food reaches the stomach

   (A) Pedicle phase

   (B) Cephalic phase

   (C) Intestinal phase

   (D) Gastric phase

43. Appetite centre present in

   (A) Stomach

   (B) Intestine

   (C) Hypothalamus

   (D) Liver

44. How much gastric acid secreted in cephalic phase?

   (A) 60 %

   (B) 80 %

   (C) 20 %

   (D) 90 %

45. In which phase gastric secretion occurs when food enters the stomach

   (A) Gastric phase

   (B) Medullar phase

   (C) Cephalic phase

   (D) Intestinal phase

46. Gastrin secretion is suppressed when the pH in the pylorus falls to about

   (A) 7.5

   (B) 1.5

   (C) 9.5

   (D) 8.5

47. How much gastric acid secreted in gastric phase?

   (A) 20 %

   (B) 15 %

   (C) 30 %

   (D) 70 %

48. Which phase occurs when the chyme reaches the duodenum

   (A) Gastric phase

   (B) Cephalic phase

   (C) Intestinal phase

   (D) Medullar phase

49. Which hormone produced by endocrine cells in the intestinal mucosa

   (A) Melatonin

   (B) Thyroxine

   (C) Insulin

   (D) Secretin

50. Production and secretion of intrinsic factor needed for absorption of

   (A) Vitamin A

   (B) Vitamin B12

   (C) Vitamin D

   (D) Vitamin C

Answer Key

Digestive System (Part-04)

Question	Answer	Question	Answer
01	A = Stomach	26	B = 1.5
02	C = Spleen	27	D = Cardiac tubular glands
03	B = Liver	28	A = Pyloric glands
04	D = Oesophagus	29	C = G cells
05	A = Small intestine	30	A = Loose areolar connective tissue
06	C = Cardiac sphincter	31	C = Myenteric plexus
07	B = Pyloric sphincter	32	C = Meissner's plexus
08	B = 50 mL	33	A = Parietal cells
09	C = 1200 – 1500 mL	34	B = 2 litres
10	B = Lesser curvature	35	D = All of the above
11	A = Greater curvature	36	D = All of the above
12	A = Cardia	37	A = 1.5 to 3.5
13	C = Fundus	38	B = Pepsin
14	B = Body	39	C = Polypeptides
15	D = Pylorus	40	B = Vagal stimulation
16	C = Both (A) and (B)	41	D = Pedicle phase
17	A = Longitudinal fibres	42	B = Cephalic phase
18	B = Circular fibres	43	C = Hypothalamus
19	D = Oblique fibres	44	C = 20 %
20	A = Rugae	45	A = Gastric phase
21	C = Parietal cells	46	B = 1.5
22	C = Left gastric artery	47	D = 70 %
23	A = Hepatic portal vein	48	C = Intestinal phase
24	C = Chief cells	49	D = Secretin
25	A = Parietal cells	50	B = Vitamin B12

Part-05

1. Which of the following is continuous with the stomach at the pyloric sphincter?

    (A) Oesophagus

    (B) Small intestine

    (C) Kidney

    (D) Pharynx

2. The diameter of small intestine is about

    (A) 7 cm

    (B) 8 cm

    (C) 2.5 cm

    (D) 10 cm

3. How long the small intestine

    (A) 5 metres

    (B) 10 metres

    (C) 15 metres

    (D) 20 metres

4. Small intestine has absorptive area over

    (A) 500 m²

    (B) 250 m²

    (C) 600 m²

    (D) 700 m²

5. Small intestine leads into the large intestine at the

    (A) Tricuspid valve

    (B) Bicuspid valve

    (C) Cardiac sphincter

    (D) Ileocecal valve

6. The first part of the small intestine is

    (A) Duodenum

    (B) Jejunum

    (C) Ileum

    (D) Pedicle

7. How long the duodenum is

    (A) 40 cm

    (B) 25 cm

    (C) 50 cm

    (D) 60 cm

8. The middle section of the small intestine

    (A) Ileum

    (B) Duodenum

    (C) Jejunum

    (D) Cisternae

9. How long the jejunum is

    (A) 4 metres

    (B) 2 metres

    (C) 5 metres

    (D) 6 metres

10. The last part of small intestine is
    - (A) Ileum
    - (C) Duodenum
    - (B) Jejunum
    - (D) Pedicle

11. How long the ileum is
    - (A) 7 metres
    - (C) 3 metres
    - (B) 1 metre
    - (D) 5 metres

12. CCK cells secretes
    - (A) Secretin
    - (C) Lysozyme
    - (B) Mucous
    - (D) Cholecystokinin

13. Mucous is secreted by
    - (A) Goblet cells
    - (C) S cells
    - (B) K cells
    - (D) CCK cells

14. S cells secretes
    - (A) Cholecystokinin
    - (C) Lysozyme
    - (B) Mucous
    - (D) Secretin

15. Lysozyme is secreted by
    - (A) S cells
    - (C) Paneth cells
    - (B) K cells
    - (D) CCK cells

16. Which cells absorb and digest nutrients
    - (A) CCK cells
    - (C) K cells
    - (B) Absorptive cells
    - (D) Paneth cells

17. Which cells secrete alkaline mucous
    - (A) Brunner's gland
    - (C) K cells
    - (B) S cells
    - (D) Paneth cells

18. The surface area of small intestine mucosa is greatly increased by
    - (A) Circular folds
    - (C) Microvilli
    - (B) Villi
    - (D) All of the above

19. The permanent folds of the mucosal and submucosal layers of the small intestine
    - (A) Spherical folds
    - (C) Rectangular folds
    - (B) Circular folds
    - (D) Round folds

20. The finger – like projections present on the mucosal epithelium of small intestine
    - (A) Flagella
    - (C) Villi
    - (B) Cisternae
    - (D) Pedicle

21. The villi is lined by columnar cells called
    - (A) Osteocytes
    - (B) Enterocytes
    - (C) Astrocytes
    - (D) Oligodendrocytes

22. Enterocytes give rise to many projections called
    - (A) Microvilli
    - (B) Minivilli
    - (C) Microvilli
    - (D) Sub villi

23. Microvilli is also called
    - (A) Brush border
    - (B) Band border
    - (C) Tail border
    - (D) Tape border

24. How many microvilli are estimated to be present per square millimetre of the small intestine
    - (A) 1000 million
    - (B) 200 million
    - (C) 600 million
    - (D) 900 million

25. Size of microvilli is about
    - (A) 9 μm
    - (B) 12 μm
    - (C) 1 μm
    - (D) 11 μm

26. How long the villi
    - (A) 6 mm
    - (B) 1 mm
    - (C) 7 mm
    - (D) 9 mm

27. Proximal to the major duodenal papilla is supplied by the
    - (A) Facial artery
    - (B) Renal artery
    - (C) Gastroduodenal artery
    - (D) Pancreatic renal artery

28. Distal to the major duodenal papilla is supplied by the
    - (A) Gastrohepatic artery
    - (B) Pancreaticoduodenal artery
    - (C) Renal artery
    - (D) Faciotemporal artery

29. The arterial supply to the jejunoileum is from the
    - (A) Superior mesenteric artery
    - (B) Renal artery
    - (C) Facial artery
    - (D) Pulmonary artery

30. The innermost layer of small intestine which contains the epithelium, lamina propria and muscularis mucosae
    - (A) Submucosa
    - (B) Mucosa
    - (C) Muscularis externa
    - (D) Adventitia

31. The connective tissue layer of small intestine which contains blood vessel, lymphatics and submucosal plexus

(A) Mucosa

(B) Muscularis externa

(C) Submucosa

(D) Adventitia

32. The layer of small intestine which consists two smooth muscle layers; outer longitudinal layer and inner circular layer

(A) Adventitia

(B) Submucosa

(C) Mucosa

(D) Muscularis externa

33. The outermost layer of small intestine is

(A) Medulla

(B) Laminae

(C) Adventitia

(D) Mucosa

34. How much intestinal juice is secreted daily by the glands of the small intestine

(A) 200 mL

(B) 1500 mL

(C) 3000 mL

(D) 3500 mL

35. The type of movements of the small intestine that carry out digestion in the small intestine mechanically

(A) Mixing contractions

(B) Propulsive movements

(C) Both (A) and (B)

(D) None of the above

36. The frequency of segmentation contractions in all parts of the small intestine is about

(A) 50 /min

(B) 60 /min

(C) 40 /min

(D) 12 /min

37. The chyme is propelled towards the anus due to peristalsis wave at the eaten of about

(A) 80 mm/min

(B) 10 mm/min

(C) 40 mm/min

(D) 60 mm/min

38. The time taken by chyme to reach caccum from duodenum is about

(A) 6 – 7 hrs

(B) 7 – 8 hrs

(C) 3 – 5 hrs

(D) 8 – 9 hrs

39. The carbohydrates – digesting enzyme is

(A) Nucleosides

(B) Phosphatase

(C) Maltase

(D) Peptidase

40. The protein - digesting enzyme is
   (A) Peptidase
   (B) Maltase
   (C) Sucrase
   (D) Lactase

41. Nucleotide - digesting enzyme is
   (A) Maltase
   (B) Sucrase
   (C) Peptidase
   (D) Nucleosidases

42. Carbohydrates are break down into
   (A) Amino acids
   (B) Fatty acids
   (C) Monosaccharides
   (D) Glycerol

43. Proteins are break down into
   (A) Amino acids
   (B) Fatty acids
   (C) Glycerol
   (D) Monosaccharides

44. Most of the digestive enzymes in the small intestine are contained in the
   (A) Osteocytes
   (B) Enterocytes
   (C) Oocytes
   (D) Astrocytes

45. Secretion of Brunner's gland is increased by
   (A) Vagus stimulation
   (B) Accessory stimulation
   (C) Optic stimulation
   (D) Auditory stimulation

46. Which hormone play an important role in increasing the movements of the villi
   (A) Melatonin
   (B) Villikinin
   (C) Thyroxine
   (D) Melanin

47. The diameter of large intestine is about
   (A) 10 cm
   (B) 18 cm
   (C) 6 cm
   (D) 14 cm

48. The length of large intestine is about
   (A) 300 cm
   (B) 150 cm
   (C) 500 cm
   (D) 450 cm

49. The blind - ended sac into which opens the lower end of ileum
   (A) Caecum
   (B) Rectum
   (C) Anus
   (D) Stomach

50. How long the caecum is
   (A) 15 – 16 cm
   (B) 20 – 22 cm
   (C) 8 – 9 cm
   (D) 1 – 2 cm

Answer Key

Digestive System (Part-05)

Question	Answer	Question	Answer
01	B = Small intestine	26	B = 1 mm
02	C = 2.5 cm	27	C = Gastroduodenal artery
03	A = 5 metres	28	B = Pancreaticoduodenal artery
04	B = 250 m^2	29	A = Superior mesenteric artery
05	D = Ileocaecal valve	30	B = Mucosa
06	A = Duodenum	31	C = Submucosa
07	B = 25 cm	32	D = Muscularis externa
08	C = Jejunum	33	C = Adventitia
09	B = 2 metres	34	B = 1500 mL
10	A = Ileum	35	Both (A) and (B)
11	C = 3 metres	36	D = 12 /min
12	D = Cholecystokinin	37	B = 10 mm/min
13	A = Goblet cells	38	C = 3 – 5 hrs
14	D = Secretin	39	C = Maltase
15	C = Paneth cells	40	A = Peptidase
16	B = Absorptive cells	41	D = Nucleosidases
17	A = Brunner's gland	42	C = Monosaccharides
18	D = All of the above	43	A = Amino acids
19	B = Circular folds	44	B = Enterocytes
20	C = Villi	45	A = Vagus stimulation
21	B = Enterocytes	46	B = Villikinin
22	C = Microvilli	47	C = 6 cm
23	A = Brush border	48	B = 150 cm
24	B = 200 million	49	A = Caecum
25	C = 1 μm	50	C = 8 – 9 cm

Part-06

1. The most proximal part of the large intestine
   - (A) Anus
   - (B) Caecum
   - (C) Duodenum
   - (D) Jejunum

2. Lymph from the caecum drains into
   - (A) Ileocolic lymph nodes
   - (B) Cervical lymph nodes
   - (C) Epitrochlear lymph nodes
   - (D) Axillary lymph nodes

3. The caecum merges with the long tube called
   - (A) Anus
   - (B) Colon
   - (C) Stomach
   - (D) Oesophagus

4. The worm – shaped tube that arises from the medial sides of caecum is called
   - (A) Cisternae
   - (B) Tibia
   - (C) Appendix
   - (D) Ileum

5. Which colon passes upwards from the caecum to the level of the liver
   - (A) Ascending colon
   - (B) Transverse colon
   - (C) Vertical colon
   - (D) Sigmoid colon

6. Which colon extends across the abdominal cavity in front of the duodenum and the stomach to the area of the spleen
   - (A) Sigmoid colon
   - (B) Ascending colon
   - (C) Transverse colon
   - (D) Descending colon

7. Which colon passes down the left side to the abdominal cavity, then curve towards the midline
   - (A) Descending colon
   - (B) Transverse colon
   - (C) Distal colon
   - (D) Vertical colon

8. How long the descending colon
   - (A) 100 cm
   - (B) 60 cm
   - (C) 70 cm
   - (D) 25 cm

9. Which colon is S – shaped curve in the pelvic cavity that continues downwards to become rectum?
   - (A) Alpha colon
   - (B) Transverse colon
   - (C) Vertical colon
   - (D) Sigmoid colon

10. How long the sigmoid colon
    (A) 10 cm
    (B) 13 cm
    (C) 40 cm
    (D) 19 cm

11. The part of large intestine connects the sigmoid colon to the anal canal
    (A) Rectum
    (B) Ileum
    (C) Jejunum
    (D) Caecum

12. Which of the following lies anterior to the sacrum and coccyx?
    (A) Ileum
    (B) Duodenum
    (C) Rectum
    (D) Stomach

13. How long the rectum is
    (A) 70 cm
    (B) 13 cm
    (C) 40 cm
    (D) 50 cm

14. The terminal opening of the GI tract situated below the root of the tail
    (A) Anus
    (B) Ileum
    (C) Caecum
    (D) Jejunum

15. How long the anal canal is
    (A) 9.3 cm
    (B) 8.7 cm
    (C) 3.8 cm
    (D) 10.9 cm

16. The muscular sphincter of anal canal is
    (A) Internal sphincter
    (B) External sphincter
    (C) Both (A) and (B)
    (D) None of the above

17. Which anal sphincter is under involuntary control?
    (A) Internal sphincter
    (B) Distal sphincter
    (C) Pedicle sphincter
    (D) External sphincter

18. Which anal sphincter is under voluntary control?
    (A) Distal sphincter
    (B) External sphincter
    (C) Pedicle sphincter
    (D) Internal sphincter

19. Which anal sphincter consists smooth muscle
    (A) Pedicle sphincter
    (B) Lateral sphincter
    (C) External sphincter
    (D) Internal sphincter

20. Which anal sphincter consists skeletal muscle
    (A) Pedicle sphincter
    (B) Internal sphincter
    (C) External sphincter
    (D) Lateral sphincter

21. The large intestine is lined by mucosa with

(A) Crypts of Lieberkuhh

(B) Cells of Langerhans

(C) Islets of Langerhans

(D) Oligodendrocytes

22. The colon helps to absorb a small volume of water from the lumen is about

(A) 1000 ml/day

(B) 400 ml/day

(C) 2000 ml/day

(D) 2500 ml/day

23. Which harmless bacteria present in large intestine

(A) E. coli

(B) S. Typhi

(C) S. aureus

(D) V. cholerae

24. Function of large intestine is

(A) Absorption of water and electrolytes

(B) Formation of faeces

(C) Absorption of vitamins

(D) All of the above

25. The accessory organ of digestive system located in the epigastric and hypochondriac region of the abdomen

(A) Pancreas

(B) Kidney

(C) Salivary glands

(D) Lungs

26. How long the pancreas is

(A) 30 cm

(B) 45 cm

(C) 15 cm

(D) 50 cm

27. The part of pancreas lies near the curve of duodenum is

(A) Body

(B) Band

(C) Tail

(D) Head

28. The part of pancreas superior to the head and lies behind the greater curvature of the stomach is called

(A) Band

(B) Root

(C) Body

(D) Head

29. The tapering part of pancreas almost reaching the spleen in front of the left kidney is called

(A) Tail

(B) Band

(C) Root

(D) Head

30. The exocrine part of stomach constitutes about the total cells of pancreas about

    (A) 10 %   (B) 99 %

    (C) 30 %   (D) 55 %

31. Exocrine cells of pancreas is glandular epithelial cells called

    (A) Cisternae   (B) Crista

    (C) Acini   (D) Pedicle

32. Exocrine cells of pancreas secrete

    (A) Pancreatic juice   (B) Renal juice

    (C) Bile juice   (D) Saliva

33. Which enzyme not contain in pancreatic juice

    (A) Trypsin   (B) Lipase

    (C) Amylase   (D) Renin

34. The pancreatic juice leaves the pancreas through a large main duct called

    (A) Pancreatic duct   (B) Renal duct

    (C) Pulmonary duct   (D) Gastric duct

35. The pancreatic duct unites with the common bile duct of the liver to form

    (A) Hepatopancreatic pedicle   (B) Renopancreatic crista

    (C) Hepatopancreatic ampulla   (D) Cervical vertebrae

36. Which of the following is proteolytic enzyme?

    (A) Trypsin   (B) Pancreatic lipase

    (C) Phospholipase A   (D) Phospholipase B

37. Which enzyme converts polysaccharides to disaccharides

    (A) Trypsin   (B) Lipase

    (C) Chymotrypsin   (D) Amylase

38. Which ducts receive secretions produced by acini and pass it on to interlobular ducts

    (A) Intervertebral ducts   (B) Intercalated ducts

    (C) Interstitial ducts   (D) Intersternal ducts

39. The functional unit of the exocrine pancreas

    (A) Mast cells   (B) Stem cells

    (C) Acinar cells   (D) Goblet cells

40. The pancreatic cells which produced, stored and release digestive enzymes

    (A) Goblet cells   (B) Stem cells

    (C) Mast cells   (D) Acinar cells

41. Accessory pancreatic duct open into
   - (A) Oesophagus
   - (B) Pharynx
   - (C) Colon
   - (D) Duodenum

42. How much pancreatic juice is secreted per day?
   - (A) 100 – 200 mL
   - (B) 1200 – 1500 mL
   - (C) 10 – 20 mL
   - (D) 200 – 300 mL

43. The pancreatic juice has pH
   - (A) 1.2 – 2.3
   - (B) 2.3 – 2.9
   - (C) 7.8 – 8.4
   - (D) 4.4 – 5.2

44. Pancreatic juice composed of water is about
   - (A) 0.5 %
   - (B) 99.5 %
   - (C) 12.4 %
   - (D) 30.5 %

45. Which nerve supplying exocrine gland of pancreas
   - (A) Vagus
   - (B) Accessory
   - (C) Olfactory
   - (D) Auditory

46. Pancreatic juice is alkaline due to high concentration of
   - (A) Calcium
   - (B) Iron
   - (C) Bicarbonate
   - (D) Chloride

47. Which organ located in the upper and right region of the abdominal cavity immediately beneath the diaphragm
   - (A) Brain
   - (B) Kidney
   - (C) Stomach
   - (D) Liver

48. The largest gland in the body
   - (A) Pancreas
   - (B) Liver
   - (C) Lungs
   - (D) Kidney

49. The weight of liver is about
   - (A) 1.2 – 2.2 Kg
   - (B) 4.4 – 5.2 Kg
   - (C) 3.9 – 4.2 Kg
   - (D) 6.2 – 6.9 Kg

50. Which organ inferior to the liver
   - (A) Stomach
   - (B) Pharynx
   - (C) Larynx
   - (D) Lungs

Answer Key

Digestive System (Part-06)

Question	Answer	Question	Answer
01	B = Caecum	26	C = 15 cm
02	A = Ileocolic lymph nodes	27	D = Head
03	B = Colon	28	C = Body
04	C = Appendix	29	A = Tail
05	A = Ascending colon	30	B = 99 %
06	C = Transverse colon	31	C = Acini
07	A = Descending colon	32	A = Pancreatic juice
08	D = 25 cm	33	D = Renin
09	D = Sigmoid colon	34	A = Pancreatic duct
10	C = 40 cm	35	C = Hepatopancreatic ampulla
11	A = Rectum	36	A = Trypsin
12	C = Rectum	37	D = Amylase
13	B = 13 cm	38	B = Intercalated ducts
14	A = Anus	39	C = Acinar cells
15	C = 3.8 cm	40	D = Acinar cells
16	C = Both (A) and (B)	41	D = Duodenum
17	A = Internal sphincter	42	B = 1200 – 1500 mL
18	B = External sphincter	43	C = 7.8 – 8.4
19	D = Internal sphincter	44	B = 99.5 %
20	C = External sphincter	45	A = Vagus
21	A = Crypts of Lieberkuhh	46	C = Bicarbonate
22	B = 400 ml/day	47	D = Liver
23	A = E. coli	48	B = Liver
24	D = All of the above	49	A =1.2 – 2.2 Kg
25	A = Pancreas	50	A = Stomach

Part-07

1. Which of the following located posterior to the liver?
   (A) Kidney
   (B) Colon
   (C) Oesophagus
   (D) Rectum

2. The portal vein, hepatic artery, parasympathetic and sympathetic nerves, hepatic ducts, lymph vessels enter and leave the liver at a point called
   (A) Portal fissure
   (B) Portal cisternae
   (C) Portal crista
   (D) Portal pedicle

3. The lobes of the liver are made of tiny functional units called
   (A) Medulla
   (B) Lobules
   (C) Trabeculi
   (D) Tubulae

4. Liver consists specialized epithelial cells called
   (A) Melanocytes
   (B) Astrocytes
   (C) Hepatocytes
   (D) Osteocytes

5. Hepatocytes secreted bile daily about
   (A) $100-200$ mL
   (B) $200-300$ mL
   (C) $300-400$ mL
   (D) $800-1000$ mL

6. Composition of bile is
   (A) Water
   (B) Mineral salts
   (C) Bile salts
   (D) All of the above

7. The anterosuperior surface of the liver
   (A) Diaphragmatic surface
   (B) Renal surface
   (C) Sphenic surface
   (D) Pancreatic surface

8. The posteroinferior surface of the liver
   (A) Dorsal surface
   (B) Visceral surface
   (C) Ventral surface
   (D) Proximal surface

9. Which space located between the diaphragm and the anterior and superior aspects of the liver
   (A) Subhepatic space
   (B) Sublateral space
   (C) Subphrenic space
   (D) Distal space

10. The subdivision of the supracolic compartment, this peritoneal space is located between the inferior surface of the liver and the transverse colon
   (A) Subhepatic surface
   (B) Sublateral surface
   (C) Subdistal surface
   (D) Subventral surface

11. A potential space between the visceral surface of the liver and the right kidney
   (A) Sublateral space
   (B) Morison's pouch
   (C) Subdistal space
   (D) Subventrical space

12. The sickle – shaped ligament attaches the anterior surface of the liver to the anterior abdominal wall
   (A) Falciform ligament
   (B) Lesser omentum
   (C) Stratified ligament
   (D) Stratum corneum

13. The ligament attaches the superior surface of the liver to the inferior surface of the diaphragm and demarcates the bare area of the liver
   (A) Renal ligament
   (B) Coronary ligament
   (C) Conchae ligament
   (D) Phalanges ligament

14. Which attaches the liver to the lesser curvature of the stomach and first part of duodenum
   (A) Greater curvature
   (B) Shorter curvature
   (C) Lesser omentum
   (D) Smaller curvature

15. The liver is covered by a fibrous layer known as
   (A) Glisson's capsule
   (B) Deltoid capsule
   (C) Obturators capsule
   (D) Soleus capsule

16. Which lobe located on the upper aspect of the visceral surface
   (A) Cisternae lobe
   (B) Caudate lobe
   (C) Tertiary lobe
   (D) Pedicle lobe

17. Which lobe located on the lower aspects of the visceral surface
   (A) Quadrate lobe
   (B) Tertiary lobe
   (C) Proximal lobe
   (D) Distal lobe

18. In between the hepatocytes, small ducts are present to receive the bile secreted by hepatocytes. These small ducts are called
   (A) Bile canaliculi
   (B) Bile foramina
   (C) Bile vertebral
   (D) Bile column

19. The special types of cells are also present in between the hepatic sinusoids called

    (A) Mast cells
    (B) Kupffer cells
    (C) Stem cells
    (D) Goblets cells

20. The liver produced the plasma proteins contained in the bloodstream about

    (A) 10 %
    (B) 20 %
    (C) 90 %
    (D) 14 %

21. The yellow bile pigment produced through the breakdown of RBCs

    (A) Bilirubin
    (B) Urea
    (C) Glucose
    (D) Uric acids

22. Which bilirubin is insoluble in water?

    (A) Conjugated bilirubin
    (B) Functional bilirubin
    (C) Unconjugated bilirubin
    (D) Non functional bilirubin

23. Which bilirubin is soluble in water?

    (A) Non-functional bilirubin
    (B) Conjugated bilirubin
    (C) Functional bilirubin
    (D) Non-functional bilirubin

24. The breakdown of glycogen to glucose

    (A) Lipogenesis
    (B) Glycogenesis
    (C) Glycogenolysis
    (D) Glycogenesis

25. Formation of glucose from non – carbohydrate sources

    (A) Glucogenesis
    (B) Lipogenesis
    (C) Glycogenesis
    (D) Glycogenolysis

26. The key regulatory enzyme in glycogenesis is

    (A) Glycogen synthase
    (B) Glycogen maltase
    (C) Glycogen lipase
    (D) Glycogen ligase

27. Glucose is converted to glucose – 6 – phosphate by

    (A) Glucolipase
    (B) Glucomaltase
    (C) Glucokinase
    (D) Glucoamylase

28. Triglycerides are hydrolysed into fatty acids and glycerol by

    (A) Triglyceride lactase
    (B) Triglyceride sucrase
    (C) Triglyceride maltase
    (D) Triglyceride lipase

29. The urea cycle occurs both within the mitochondria and cytoplasm of the

    (A) Hepatocytes
    (B) Astrocytes
    (C) Oligodendrocytes
    (D) Osteocytes

30. Which organ is important in the metabolic activation of Vitamin D
    (A) Lungs
    (B) Kidney
    (C) Liver
    (D) Stomach

31. Liver acts as reservoir of blood and stores blood about
    (A) 100 mL
    (B) 1200 mL
    (C) 650 mL
    (D) 1500 mL

32. How much glycogen stored in the liver?
    (A) 1000 g
    (B) 100 g
    (C) 700 g
    (D) 800 g

33. Vitamin A is also called
    (A) Retinol
    (B) Tocopherol
    (C) Niacin
    (D) Pyridoxine

34. Function of vitamin E is
    (A) Antioxidant
    (B) Prevents free radical
    (C) Protect Vitamin A
    (D) All of the above

35. Vitamin B12 is also called
    (A) Thiamine
    (B) Niacin
    (C) Cobalamin
    (D) Tocopherol

36. The destruction of RBCs also occurs in
    (A) Brain
    (B) Kidney
    (C) Liver
    (D) Lungs

37. The hepatic artery which is a branch of coeliac trunk supplies the total
    blood about
    (A) 80 – 90 %
    (B) 20 – 25 %
    (C) 70 – 80 %
    (D) 60 – 70 %

38. Portal vein which collect blood from the mesenteric and splenic vascular
    bed supplies total blood about
    (A) 10 – 15 %
    (B) 20 – 25 %
    (C) 75 – 80 %
    (D) 30 – 35 %

39. How long the hepatic duct is
    (A) 10 cm
    (B) 20 cm
    (C) 26 cm
    (D) 4 cm

40. The pear – shaped sac attached to the posterior surface of the liver by
    connective tissue
    (A) Gall bladder
    (B) Stomach
    (C) Spleen
    (D) Thyroid

41. How long the common bile duct
    - (A) 20 cm
    - (B) 30 cm
    - (C) 8 cm
    - (D) 34 cm

42. Gall bladder has capacity to store bile about
    - (A) 30 – 50 mL
    - (B) 100 – 200 mL
    - (C) 200 – 250 mL
    - (D) 90 – 100 mL

43. How long the gall bladder is
    - (A) 70 – 80 cm
    - (B) 7 – 10 cm
    - (C) 40 – 45 cm
    - (D) 80 – 90 cm

44. The bile secreted by hepatocytes in the liver and stored in the
    - (A) Gall bladder
    - (B) Stomach
    - (C) Pancreas
    - (D) Kidney

45. The lowest globular part, which projects beyond the inferior border of liver and is surrounded all around by peritoneum
    - (A) Fundus
    - (B) Band
    - (C) Tail
    - (D) Cristae

46. The central part of gall bladder
    - (A) Body
    - (B) Fundus
    - (C) Cristae
    - (D) Tail

47. Which artery supplies the blood to the gall bladder
    - (A) Renal artery
    - (B) Pulmonary artery
    - (C) Facial artery
    - (D) Cystic artery

48. The venous supplies the blood to the gall bladder
    - (A) Facial vein
    - (B) Renal vein
    - (C) Cystic vein
    - (D) Pulmonary vein

49. The rapid absorption of water through the mucosa of gallbladder results in the concentration of the bile up to
    - (A) 40 – 50 folds
    - (B) 12 – 15 folds
    - (C) 60 – 70 folds
    - (D) 55 – 60 folds

50. The bile released through the common bile duct into the
    - (A) Colon
    - (B) Rectum
    - (C) Caecum
    - (D) Duodenum

Answer Key

Digestive System (Part-07)

Question	Answer	Question	Answer
01	C = Oesophagus	26	A = Glycogen synthase
02	A = Portal fissure	27	C = Glucokinase
03	B = Lobules	28	D = Triglyceride lipase
04	C = Hepatocytes	29	A = Hepatocytes
05	D = 800 – 1000 mL	30	C = Liver
06	D = All of the above	31	C = 650 mL
07	A = Diaphragmatic surface	32	B = 100 g
08	B = Visceral surface	33	A = Retinol
09	C = Subphrenic space	34	D = All of the above
10	A = Subhepatic surface	35	C = Cobalamin
11	B = Morison's pouch	36	C = Liver
12	A = Falciform ligament	37	B = 20 – 25 %
13	B = Coronary ligament	38	C = 75 – 80 %
14	C = Lesser curvature	39	D = 4 cm
15	A = Glisson's capsule	40	A = Gall bladder
16	B = Caudate lobe	41	C = 8 cm
17	A = Quadrate lobe	42	A = 30 – 50 mL
18	A = Bile canaliculi	43	B = 7 – 10 cm
19	B = Kupffer cells	44	A = Gall bladder
20	C = 90 %	45	A = Fundus
21	A = Bilirubin	46	A = Body
22	C = Unconjugated bilirubin	47	D = Cystic artery
23	B = Conjugated bilirubin	48	C = Cystic vein
24	C = Glycogenolysis	49	B = 12 – 15 folds
25	A = Glucogenesis	50	D = Duodenum

Part-08

1. The synthesis of complex molecules from simpler one is called
   - (A) Catabolism
   - (B) Anabolism
   - (C) Orthobolism
   - (D) Embolism

2. The breakdown of complex molecules into simpler one is called
   - (A) Catabolism
   - (B) Orthobolism
   - (C) Parabolism
   - (D) Anabolism

3. 1 g of carbohydrate provides
   - (A) 30 kJ
   - (B) 17 kJ
   - (C) 100 kJ
   - (D) 230 kJ

4. 1 g of fat provides
   - (A) 38 kJ
   - (B) 100 kJ
   - (C) 60 kJ
   - (D) 69 kJ

5. The destructive process causing decalcification of the tooth enamel
   - (A) Dental carries
   - (B) Gingivitis
   - (C) Cleft palate
   - (D) Parotitis

6. The inflammation of the gums
   - (A) Parotitis
   - (B) Gingivitis
   - (C) Gastritis
   - (D) Hepatitis

7. Which referred to as a pus – filled structure caused by a tooth infection
   - (A) Tooth abscess
   - (B) Gingivitis
   - (C) Parotitis
   - (D) Cleft palate

8. When salivary glands fail to produce sufficient saliva
   - (A) Stye
   - (B) Cleft palate
   - (C) Xerostomia
   - (D) Emphysema

9. The birth defect of lip and mouth
   - (A) Cleft palate
   - (B) Compact palate
   - (C) Dislocated jaw
   - (D) Xerostomia

10. The acute viral infection that affects mostly the parotid glands
    - (A) Parotitis
    - (B) Nephritis
    - (C) Hepatitis
    - (D) Gastritis

11. The condition in which the stomach lining known as the mucosa is inflamed

    (A) Arthritis

    (B) Gastritis

    (C) Hepatitis

    (D) Nephritis

12. The inflammation of oesophagus is

    (A) Oesophagitis

    (B) Gastritis

    (C) Parotitis

    (D) Hepatitis

13. The sore that develops on the lining of the stomach or duodenum

    (A) Renal ulcer

    (B) Throat ulcer

    (C) Hepatic ulcer

    (D) Peptic ulcer

14. Peptic ulcer in the stomach is also called

    (A) Gastric ulcer

    (B) Hepatic ulcer

    (C) Throat ulcer

    (D) Renal ulcer

15. The bacterium that causes peptic ulcer is

    (A) Salmonella typhi

    (B) Helicobacter pylori

    (C) Bacillus anthracis

    (D) Vibrio cholerae

16. Symptoms of peptic ulcer

    (A) Poor appetite

    (B) Weight loss

    (C) Nausea and vomiting

    (D) All of the above

17. The condition in which food or stool cannot move through

    (A) Pancreatic obstruction

    (B) Renal obstruction

    (C) Intestinal obstruction

    (D) Oesophagus obstruction

18. A small clump of cells that forms on the lining of the colon or rectum

    (A) Colorectal polyp

    (B) Rectocolon pons

    (C) Appendicitis

    (D) Peritonitis

19. The painful swelling and infection of the appendix

    (A) Appendicitis

    (B) Gastritis

    (C) Parotitis

    (D) Oesophagitis

20. The bursting of appendix spreads the infection throughout the abdomen and may result in a potentially dangerous condition called

    (A) Parotitis

    (B) Peritonitis

    (C) Gastritis

    (D) Hepatitis

21. The disorder that causes inflammation of GI tract

    (A) Cushing syndrome

    (B) Atherosclerosis

    (C) Crohn's disease

    (D) Addison's disease

22. The chronic inflammatory disease of the mucosa of the colon and rectum

    (A) Hepatitis   (B) Ulcerative colitis

    (C) Nephritis   (D) Parotitis

23. The inflammation occurred in the rectum and lower part of the colon is called

    (A) Ulcerative proctitis   (B) Bronchitis

    (C) Nephritis   (D) Parotitis

24. The acute infection is caused by the yeast candida albicans, which occurs when the commensal microbe grows in white patches on the tongue and oral mucosa

    (A) Angiomas   (B) Thrush

    (C) Emphysema   (D) Haematuria

25. The condition in which peristalsis of the lower oesophagus is impaired

    (A) Emphysema   (B) Ischemia

    (C) Arthritis   (D) Achalasia

26. Typhoid fever are caused by

    (A) Salmonella typhi   (B) Vibrio cholerae

    (C) Variola virus   (D) Clostridium tetani

27. Incubation period of salmonella typhi is

    (A) 30 – 40 days   (B) 1 – 2 days

    (C) 10 – 14 days   (D) 40 – 45 days

28. After contaminated food is eaten, ingested staphylococcus aureus releases toxins that cause

    (A) Acute bronchitis   (B) Acute gastroenteritis

    (C) Acute nephritis   (D) Acute parotitis

29. Cholera is caused by

    (A) Vibrio cholerae   (B) Clostridium tetani

    (C) Salmonella typhi   (D) Bacillus anthracis

30. Which disease is caused by the protozoan Entamoeba histolytica?

    (A) Amoebiasis   (B) Hernia

    (C) Emphysema   (D) Splenomegaly

31. The protrusion of an organ or part of an organ through a weak point or aperture in the surround structure

    (A) Amoebiasis   (B) Hernias

    (C) Emphysema   (D) Stye

32. The protrusion of a part of the fundus of the stomach through the oesophageal opening in the diaphragm

   (A) Temporal hernia

   (B) Umbilical hernia

   (C) Hiatus hernia

   (D) Inguinal hernia

33. The weak point is the umbilicus, where the umbilical blood vessels from the placenta entered the fetus before birth

   (A) Umbilical hernia

   (B) Temporal hernia

   (C) Incisional hernia

   (D) Inguinal hernia

34. Which hernia is caused by repeated stretching of fibrous tissue formed after previous abdominal cavity?

   (A) Hiatus hernia

   (B) Incisional hernia

   (C) Inguinal hernia

   (D) Femoral hernia

35. Which occurs when a loop of bowel twists occluding its lumen and resulting in intestinal obstruction

   (A) Presbyopia

   (B) Volvulus

   (C) Stye

   (D) Presbycusis

36. The condition in which the length of intestine is investigated into itself, causing intestinal obstruction

   (A) Intussusception

   (B) Presbycusis

   (C) Stye

   (D) Presbyopia

37. The yellowing of the skin and mucous membrane is a sign of abnormal bilirubin metabolism and excretion

   (A) Otitis

   (B) Cataracts

   (C) Jaundice

   (D) Bronchiectasis

38. Acute inflammation occurs when a gallstone becomes impacted in the cystic duct

   (A) Acute cholecystitis

   (B) Acute otitis

   (C) Acute bronchiectasis

   (D) Acute blepharitis

39. The inflammation of bile ducts caused by bacterial infection and is typically accompanied by abdominal pain, fever and jaundice

   (A) Blepharitis

   (B) Cholangitis

   (C) Bronchitis

   (D) Thyroiditis

40. The term used to denote swallowing due to any cause

   (A) Dysphagia

   (B) Jaundice

   (C) Presbycusis

   (D) Presbyopia

41. The inflammation of liver is called
    (A) Thyroiditis
    (B) Arthritis
    (C) Hepatitis
    (D) Bronchitis

42. Hepatitis is caused by
    (A) Bacteria
    (B) Virus
    (C) Fungus
    (D) Protozoa

43. The incubation period of hepatitis B is between
    (A) 50 – 180 days
    (B) 3 – 6 days
    (C) 14 – 20 days
    (D) 30 – 35 days

44. The condition causes immune system to attack the liver, resulting in inflammation
    (A) Biliary cirrhosis
    (B) Autoimmune hepatitis
    (C) Autoimmune gastritis
    (D) Autoimmune nephritis

45. The high blood pressure in the portal vein, which supplies the liver with blood from the intestine and spleen called
    (A) Portal hypertension
    (B) Portal hypotension
    (C) Renal hypertension
    (D) Pulmonary hypertension

46. The fluid build-up in the abdominal cavity caused by fluids leaks from the surface of the liver and intestine
    (A) Tetany
    (B) Atheroma
    (C) Arthritis
    (D) Ascites

47. The condition characterized by inflammation and itching of the GI tract
    (A) Blepharitis
    (B) Gastroenteritis
    (C) Bronchitis
    (D) Thyroiditis

48. The inflamed or swollen condition of the vascular structure in the anal canal and may cause bleeding
    (A) Haemorrhoids
    (B) Presbycusis
    (C) Jaundice
    (D) Presbyopia

49. The condition of increased frequency and loose or liquid stools caused by increased motility and decrease in absorption by the intestine
    (A) Diarrhoea
    (B) Presbyopia
    (C) Otitis
    (D) Stye

50. The digestive disease that damages the small intestine and interfere with absorption of nutrients from food
    (A) Hepatitis
    (B) Atheroma
    (C) Celiac disease
    (D) Embolism

Answer Key

Digestive System (Part-08)

Question	Answer	Question	Answer
01	B = Anabolism	26	A = Salmonella typhi
02	A = Catabolism	27	C = 10 – 14 days
03	B = 17 kJ	28	B = Acute gastroenteritis
04	A = 38 kJ	29	A = Vibrio cholerae
05	A = Dental carries	30	A = Amoebiasis
06	B = Gingivitis	31	B = Hernias
07	A = Tooth abscess	32	C = Hiatus hernia
08	C = Xerostomia	33	A = Umbilical hernia
09	A = Cleft palate	34	B = Incisional hernia
10	A = Parotitis	35	B = Volvulus
11	B = Gastritis	36	A = Intussusception
12	A = Oesophagus	37	C = Jaundice
13	D = Peptic ulcer	38	A = Acute cholecystitis
14	A = Gastric ulcer	39	B = Cholangitis
15	B = Helicobacter pylori	40	A = Dysphagia
16	D = All of the above	41	C = Hepatitis
17	C = Intestinal obstruction	42	B = Virus
18	A = Colorectal polyp	43	A = 50 – 180 days
19	A = Appendicitis	44	B = Autoimmune hepatitis
20	B = Peritonitis	45	A = Portal hypertension
21	C = Crohn's disease	46	D = Ascites
22	B = Ulcerative colitis	47	B = Gastroenteritis
23	A = Ulcerative proctitis	48	A = Haemorrhoids
24	B = Thrush	49	A = Diarrhoea
25	D = Achalasia	50	C = Celiac disease

Notes

Unit - IX

Respiratory System and Urinary System

Part-01

1. The study of the respiratory system is known as
   - (A) Pulmonology
   - (B) Cardiology
   - (C) Neurology
   - (D) Nephrology

2. The highest recorded sneeze speed is
   - (A) 60 km/h
   - (B) 165 km/h
   - (C) 100 km/h
   - (D) 90 km/h

3. If capillaries of lungs placed end to end it would extend
   - (A) 100 km
   - (B) 1600 km
   - (C) 200 km
   - (D) 500 km

4. A person at rest usually breathes
   - (A) 12 – 15 times/ min
   - (B) 30 – 35 times/ min
   - (C) 40 – 45 times/ min
   - (D) 35 – 40 times/ min

5. Which system consists of the organs that exchange the gases between the atmosphere and the blood
   - (A) Urinary system
   - (B) Nervous system
   - (C) Respiratory system
   - (D) Gastrointestinal system

6. Which of the following is not a part of respiratory system?
   - (A) Nasal cavity
   - (B) Pharynx
   - (C) Larynx
   - (D) Loop of Henle

7. The first respiratory organ is
   - (A) Tongue
   - (B) Nose
   - (C) Iris
   - (D) Retina

8. The chief organ of the respiratory system is
   - (A) Heart
   - (B) Liver
   - (C) Lungs
   - (D) Kidney

9. The outer portion of the nose that appears on the face
   (A) External nose
   (B) Internal nose
   (C) Temporal nose
   (D) Parietal nose

10. External nose is not formed by bone are
   (A) Frontal
   (B) Tibia
   (C) Nasal
   (D) Maxilla

11. The external nose has two openings known as
   (A) Tongue
   (B) Lips
   (C) Nostrils
   (D) Iris

12. The skeletal of external nose is made up of
   (A) Bony component
   (B) Cartilaginous component
   (C) Both (A) and (B)
   (D) None of the above

13. Which component of external nose located superiorly
   (A) Bony component
   (B) Cartilaginous component
   (C) Ligamentous component
   (D) Soleus component

14. Which component of the external nose located inferiorly
   (A) Ligamentous component
   (B) Cartilaginous component
   (C) Bony component
   (D) Flexor component

15. The bony component is comprised of contributions from
   (A) Alar cartilage
   (B) Septal cartilage
   (C) Nasal bones
   (D) Lateral cartilage

16. How many lateral cartilages comprised in cartilaginous component of external nose?
   (A) Three
   (B) Two
   (C) Five
   (D) Six

17. How many septal cartilages comprised in cartilaginous component of external nose?
   (A) One
   (B) Three
   (C) Four
   (D) Five

18. Small muscles of external nose are innervated by branches of the
   (A) Auditory nerve
   (B) Optic nerve
   (C) Vagus nerve
   (D) Facial nerve

19. Which muscle originates in the fascia overlying the nasal bone and lateral cartilage, inserting into the inferior forehead
   (A) Procerus
   (B) Soleus
   (C) Sartorius
   (D) Obliquus

20. The skin of the external nose receives arterial supply from the branches of the
    (A) Renal arteries
    (B) Maxillary arteries
    (C) Pulmonary arteries
    (D) Clavicle arteries

21. The external nose venous drainage is into the
    (A) Facial vein
    (B) Pulmonary vein
    (C) Clavicle vein
    (D) Renal vein

22. The roof of internal nose is formed by
    (A) Ethmoid bone
    (B) Nasal bone
    (C) Sphenoid bone
    (D) All of the above

23. Which bone is not found in lateral walls of the internal nose?
    (A) Maxilla bone
    (B) Lacrimal bone
    (C) Tibial bone
    (D) Palatine bone

24. The nose is lined with
    (A) Ciliated columnar epithelium
    (B) Simple cuboidal epithelium
    (C) Simple squamous epithelium
    (D) Stratified squamous epithelium

25. Ciliated columnar epithelium of nose contains
    (A) Mast cells
    (B) Stem cells
    (C) Goblet cells
    (D) Astrocytes

26. The lateral walls of the nose are formed by
    (A) Medulla
    (B) Fundus
    (C) Turbinates
    (D) Caecum

27. The cavities in the bones of the face and the skull bones that contain air and provide a chamber of resonation for sound upon the speaking and singing
    (A) Paranasal sinuses
    (B) Orthonasal sinuses
    (C) Metanasal sinuses
    (D) Pedicle sinuses

28. The sinus which opens in the lateral walls of the internal nose
    (A) Frontal sinuses
    (B) Temporal sinuses
    (C) Parietal sinuses
    (D) Maxillary sinuses

29. Which sinus open into the roof of the internal nose
    (A) Parietal sinuses
    (B) Temporal sinuses
    (C) Frontal sinuses
    (D) Maxillary sinuses

30. Which sinus open in the upper part of the lateral walls of the internal nose
    - (A) Mandible sinuses
    - (B) Ethmoid sinuses
    - (C) Parietal sinuses
    - (D) Temporal sinuses
31. The right and left nasal cavities are separated by
    - (A) Nasal septum
    - (B) Nasal fundus
    - (C) Nasal soleus
    - (D) Nasal surae
32. Which of the following is an olfactory and respiratory organ?
    - (A) Tongue
    - (B) Nose
    - (C) Teeth
    - (D) Eye
33. The most superior part of the respiratory tract is
    - (A) Ventral cavity
    - (B) Nasal crista
    - (C) Nasal cavity
    - (D) Renal cavity
34. The area surrounding the anterior external opening to the nasal cavity
    - (A) Vestibule
    - (B) Pedicle
    - (C) Lamellae
    - (D) Fundus
35. The respiratory region is lined by
    - (A) Simple cuboidal epithelium
    - (B) Ciliated pseudostratified epithelium
    - (C) Simple columnar epithelium
    - (D) Stratified squamous epithelium
36. The region located at the apex of the nasal cavity
    - (A) Vagus region
    - (B) Auditory region
    - (C) Optic region
    - (D) Olfactory region
37. The extension from each side of lateral walls of the nasal cavity forms the shelf – like projections called
    - (A) Conchae
    - (B) Cisternae
    - (C) Caecum
    - (D) Compact
38. The conchae further divide each part of the nasal cavity into three hollow passages called
    - (A) Caecum
    - (B) Meatuses
    - (C) Dorsal
    - (D) Fundus
39. The meatus between the inferior concha and floor of the nasal cavity
    - (A) Distal meatus
    - (B) Middle meatus
    - (C) Inferior meatus
    - (D) Superior meatus

40. The meatus between the inferior and middle concha
    (A) Middle meatus
    (B) Inferior meatus
    (C) Distal meatus
    (D) Vertical meatus

41. The meatus between the middle and superior concha
    (A) Vertical meatus
    (B) Superior meatus
    (C) Distal meatus
    (D) Middle meatus

42. The middle ethmoidal sinuses empty out onto a structure called
    (A) Ethmoidal bulla
    (B) Ethmoidal fundus
    (C) Ethmoidal compact
    (D) Ethmoidal chondral

43. Which plate is part of the ethmoid bone?
    (A) Crucial plate
    (B) Cribriform plate
    (C) Actin plate
    (D) Medullary plate

44. The ethmoid artery is branch of the
    (A) Auditory artery
    (B) Renal artery
    (C) Ophthalmic artery
    (D) Pulmonary artery

45. The non-respiratory function of nose is
    (A) Voice
    (B) Breathing
    (C) Air conditioning
    (D) Cleansing

46. Nose is the organ of
    (A) Taste
    (B) Smell
    (C) Hearing
    (D) Vision

47. Smell is detected by
    (A) Auditory receptors
    (B) Optic receptors
    (C) Olfactory receptors
    (D) Cutaneous receptors

48. The rich blood supply to the nasal mucosa is formed by
    (A) Endothelial cells
    (B) Exothelial cells
    (C) Extracellular cells
    (D) Exocrine cells

49. In frontal sinuses sensation is supplied by
    (A) Supraorbital nerve
    (B) Sural nerve
    (C) Fibular nerve
    (D) Obturator nerve

50. Sphenoid sinuses receive blood supply from pharyngeal branches of the
    (A) Renal arteries
    (B) Clavicle arteries
    (C) Maxillary arteries
    (D) Gastric arteries

Answer Key

Respiratory System and Urinary System (Part-01)

Question	Answer	Question	Answer
01	A = Pulmonary	26	C = Turbinates
02	B = 165 km/h	27	A = Paranasal sinuses
03	B = 1600 km	28	D = Maxillary sinuses
04	A = 12 – 15 times/min	29	C = Frontal sinuses
05	C = Respiratory system	30	B = Ethmoid sinuses
06	D = Loop of Henle	31	A = Nasal septum
07	B = Nose	32	B = Nose
08	C = Lungs	33	C = Nasal cavity
09	A = External nose	34	A = Vestibule
10	B = Tibia	35	B = Stratified pseudostratified epithelium
11	C = Nostrils	36	D = Olfactory region
12	C = Both (A) and (B)	37	A = Conchae
13	A = Bony component	38	B = Meatuses
14	B = Cartilaginous component	39	C = Inferior meatus
15	C = Nasal bones	40	A = Middle meatus
16	B = Two	41	B = Superior meatus
17	A = One	42	A = Ethmoidal bulla
18	D = Facial nerve	43	B = Cribriform plate
19	A = Procerus	44	C = Ophthalmic artery
20	B = Maxillary arteries	45	A = Voice
21	A = Facial vein	46	B = Smell
22	D = All of the above	47	C = Olfactory receptors
23	C = Tibial bone	48	A = Endothelial cells
24	A = Ciliated columnar epithelium	49	A = Supraorbital nerve
25	C = Goblet cells	50	C = Maxillary arteries

Part-02

1. How long the pharynx is
   - (A) 12 – 15 cm
   - (B) 20 – 25 cm
   - (C) 30 – 35 cm
   - (D) 25 – 30 cm

2. Which connects the nasal and oral cavities to the larynx and oesophagus
   - (A) Aorta
   - (B) Fissure
   - (C) Pharynx
   - (D) Fundus

3. Which serves as the common passageway for food and air
   - (A) Diaphragm
   - (B) Pharynx
   - (C) Fissure
   - (D) Aorta

4. Pharynx is inferiorly continuous with the
   - (A) Skull
   - (B) Tongue
   - (C) Oesophagus
   - (D) Teeth

5. Pharynx extends from the posterior nares and runs behind the mouth ana larynx to the level of
   - (A) Sixth cervical vertebrae
   - (B) Fourth coccyx vertebrae
   - (C) Fifth sacrum vertebrae
   - (D) Seventh lumbar vertebrae

6. Which attached anteriorly to the oral cavity, larynx and nasal cavity
   - (A) Fundus walls
   - (B) Pelvic walls
   - (C) Pharyngeal walls
   - (D) Abdominal walls

7. Which of the following lies at the back of the posterior conchae of the nasal and above the level of the soft palate?
   - (A) Nasopharynx
   - (B) Oropharynx
   - (C) Laryngopharynx
   - (D) Parapharynx

8. The posterosuperior nasopharynx contains the
   - (A) Adenoid tonsils
   - (B) Lingual tonsils
   - (C) Pedicle tonsils
   - (D) Ventral tonsils

9. Which separates the nasopharynx from the oropharynx?
   - (A) Band palate
   - (B) Soft palate
   - (C) Long palate
   - (D) Short palate

10. The lateral walls of the nasopharynx have the opening of

    (A) Uterine tubes
    (B) Temporal tubes
    (C) Pharyngotympanic tubes
    (D) Pharyngoparietal tubes

11. Which of the following lies posteriorly to the oral cavity, inferiorly to the soft palate to the epiglottis?

    (A) Metapharynx
    (B) Oropharynx
    (C) Laryngopharynx
    (D) Parapharynx

12. Which has only one opening from the mouth

    (A) Oropharynx
    (B) Nasopharynx
    (C) Parapharynx
    (D) Metapharynx

13. Which of the following extends from the oropharynx above tot the oesophagus at the level of the sixth thoracic vertebrae?

    (A) Oropharynx
    (B) Parapharynx
    (C) Laryngopharynx
    (D) Metapharynx

14. Anterior wall of the laryngopharynx of the

    (A) Laryngeal inlet
    (B) Pelvic inlet
    (C) Pubis inlet
    (D) Iliac inlet

15. The muscle of pharynx is mostly innervated by the

    (A) Auditory nerve
    (B) Vagus nerve
    (C) Accessory nerve
    (D) Oculomotor nerve

16. The group of muscles of pharynx are

    (A) Soleus muscles
    (B) Gracilis muscles
    (C) Pharyngeal muscles
    (D) Sartorius muscle

17. Which of the following lined by ciliated columnar epithelium?

    (A) Oropharynx
    (B) Laryngopharynx
    (C) Nasopharynx
    (D) Metapharynx

18. Muscle coat is made of striped muscle which are in pharynx

    (A) Outer circular layer
    (B) Inner longitudinal layer
    (C) Both (A) and (B)
    (D) None of the above

19. Which coat is formed by bucopharyngeous fascia?

    (A) Areolar coat
    (B) Adipose coat
    (C) Muscle coat
    (D) Serous coat

20. The uppermost pharyngeal constrictor is
    (A) Superior pharyngeal constrictor
    (B) Middle pharyngeal constrictor
    (C) Inferior pharyngeal constrictor
    (D) Distal pharyngeal constrictor

21. The constrictor located in the laryngopharynx is
    (A) Superior pharyngeal constrictor
    (B) Ventricle pharyngeal constrictor
    (C) Middle pharyngeal constrictor
    (D) Proximal pharyngeal constrictor

22. The component of inferior pharyngeal constrictor
    (A) Thyropharyngeus   (B) Cricopharyngeus
    (C) Both (A) and (B)   (D) None of the above

23. Which arises from the styloid process of the temporal bone, inserts into the pharynx
    (A) Palatopharyngeus   (B) Stylopharyngeus
    (C) Salpingopharyngeus   (D) Adductor longus

24. The pharynx receives sensory innervation from the
    (A) Glossopharyngeal nerve   (B) Saphenous nerve
    (C) Sural nerve   (D) Pudendal nerve

25. Arterial supply to the pharynx is via branches of the
    (A) Renal artery   (B) Gastric artery
    (C) External carotid   (D) Tibial artery

26. Venous drainage in pharynx is achieved by
    (A) Deep femoral venous   (B) Deep palmar arch
    (C) Pharyngeal venous plexus   (D) Ulnar venous

27. Function of pharynx is
    (A) Speech   (B) Warming and humidifying
    (C) Protection   (D) All of the above

28. Which of the following is called 'voice box'?
    (A) Larynx   (B) Bronchus
    (C) Epiglottis   (D) Pharynx

29. Which of the following located laterally to the larynx?
    (A) Lobe of the adrenal gland (B) Lobe of the thyroid gland
    (C) Lobe of the pineal gland   (D) Lobe of the spleen

30. Inferiorly trachea is continuous with the
    (A) Oesophagus
    (B) Tongue
    (C) Trachea
    (D) Teeth

31. Which of the following present from the inferior surface of the epiglottis to the vestibular folds?
    (A) Metaglottis
    (B) Supraglottis
    (C) Paraglottis
    (D) Orthoglottis

32. How many irregular shaped cartilages attached to each other by ligament and membranes of the larynx
    (A) Eleven
    (B) Fourteen
    (C) Fifteen
    (D) Nine

33. How many thyroids cartilage present in larynx?
    (A) 5
    (B) 6
    (C) 1
    (D) 8

34. How many arytenoid cartilages present in larynx?
    (A) 8
    (B) 2
    (C) 6
    (D) 4

35. Which cartilage is the most prominent of the laryngeal cartilages of larynx?
    (A) Thyroid cartilage
    (B) Corniculate cartilage
    (C) Cuboidal cartilage
    (D) Compact cartilage

36. Which cartilage forms most of the anterior and lateral walls of the larynx
    (A) Adrenal cartilage
    (B) Cuboidal cartilage
    (C) Thyroid cartilage
    (D) Corniculate cartilage

37. The anterior wall of thyroid cartilage projects into the soft tissues in front of the throat forming the laryngeal prominence is known as
    (A) Adam's apple
    (B) Adam's food
    (C) Adam's crista
    (D) Adam's fluid

38. The upper part of the thyroid cartilage is lined with
    (A) Stratified squamous epithelium
    (B) Simple columnar epithelium
    (C) Simple cuboidal epithelium
    (D) Stratified cuboidal epithelium

39. Which cartilage is lies below the thyroid cartilage and composed of hyaline cartilage?

    (A) Columnar cartilage

    (B) Cricoid cartilage

    (C) Compact cartilage

    (D) Cuboidal cartilage

40. Which give attachment to the vocal cords and to muscles and are lined with ciliated columnar epithelium

    (A) Arytenoid cartilages

    (B) Tendon cartilages

    (C) Temporal cartilages

    (D) Cuboidal cartilages

41. The two roughly pyramid – shaped hyaline cartilages situated on top of the broad part of the cricoid cartilage

    (A) Tendon cartilages

    (B) Adrenal cartilages

    (C) Thyroid cartilages

    (D) Arytenoid cartilages

42. The leaf – shaped fibroelastic attached by a flexible stalk of cartilage to the inner surface of the anterior wall of the thyroid cartilage

    (A) Epiglottis

    (B) Stomach

    (C) Tongue

    (D) Bronchus

43. Which acts as a lid and closes the larynx during swallowing of food or drink

    (A) Oesophagus

    (B) Epiglottis

    (C) Tongue

    (D) Stomach

44. How many epiglottises are there?

    (A) 2

    (B) 4

    (C) 1

    (D) 3

45. The apex of the arytenoid cartilages of larynx articulates with the

    (A) Corniculate cartilage

    (B) Cuboidal cartilage

    (C) Thyroid cartilage

    (D) Adrenal cartilage

46. The corniculate cartilages articulate with the apices of the

    (A) Arytenoid cartilages

    (B) Tendon cartilages

    (C) Cuboidal cartilages

    (D) Thyroid cartilages

47. Which cartilages are the conical – shaped two small elastic cartilages present at the apices of the arytenoid cartilages?

    (A) Columnar cartilages

    (B) Cuboidal cartilages

    (C) Corniculate cartilages

    (D) Cruciform cartilages

48. Which cartilages are the club – shaped two fibroelastic cartilages present on the anterior side of the corniculate cartilages?

(A) Cuneiform cartilages

(B) Cricoid cartilages

(C) Tendon cartilages

(D) Thyroid cartilages

49. In which cartilage of larynx, the upper respiratory system ends

(A) Adrenal cartilage

(B) Cricoid cartilage

(C) Thyroid cartilage

(D) Tenoid cartilage

50. Which organ are responsible for sound/voice production?

(A) Tongue

(B) Vocal folds

(C) Lungs

(D) All of the above

Answer Key

Respiratory System and Urinary System (Part-02)

Question	Answer	Question	Answer
01	A = 12 – 15 cm	26	C = Pharyngeal venous plexus
02	C = Pharynx	27	D = All of the above
03	B = Pharynx	28	A = Larynx
04	C = Oesophagus	29	B = Lobe of the thyroid gland
05	A = Sixth cervical vertebrae	30	C = Trachea
06	C = Pharyngeal walls	31	B = Supraglottis
07	A = Nasopharynx	32	C = Nine
08	A = Adenoid tonsils	33	C = 1
09	B = Soft palate	34	B = 2
10	C = Pharyngotympanic tubes	35	A = Thyroid cartilage
11	B = Oropharynx	36	C = Thyroid cartilage
12	A = Oropharynx	37	A = Adam's apple
13	C = Laryngopharynx	38	A = Stratified squamous epithelium
14	A = laryngeal inlet	39	B = Cricoid cartilage
15	B = Vagus nerve	40	A = Arytenoid cartilages
16	C = Pharyngeal muscles	41	D = Arytenoid cartilages
17	C = Nasopharynx	42	A = Epiglottis
18	C = Both (A) and (B)	43	B = Epiglottis
19	A = Areolar coat	44	C = 1
20	A = Superior pharyngeal constrictor	45	A = Corniculate cartilage
21	C = Middle pharyngeal constrictor	46	A = Arytenoid cartilages
22	C = Both (A) and (B)	47	C = Arytenoid cartilages
23	B = Stylopharyngeus	48	A = Cuneiform cartilages
24	A = Glossopharyngeal nerve	49	B = Cricoid cartilage
25	C = External carotid	50	D = All of the above

Part-03

1. The windpipe is continuation of the larynx are
   (A) Oesophagus
   (B) Trachea
   (C) Aorta
   (D) Ventricles
2. How long the trachea is
   (A) 20 – 30 cm
   (B) 25 – 30 cm
   (C) 10 – 12 cm
   (D) 40 – 45 cm
3. The diameter of trachea is
   (A) 2 – 2.5 cm
   (B) 5 – 5.5 cm
   (C) 6 – 7 cm
   (D) 7 – 7.5 cm
4. Trachea is extending to the
   (A) 5th thoracic vertebrae
   (B) 5th coccyx vertebrae
   (C) 4th lumbar vertebrae
   (D) 10th lumbar vertebrae
5. Trachea is separated into left and right
   (A) Diaphragm
   (B) Oesophagus
   (C) Bronchi
   (D) Fundus
6. Which of the following lies posterior to the trachea?
   (A) Stomach
   (B) Liver
   (C) Oesophagus
   (D) Tongue
7. How many C – shaped rings present in trachea
   (A) 30 – 40
   (B) 16 – 20
   (C) 50 – 55
   (D) 55 – 60
8. The ring of trachea is made up of
   (A) Hyaline cartilages
   (B) Hollow cartilages
   (C) Fibrous cartilages
   (D) Elastic cartilages
9. The free ends of tracheal rings are supported by
   (A) Soleus muscle
   (B) Trachealis muscle
   (C) Gracilis muscle
   (D) Sartorius muscle
10. The inner wall of the mucosal layer of trachea is composed of
    (A) Ciliated columnar epithelium
    (B) Simple cuboidal epithelium
    (C) Stratified cuboidal epithelium
    (D) Stratified squamous epithelium

11. The middle layer is the submucosal layer, and the cartilaginous layer is arranged in

    (A) Spherical manner   (B) Helical manner

    (C) Round manner   (D) Circular manner

12. The submucosal layer of trachea is made up of

    (A) Cardiac tissue   (B) Dense tissue

    (C) Areolar tissue   (D) Adipose tissue

13. The main arterial blood supply to the trachea is

    (A) Inferior thyroid arteries   (B) Bronchial arteries

    (C) Both (A) and (B)   (D) None of the above

14. The airway passage in the respiratory tract, which conducts air into the lungs

    (A) Bronchi   (B) Oesophagus

    (C) Tongue   (D) Ear canal

15. How many lobes subdivided from the right bronchus?

    (A) Two   (B) Four

    (C) Three   (D) Five

16. How long the right bronchus

    (A) 4.5 cm   (B) 2.5 cm

    (C) 6.5 cm   (D) 8.5 cm

17. How many lobes subdivided from the left bronchus?

    (A) Three   (B) Two

    (C) Four   (D) Six

18. How long the left bronchus is

    (A) 5 cm   (B) 8 cm

    (C) 10 cm   (D) 11 cm

19. The lobes of bronchi are divided into

    (A) Segmental bronchi   (B) Parietal bronchi

    (C) Temporal bronchi   (D) Occipital bronchi

20. Segmental bronchi are also called as

    (A) Primary bronchi   (B) Secondary bronchi

    (C) Quaternary bronchi   (D) Tertiary bronchi

21. Each of the bronchus supplies a

   (A) Bronchopulmonary section
   (B) Bronchorenal section
   (C) Bronchospleen section
   (D) Gastrobronchus section

22. The bronchopulmonary section is a division of a lung separated from the rest of the lung by a

   (A) Epithelial tissue
   (B) Connective tissue
   (C) Nervous tissue
   (D) Cardiac tissue

23. Bronchi is subdivided into

   (A) Pedicles
   (B) Bronchioles
   (C) Oesophagus
   (D) Sternal

24. The arterial supply to the walls of bronchi and smaller air passages is through

   (A) Bronchial arteries
   (B) Renal arteries
   (C) Gastric arteries
   (D) Splenic arteries

25. The venous drainage of bronchi is into the

   (A) Renal veins
   (B) Bronchial veins
   (C) Splenic veins
   (D) Tibial veins

26. The nerve stimulates the contraction of smooth muscle in the bronchial tree

   (A) Vagus nerve
   (B) Accessory nerve
   (C) Auditory nerve
   (D) Optic nerve

27. The tracheobronchial tree consists of

   (A) Trachea
   (B) Bronchi
   (C) Branches of bronchi
   (D) All of the above

28. How many times the air passages between trachea and alveoli divide to form the extensive tracheobronchial tree

   (A) 53 times
   (B) 23 times
   (C) 63 times
   (D) 73 times

29. How many generation divisions of tracheobronchial tree

   (A) 23 generation
   (B) 33 generation
   (C) 43 generation
   (D) 53 generation

30. Which bronchi are division of the principle bronchus, form the 2nd generation?

   (A) Vomer bronchi
   (B) Pedicle bronchi
   (C) Fundus bronchi
   (D) Lobar bronchi

31. Which bronchi are further division of each lobar bronchus, forms the 3rd generation?

    (A) Segmental bronchi

    (B) Pedimental bronchi

    (C) Condimental bronchi

    (D) Tegmental bronchi

32. Which bronchiole is the name given to 16th generation of the divisions?

    (A) Cuboidal bronchiole

    (B) Cuticle bronchiole

    (C) Terminal bronchiole

    (D) Tegmental bronchiole

33. Which bronchiole is the name given to 17th to 22nd generation of the divisions?

    (A) Cuticle bronchiole

    (B) Respiratory bronchiole

    (C) Tegmental bronchiole

    (D) Cuticle bronchiole

34. Which of the following end in the alveoli which form the 23rd generation?

    (A) Salivary ducts

    (B) Lacrimal ducts

    (C) Alveolar ducts

    (D) Synovial ducts

35. The air passages are formed by the first 16 generations of passages and it only transports gases from and to the anterior called

    (A) Conducting zone

    (B) Transmitting zone

    (C) Penetrating zone

    (D) Implanting zone

36. The total capacity of conducting zone is approximately

    (A) 250 mL

    (B) 150 mL

    (C) 300 mL

    (D) 350 mL

37. The remaining 7 generations of tracheobronchial tree which includes the respiratory bronchioles, alveolar ducts and alveoli form the

    (A) Implanting zone

    (B) Penetrating zone

    (C) Respiratory zone

    (D) Implanting zone

38. How many alveolar ducts are there?

    (A) 2 – 11

    (B) 12 – 21

    (C) 22 – 24

    (D) 26 – 31

39. How many alveolar sacs associated with each alveolar duct?

    (A) 10 – 15

    (B) 5 – 6

    (C) 16 – 20

    (D) 21 – 24

40. The basic anatomical unit of gas exchange in the lung

    (A) Neuron

    (B) Nephron

    (C) Alveolus

    (D) Soleus

41. The volume of respiratory zone is approximately

(A) 4 L

(B) 9 L

(C) 10 L

(D) 12 L

42. The trachea and bronchi is interspersed by

(A) Mast cells

(B) Goblet cells

(C) Stem cells

(D) Astrocytes

43. How many alveoli contain the paired human lungs?

(A) 600 million

(B) 1000 million

(C) 1600 million

(D) 1800 million

44. The average diameter of adult alveolus is around

(A) $10 - 20 \ \mu m$

(B) $200 - 300 \ \mu m$

(C) $500 - 600 \ \mu m$

(D) $1000 - 2000 \ \mu m$

45. Which of the following is Type I alveolar cells?

(A) Cuboidal alveolar cells

(B) Columnar alveolar cells

(C) Squamous alveolar cells

(D) Cardiac alveolar cells

46. Which of the following is Type II alveolar cells?

(A) Great alveolar cells

(B) Short alveolar cells

(C) Lesser alveolar cells

(D) Cuboidal alveolar cells

47. Which of the following is Type III alveolar cells?

(A) Short alveolar cells

(B) Columnar alveolar cells

(C) Macrophages

(D) Cuboidal alveolar cells

48. Which alveolar cells form the alveolar wall structure

(A) Type I

(B) Type II

(C) Type III

(D) Type IV

49. Which alveolar cells cause increased permeability of gaseous exchange

(A) Lesser alveolar cells

(B) Great alveolar cells

(C) Cuboidal alveolar cells

(D) Columnar alveolar cells

50. Which type of alveolar cells kill/destroy foreign particles

(A) Type IV

(B) Type VI

(C) Type I

(D) Type III

Answer Key

Respiratory System and Urinary System (Part-03)

Question	Answer	Question	Answer
01	B = Trachea	26	A = Vagus nerve
02	C = 10 – 12 cm	27	D = All of the above
03	A = 2 – 2.5 cm	28	B = 23 times
04	A = 5th thoracic vertebrae	29	A = 23 generation
05	C = Bronchi	30	D = Lobar bronchi
06	C = Oesophagus	31	A = Segmental bronchi
07	B = 16 – 20	32	C = Terminal bronchiole
08	A = Hyaline cartilages	33	B = Respiratory bronchiole
09	B = Trachealis muscle	34	C = Alveolar ducts
10	A = Ciliated columnar epithelium	35	A = Conducting zone
11	B = Helical manner	36	B = 150 mL
12	C = Areolar tissue	37	C = Respiratory zone
13	C = Both (A) and (B)	38	A = 2 – 11
14	A = Bronchi	39	B = 5 – 6
15	C – Three	40	C = Alveolus
16	B = 2.5 cm	41	A = 4 L
17	B = Two	42	B = Goblet cells
18	A = 5 cm	43	A = 600 million
19	A = Segmental bronchi	44	B = 200 – 300 μm
20	D = Tertiary bronchi	45	C = Squamous alveolar cells
21	A = Bronchopulmonary section	46	A = Great alveolar cells
22	B = Connective tissue	47	C = Macrophages
23	B = Bronchioles	48	A = Type I
24	A = Bronchial arteries	49	B = Great alveolar cells
25	B = Bronchial veins	50	D = Type III

Part-04

1. The two cone – shaped organ, one lying on each side of the midline in the thoracic cavity
   - (A) Stomach
   - (B) Lungs
   - (C) Kidney
   - (D) Spleen
2. Apex is rounded and rises into the root of the neck, about
   - (A) 50 mm
   - (B) 75 mm
   - (C) 25 mm
   - (D) 5 mm
3. The concave and semilunar in shape, and lies on the upper (thoracic) surface of the diaphragm
   - (A) Base
   - (B) Band
   - (C) Tail
   - (D) Roof
4. The broad outer surface of the lungs that lies directly against the costal cartilages, the ribs and the intercostal muscles
   - (A) Costal surface
   - (B) Planta surface
   - (C) Tarsus surface
   - (D) Suture surface
5. The surface of each lung faces the other directly across the space between the lungs, the mediastinum is
   - (A) Distal surface
   - (B) Medial surface
   - (C) Sural surface
   - (D) Medulla surface
6. The large, depressed area that lies near the center of the medial surface of lungs
   - (A) Hyline
   - (B) Hilum
   - (C) Fundus
   - (D) Tibial
7. The mediastinum contains
   - (A) Heart
   - (B) Great vessels
   - (C) Trachea
   - (D) All of the above
8. How many lobes are divided by right lung?
   - (A) Four
   - (B) Five
   - (C) Three
   - (D) Two

9. How many lobes are divided by left lung?
    (A) Three
    (B) Two
    (C) Five
    (D) Four
10. The root of the lung extends inferiorly as a narrow fold
    (A) Pulmonary tendon
    (B) Pulmonary ligament
    (C) Pulmonary cartilage
    (D) Pulmonary sutures
11. The border of the lung is formed by the convergence of the mediastinal and costal surfaces
    (A) Anterior border
    (B) Distal border
    (C) Proximal border
    (D) Posterior border
12. The border separates the base of the lung from the costal and mediastinal surfaces
    (A) Distal border
    (B) Inferior border
    (C) Posterior border
    (D) Proximal border
13. Which runs from the inferior border of the lung in a super posterior direction, until it meets the posterior lung border
    (A) Oblique fissures
    (B) Temporal fissures
    (C) Horizontal fissures
    (D) Distal fissures
14. Which runs horizontally from the sternum, at the level of the 4th rib, to meet the oblique fissure
    (A) Proximal fissures
    (B) Distal fissures
    (C) Horizontal fissures
    (D) Lateral fissures
15. The divisions between the lobes of lungs are called
    (A) Fissures
    (B) Pons
    (C) Fundus
    (D) Pedicle
16. The pleura is enclosed by sacs of
    (A) Synovial membrane
    (B) Meninges membrane
    (C) Pedicle membrane
    (D) Serous membrane
17. The serous membrane of pleura contains small amount of fluid called
    (A) Pleural fluid
    (B) Lacrimal fluid
    (C) Synovial fluid
    (D) Cerebrospinal fluid
18. Which of the following adhere to the lung, covering each lobe and passing into the fissures that separates them?
    (A) Distal pleura
    (B) Visceral pleura
    (C) Temporal pleura
    (D) Parietal pleura

19. Which of the following adhere to the inside of the chest wall and the upper surface of the diaphragm?

(A) Temporal pleura

(B) Parietal pleura

(C) Occipital pleura

(D) Lacrimal pleura

20. The only potential space and contains no air, so the pressure within is negative to atmospheric pressure

(A) Pleural cavity

(B) Ilium cavity

(C) Pelvic cavity

(D) Cranial Cavity

21. In health, the space between the pleural layers, the pleural space, contains on average between

(A) 20 – 30 mL

(B) 80 – 90 mL

(C) 7 – 10 mL

(D) 100 – 120 mL

22. The pulmonary trunk divided into the

(A) Right pulmonary arteries

(B) Left pulmonary arteries

(C) Both (A) and (B)

(D) None of the above

23. The walls of the alveoli and the capillaries each consist of only one layer of

(A) Flattened epithelial cells

(B) Round epithelial cells

(C) Spherical epithelial cells

(D) Circular epithelial cells

24. The pulmonary capillaries merge into a network of

(A) Pulmonary vacuoles

(B) Pulmonary venules

(C) Pulmonary cuboids

(D) Pulmonary column

25. How many bronchioles are there in each lung?

(A) 50,000

(B) 60,000

(C) 30,000

(D) 80,000

26. The ultimate pulmonary unit from the respiratory bronchiole to alveoli is called

(A) Acinus

(B) Nephron

(C) Neuron

(D) Soleus

27. The dome – shaped muscular structure separating the thoracic and abdominal cavities

(A) Esophagus

(B) Diaphragm

(C) Uterus

(D) Spleen

28. The diaphragm is located at the inferior most aspect of the ribcage filling the

    (A) Distal thoracic aperture
    (B) Proximal coccyx aperture
    (C) Inferior thoracic aperture
    (D) Lateral lumbar aperture

29. The parts of the diaphragm that arise from the vertebrae are tendinous in structure and are known as

    (A) Crura
    (B) Crista
    (C) Cisternae
    (D) Cuticle

30. How many crura are there in diaphragm

    (A) Three
    (B) Four
    (C) Six
    (D) Two

31. Which of the following arises from L1 – L3 and their intervertebral disc

    (A) Right crus
    (B) Left crista
    (C) Right crista
    (D) Left crus

32. Which of the following arises from the L1 – L2 and their intervertebral disc

    (A) Right crus
    (B) Left crus
    (C) Right crista
    (D) Left crista

33. The muscle fibres of the diaphragm combine to form a

    (A) Central tendon
    (B) Distal tendon
    (C) Lateral tendon
    (D) Corner tendon

34. Either side of the pericardium the diaphragm ascends to form

    (A) Bands
    (B) Tails
    (C) Domes
    (D) Roots

35. When the diaphragm is relaxed, the central level is at the level of the

    (A) 8th thoracic vertebrae
    (B) 5th coccyx vertebrae
    (C) 8th coccyx vertebrae
    (D) 8th lumbar vertebrae

36. When the diaphragm is contracts, its muscle fibres shorten and the central tendon is pulled downwards to the level of the

    (A) 7th coccyx vertebrae
    (B) 9th coccyx vertebrae
    (C) 9th thoracic vertebrae
    (D) 9th lumbar vertebrae

37. The halves of the diaphragm receive motor innervation from the

    (A) Auditory nerve
    (B) Phrenic nerve
    (C) Femoral nerve
    (D) Obturator nerve

38. The majority of the arterial supply to the diaphragm is delivered via the
   - (A) Inferior phrenic arteries
   - (B) Lateral femoral arteries
   - (C) Inferior renal arteries
   - (D) Distal facial arteries

39. How many pairs of intercostal muscle are in each of the intercoastal spaces, arranges from superficial to deep?
   - (A) 19 pairs
   - (B) 21 pairs
   - (C) 23 pairs
   - (D) 11 pairs

40. Which extend downwards and forwards from the lower border of the rib above to the upper border of the rib below
   - (A) External intercostal muscles
   - (B) Internal iliopsoas muscle
   - (C) Internal soleus muscle
   - (D) Internal sartorius muscle

41. Which extent downwards and backwards from the lower of the rib above to the upper border of the rib bellow
   - (A) External semitendinosus muscle
   - (B) External gastrocnemius muscle
   - (C) Internal intercostal muscle
   - (D) Internal sartorius muscle

42. The exchange of gases between the alveoli and the pulmonary capillaries
   - (A) Pulmonary gas exchange
   - (B) Renal gas exchange
   - (C) Gastric gas exchange
   - (D) Hepatic gas exchange

43. The gaseous exchange between the tissue capillaries and the cells of the tissues
   - (A) Central gas exchange
   - (B) Peripheral gas exchange
   - (C) Somatic gas exchange
   - (D) Proximal gas exchange

44. The oxygen consumption by the brain is
   - (A) $11.0 \, mLO_2$ / min per 100 g
   - (B) $50.0 \, mLO_2$ / min per 100 g
   - (C) $55.0 \, mLO_2$ / min per 100 g
   - (D) $3.0 \, mLO_2$ / min per 100 g

45. The oxygen consumption by the skeletal muscle (during contraction) is
   - (A) $70.0 \, mLO_2$ / min per 100 g
   - (B) $10.0 \, mLO_2$ / min per 100 g
   - (C) $50.0 \, mLO_2$ / min per 100 g
   - (D) $3.0 \, mLO_2$ / min per 100 g

46. A healthy adult person ventilates about
    (A) 30 – 40 times per minute
    (B) 12 – 15 times per minute
    (C) 50 – 55 times per minute
    (D) 55 – 60 times per minute

47. The total volume of gas entering the lungs per minute from the outside
    (A) Minute ventilation
    (B) Second ventilation
    (C) Alveolar ventilation
    (D) Dead space ventilation

48. The volume of gas that reaches the areas of lungs where gas exchange occurs per unit time
    (A) Minute ventilation
    (B) Second ventilation
    (C) Alveolar ventilation
    (D) Dead space ventilation

49. The volume of gas that always remains in the airways per unit time
    (A) Dead space ventilation
    (B) Band space ventilation
    (C) Second ventilation
    (D) Minute ventilation

50. The rate of ventilation changes with
    (A) Age
    (B) Exercise
    (C) Disease
    (D) All of the above

Answer Key

Respiratory System and Urinary System (Part-04)

Question	Answer	Question	Answer
01	B = Lungs	26	A = Acinus
02	C = 25 mm	27	B = Diaphragm
03	A = Base	28	C = Inferior thoracic aperture
04	A = Costal surface	29	A = Crura
05	B = Medial surface	30	D = Two
06	B = Helium	31	A = Right crus
07	D = All of the above	32	B = Left crus
08	C = Three	33	A = Central tendon
09	B = Two	34	C = Domes
10	B = Pulmonary ligament	35	A = 8th thoracic vertebrae
11	A = Anterior border	36	C = 9th thoracic vertebrae
12	B = Inferior border	37	B = Phrenic nerve
13	A = Oblique fissures	38	A = Inferior phrenic arteries
14	C = Horizontal fissures	39	D = 11 pairs
15	A = Fissures	40	A = External intercostal muscles
16	D = Serous membrane	41	C = Internal intercostal muscles
17	A = Pleural fluid	42	A = Pulmonary gas exchange
18	B = Visceral pleura	43	B = Peripheral gas exchange
19	B = Parietal pleura	44	D = 3.0 mLO_2/min per 100 g
20	A = Pleural cavity	45	C = 50.0 mLO_2/min per 100 g
21	C = 7 – 10 mL	46	B = 12 – 15 times per minute
22	C = Both (A) and (B)	47	A = Minute ventilation
23	A = Flattened epithelial cells	48	C = Alveolar ventilation
24	B = Pulmonary venules	49	A = Dead space ventilation
25	C = 30,000	50	D = All of the above

Part-05

1. Minute respiratory volume is around
   (A) 6 / L min
   (C) 15 / L min
   (B) 12 / L min
   (D) 21 / L min

2. Type of dead space is
   (A) Anatomic dead space
   (C) Both (A) and (B)
   (B) Physiological dead space
   (D) None of the above

3. Physiological dead space volume is
   (A) 200 mL
   (C) 150 mL
   (B) 250 mL
   (D) 400 mL

4. The alveolar ventilation rate is
   (A) 9.25 litres per minute
   (C) 10.2 litres per minute
   (B) 5.25 litres per minute
   (D) 13.3 litres per minute

5. How many complete respiratory cycles per minute in normal quite breathing
   (A) 27
   (C) 15
   (B) 35
   (D) 30

6. The process of diffusing oxygen from the blood, into the interstitial fluids and into the cells
   (A) External respiration
   (C) Digestion
   (B) Internal respiration
   (D) Urination

7. A cycle of respiration occurs
   (A) 12 – 18 times / min
   (C) 28 – 30 times / min
   (B) 30 – 40 times / min
   (D) 50 – 55 times / min

8. In which process the intercostal muscle and diaphragm contract, which descends the diaphragm and raises the rib cage outwards
   (A) Expiration
   (C) Inspiration
   (B) Digestion
   (D) Urination

9. In which process the volume of the thoracic cavity increases and the lung stretches
   (A) Expiration
   (C) Urination
   (B) Inspiration
   (D) Digestion

10. At resting condition, the inspiration lasts for about
    (A) 10 sec
    (B) 20 sec
    (C) 16 sec
    (D) 2 sec

11. The expansion of the lungs against the lung and chest elastic forces
    (A) Airway resistance work
    (B) Tissue resistance work
    (C) Compliance work
    (D) Reflection work

12. The work required to overcome the viscosity of the lungs and chest wall structures
    (A) Tissue resistance work
    (B) Airway resistance work
    (C) Reflection work
    (D) Compliance work

13. The work required to overcome resistance for movement of air into the lungs
    (A) Tissue resistance work
    (B) Airway resistance work
    (C) Compliance work
    (D) Elastic work

14. The process in which the intercostal muscles relax, the diaphragm moves upward and the ribcage descends down
    (A) Expiration
    (B) Digestion
    (C) Urination
    (D) Inspiration

15. In which process the volume of the thoracic cavity decreases, thereby enabling the lungs and chest wall to recoil, and the intrapulmonary volume also decreases
    (A) Urination
    (B) Inspiration
    (C) Expiration
    (D) Digestion

16. At resting condition, expiration lasts for about
    (A) 10 sec
    (B) 13 sec
    (C) 4 sec
    (D) 14 sec

17. An adult healthy human male has total lung capacity for air is about
    (A) 13 L
    (B) 14 L
    (C) 10 L
    (D) 6 L

18. In mammals, the mechanism of breathing is called
    (A) Tidal breathing
    (B) Virtual breathing
    (C) Interconnected breathing
    (D) Intrinsic breathing

19. The amount of air that is breathed in and out of the lungs during in each cycle of breathing
    (A) Extrinsic volume
    (B) Intrinsic volume
    (C) Intracellular volume
    (D) Tidal volume

20. The value of tidal volume in male is

    (A) 850 mL
    (B) 500 mL
    (C) 650 mL
    (D) 950 mL

21. The value of tidal volume in female is

    (A) 90 mL
    (B) 120 mL
    (C) 390 mL
    (D) 890 mL

22. The volume of air left in the lungs after a maximal forced exhalation is called

    (A) Reflected volume
    (B) Residual volume
    (C) Suitable volume
    (D) Functional volume

23. The value of residual volume in male

    (A) 1.2 L
    (B) 4.6 L
    (C) 5.5 L
    (D) 3.9 L

24. The value of residual volume in female

    (A) 3.5 L
    (B) 0.93 L
    (C) 0.19 L
    (D) 5.5 L

25. The maximum amount of air that can be expelled from the lungs during maximal expiration

    (A) Expiratory reserve volume
    (B) Efficient reverse value
    (C) Interfacial reverse volume
    (D) Interfacial reflected volume

26. The value of expiratory reserve volume in male is

    (A) 5.5 L
    (B) 1.2 L
    (C) 9.5 L
    (D) 7.4 L

27. The value of inspiratory reserve volume in female is

    (A) 0.13 L
    (B) 0.34 L
    (C) 0.9 L
    (D) 4.2 L

28. The extra volume of air that can be inspired over and above the normal tidal volume when a person inspires with total force

    (A) Intracellular reverse volume
    (B) Inspiratory reserve volume
    (C) Infraction reverse value
    (D) Efficient reverse capacity

29. The value of inspiratory reserve volume in female is
   (A) 2.3 L
   (B) 9.3 L
   (C) 8.9 L
   (D) 6.9 L

30. The value of inspiratory reserve volume in male is
   (A) 8.0 L
   (B) 9.0 L
   (C) 7.0 L
   (D) 3.0 L

31. Which of the following is expressed as a series of volumes in specific time intervals?
   (A) Forced vital capacity
   (B) Forced variation capacity
   (C) Functional variation capacity
   (D) Functional vital combination

32. The maximum volume to which the lungs can be expanded with the most possible effort
   (A) Total lung capacity
   (B) Transfer lung combination
   (C) Target lung combination
   (D) Transmit lung capacity

33. The value of total lung capacity in male is
   (A) 9.8 L
   (B) 8.8 L
   (C) 5.8 L
   (D) 7.9 L

34. The value of total lung capacity in female is
   (A) 9.7 L
   (B) 4.7 L
   (C) 8.9 L
   (D) 8.7 L

35. The maximum volume of air that can be moved into and out of the lungs
   (A) Variation capacity
   (B) Vital capacity
   (C) Target lung capacity
   (D) Total lung combination

36. The value of vital capacity in male is
   (A) 4.6 L
   (B) 9.6 L
   (C) 8.6 L
   (D) 7.9 L

37. The value of vital capacity in female is
   (A) 9.6 L
   (B) 8.5 L
   (C) 8.6 L
   (D) 3.6 L

38. The amount of air that is left in the air passages and alveoli at the end of normal quiet breathing
   (A) Functional residual capacity
   (B) Total lung combination
   (C) Functional reflected combination
   (D) Target lung capacity

39. The value of functional residual capacity in female is
    - (A) 1.9 L
    - (B) 9.8 L
    - (C) 8.9 L
    - (D) 7.9 L

40. The value of functional residual capacity in male is
    - (A) 9.4 L
    - (B) 8.9 L
    - (C) 2.4 L
    - (D) 8.4 L

41. The expression of functional residual capacity is
    - (A) Tidal volume – inspiratory reverse volume
    - (B) Expiratory reverse volume + residual volume
    - (C) Tidal volume – residual volume
    - (D) Residual volume + tidal volume

42. The amount of air that can be inspired with maximum effort
    - (A) Inspiratory capacity
    - (B) Target lung capacity
    - (C) Total lung combination
    - (D) Functional reflected capacity

43. The value of inspiratory capacity in male is
    - (A) 9.5 L
    - (B) 8.5 L
    - (C) 3.5 L
    - (D) 7.8 L

44. The value of inspiratory capacity in female is
    - (A) 2.7 L
    - (B) 9.7 L
    - (C) 6.7 L
    - (D) 7.7 L

45. The expression of inspiratory capacity is
    - (A) Tidal volume + inspiratory reserve volume
    - (B) Expiratory reverse volume + residual volume
    - (C) Tidal volume – residual volume
    - (D) Expiratory reverse volume – residual volume

46. Which of the following measures the mechanical function of the lung, chest walls and respiratory muscles?
    - (A) Spirometry
    - (B) Hysteroscopy
    - (C) Laparoscopy
    - (D) Microscopy

47. The instrument which measures spirometry is called
    - (A) Laparometer
    - (B) Spirometer
    - (C) Hysterometer
    - (D) Microscope

48. In spirometry, the common parameters evaluated include
    - (A) Vital capacity
    - (B) Forced vital capacity
    - (C) Forced expiratory volume
    - (D) All of the above

49. Which of the following is used to measure total lung capacity?
    - (A) Helium dilution
    - (B) Cobalt dilution
    - (C) Carbon dilution
    - (D) Sodium dilution

50. Relative contraindications for spirometry testing include
    - (A) Pneumothorax
    - (B) Angina pectoris
    - (C) Myocardial infraction
    - (D) All of the above

Answer Key

Respiratory System and Urinary System (Part-05)

Question	Answer	Question	Answer
01	A = 6 / L min	26	B = 1.2 L
02	C = Both (A) and (B)	27	C = 0.9 L
03	C = 150 mL	28	B = Inspiratory reverse volume
04	B = 5.25 litres per minute	29	A = 2.3 L
05	C = 15	30	D = 3.0 L
06	B = Internal respiration	31	A = Forced vital capacity
07	A = 12 – 18 times / min	32	A = Total lung capacity
08	C = Inspiration	33	C = 5.8 L
09	B = Inspiration	34	B = 4.7 L
10	D = 2 sec	35	B = Vital capacity
11	C = Compliance work	36	A = 4.6 L
12	A = Tissue resistance work	37	D = 3.6 L
13	B = Airway resistance work	38	A = Functional residual capacity
14	A = Expiration	39	A = 1.9 L
15	C = Expiration	40	C = 2.4 L
16	C = 4 sec	41	B = Expiratory reserve volume + residual volume
17	D = 6 L	42	A = Inspiratory capacity
18	A = Tidal breathing	43	C = 3.5 L
19	D = Tidal volume	44	A = 2.7 L
20	B = 500 mL	45	A = Tidal volume + inspiratory reverse volume
21	C = 390 mL	46	A = Spirometry
22	B = Residual volume	47	B = Spirometer
23	A = 1.2 L	48	D = All of the above
24	B = 0.93 L	49	A = Helium dilution
25	A = Expiratory reserve volume	50	D = All of the above

Part-06

1. The maximum speed of air achieved during the maximally forced expiration after full inspiration
   - (A) Position expiratory rate
   - (B) Peak expiratory flow
   - (C) Peak respiratory rate
   - (D) Second respiratory flow

2. The evaluation of the maximum amount of air that can be inhaled and exhaled per minute
   - (A) Maximum voluntary ventilation
   - (B) Minimum involuntary rate
   - (C) Minimum respiratory flow
   - (D) Minimum involuntary flow

3. The measure of ability of the lungs to transfer gas
   - (A) Diffusing capacity
   - (B) Deflection volume
   - (C) Deflection rate
   - (D) Reflection capacity

4. The term in the human respiratory system for normal, good and unlabored breathing
   - (A) Endocarditis
   - (B) Eupnoea
   - (C) Angina
   - (D) Ascites

5. The type of breathing is
   - (A) Costal breathing
   - (B) Diaphragmatic breathing
   - (C) Both (A) and (B)
   - (D) None of the above

6. Which breathing characterized by an outwards, upwards movement of the chest wall
   - (A) Sternal breathing
   - (B) Costal breathing
   - (C) Diaphragmatic breathing
   - (D) Fundus breathing

7. In which breathing, the expansion is centered at the midpoint and thus it aerates mostly the midportion of the lung
   - (A) Costal breathing
   - (B) Fundus breathing
   - (C) Sternal breathing
   - (D) Suture breathing

8. Which breathing involved the diaphragm, a dome – shaped sheet of muscle that separates the chest cavity from the abdomen
   - (A) Suture breathing
   - (B) Sternal breathing
   - (C) Diaphragmatic breathing
   - (D) Fundus breathing

9. Expired air consists mainly of
    (A) Carbon dioxide
    (B) Oxygen
    (C) Nitrogen
    (D) All of the above

10. The condition in which spasmodic contraction of the muscles that helps expel air forcefully through the mouth and nose
    (A) Sneezing
    (B) Laughing
    (C) Crying
    (D) Coughing

11. The act of sudden and sometimes repetitively occurring reflex, which is useful in clearing the breathing passages from foreign particles
    (A) Laughing
    (B) Coughing
    (C) Crying
    (D) Sighing

12. The reflex and deep simultaneous inhalation of air and stretching of the eardrums, followed by exhalation of breath
    (A) Yawning
    (B) Coughing
    (C) Crying
    (D) Laughing

13. The long and deep inhalation simultaneously followed by a short, audible and forceful exhalation of air arising from emotional changes and tiredness
    (A) Yawning
    (B) Crying
    (C) Laughing
    (D) Sighing

14. The convulsive gasping while aloud so that a series of convulsive inhalations is followed by a single relatively long exhalation
    (A) Sneezing
    (B) Sobbing
    (C) Laughing
    (D) Crying

15. The involuntary spasmodic contraction of the diaphragm that usually repeats several times a minute
    (A) Hiccupping
    (B) Crying
    (C) Laughing
    (D) Coughing

16. Which center stimulate and cause contraction of expiratory muscles and expiration
    (A) Lateral respiratory group
    (B) Distal respiratory group
    (C) Ventral respiratory group
    (D) Proximal respiratory group

17. Which centre stimulate and cause contraction of inspiratory muscles and prolonged inspiration

   (A) Proximal respiratory group
   (B) Dorsal respiratory group
   (C) Distal respiratory group
   (D) Lateral respiratory group

18. Which regulates the activity of inspiratory center by sending inhibitory impulses to the inspiratory area

   (A) Pneumotaxic center
   (B) Insular cortex
   (C) Broca's area
   (D) Dorsal posterior insula

19. Which centre sends stimulatory impulses to the inspiratory area to accelerate the depth of inspiration

   (A) Broca's area
   (B) Insular cortex
   (C) Apneustic centre
   (D) Dorsal posterior insula

20. Which receptor stimulated by changes in the chemical composition of their immediate environment

   (A) Chemoreceptors
   (B) Baroreceptors
   (C) Nociceptors
   (D) Thermoreceptors

21. Chemoreceptors are located in the

   (A) Diaphragm
   (B) Medulla oblongata
   (C) Spinal cord
   (D) Hypothalamus

22. Which receptors are located in the walls of the aortic arch and carotid arteries?

   (A) Peripheral chemoreceptors
   (B) Cutaneous chemoreceptors
   (C) Cutaneous thermoreceptors
   (D) Central nociceptors

23. Which receptor detect variations of oxygen, carbon dioxide and pH in the arterial blood

   (A) Central nociceptors
   (B) Cutaneous thermoreceptors
   (C) Peripheral chemoreceptors
   (D) Cutaneous nociceptors

24. Which receptors present in the walls of bronchi and bronchioles that respond to the stretching of the lung tissues

   (A) Mechanoreceptors
   (B) Thermoreceptors
   (C) Nociceptors
   (D) Chemoreceptors

25. The inflammation of sinus is called
    (A) Sinusitis
    (B) Arthritis
    (C) Bronchitis
    (D) Alveolitis

26. The inflammation of tonsils is called
    (A) Sinusitis
    (B) Arthritis
    (C) Tonsilitis
    (D) Alveolitis

27. The inflammation of throat is called
    (A) Alveolitis
    (B) Pharyngitis
    (C) Arthritis
    (D) Tonsilitis

28. The inflammation of larynx is called
    (A) Pharyngitis
    (B) Arthritis
    (C) Laryngitis
    (D) Tonsilitis

29. The disease occurring most commonly in children in which the area around the larynx and the trachea gets swollen, causing breathing problem
    (A) Endocarditis
    (B) Croup
    (C) Arrythmia
    (D) Dementia

30. The croup disease is caused by various viruses such as
    (A) Parainfluenza virus
    (B) Adenovirus
    (C) Influenza virus
    (D) All of the above

31. The permanent abnormal dilation of bronchi and bronchioles is called
    (A) Bronchiectasis
    (B) Meningitis
    (C) Arthritis
    (D) Nephritis

32. The common inflammatory disease of the airways associated with episodes of reversible over – reactivity of the airway smooth muscle
    (A) Cataracts
    (B) Asthma
    (C) Dementia
    (D) Sclerosis

33. The presence of air in the thoracic interstitial tissues
    (A) Presbyopia
    (B) Presbycusis
    (C) Interstitial emphysema
    (D) Cataracts

34. The group of lung diseases is caused by prolonged exposure to inhale organic dusts, which triggers a generalized inflammation and progressive fibrosis of lung tissues
    (A) Cataracts
    (B) Presbyopia
    (C) Presbycusis
    (D) Pneumoconiosis

35. The localized suppuration and necrosis within the lung substance

(A) Lung abscess

(B) Renal abscess

(C) Gastric abscess

(D) Tibia abscess

36. The infection of the upper respiratory tract caused by the anaerobic Gram – positive bacterium *Coryebacteriumdiphtheriea*

(A) Presbyopia

(B) Diphtheria

(C) Blepharitis

(D) Cataracts

37. An allergic reaction that causes the release of histamine and other mediators of inflammation from the mast cells granules and basophils

(A) Allergic rhinitis

(B) Blepharitis

(C) Labyrinthitis

(D) Otitis

38. The inflammation of epiglottis is called

(A) Arthritis

(B) Pharyngitis

(C) Nephritis

(D) Epiglottitis

39. The bacterium causing tuberculosis is

(A) Otitis

(B) Mycobacterium tuberculosis

(C) Blepharitis

(D) Motion sickness

40. The chronic lung disorder in which the alveoli may be destroyed, narrowed, collapsed, stretched, and overinflated

(A) Pulmonary emphysema

(B) Conjunctivitis

(C) Strabismus

(D) Trachoma

41. The condition in which air gets filled in the pleural cavities

(A) Trachoma

(B) Cataract

(C) Pneumothorax

(D) Otitis

42. The inflammation of the pleural membrane

(A) Pleurisy

(B) Nephritis

(C) Stye

(D) Presbyopia

43. Which infection is caused by bacteria *Streptococcuspneumoniae?*

(A) Presbyopia

(B) Pneumonia

(C) Presbycusis

(D) Labyrinthitis

44. The severe life – threatening condition caused by the blocking if pulmonary artery by blood clot called
    (A) Pulmonary embolism
    (B) Renal embolism
    (C) External otitis
    (D) Blepharitis

45. The inflammation of the bronchioles is called
    (A) Vasculitis
    (B) Arthritis
    (C) Bronchiolitis
    (D) Nephritis

46. The inflammation of the air sacs is called
    (A) Alveolitis
    (B) Nephritis
    (C) Arthritis
    (D) Pharyngitis

47. The inflammation of the lung capillaries is called
    (A) Arthritis
    (B) Pharyngitis
    (C) Vasculitis
    (D) Nephritis

48. The fluid collects in the space between lung and the chest wall
    (A) Arthritis
    (B) Pleural effusion
    (C) Blepharitis
    (D) Stye

49. COPD stands for
    (A) Chronic obstructive pulmonary disease
    (B) Chronic objection pulmonary disorder
    (C) Chronic otitis pulmonary disorder
    (D) Chronic obsessive pulmonary disorder

50. Symptoms of COPD is
    (A) Wheezing
    (B) Shortness of breath
    (C) Chest tightness
    (D) All of the above

Answer Key

Respiratory System and Urinary System (Part-06)

Question	Answer	Question	Answer
01	B = Peak expiratory flow	26	C = Tonsilitis
02	A = Maximum voluntary ventilation	27	B = Pharyngitis
03	A = Diffusing capacity	28	C = Laryngitis
04	B = Eupnoea	29	B = Croup
05	C = Both (A) and (B)	30	D = All of the above
06	B = Costal breathing	31	A = Bronchiectasis
07	A = Costal breathing	32	B = Asthma
08	C = Diaphragmatic breathing	33	C = Interstitial emphysema
09	D = All of the above	34	D = Pneumoconiosis
10	A = Sneezing	35	A = Lung abscess
11	B = Coughing	36	B = Diphtheria
12	A = Yawning	37	A = Allergic rhinitis
13	D = Sighing	38	D = Epiglottis
14	B = Sobbing	39	B = Mycobacterium tuberculosis
15	A = Hiccupping	40	A = Pulmonary emphysema
16	C = Ventral respiratory group	41	C = Pneumothorax
17	B = Dorsal respiratory group	42	A = Pleurisy
18	A = Pneumotaxic centre	43	B = Pneumonia
19	C = Apneustic centre	44	A = Pulmonary embolism
20	A = Chemoreceptors	45	C = Bronchiolitis
21	B = Medulla oblongata	46	A = Alveolitis
22	A = Peripheral chemoreceptors	47	C = Vasculitis
23	C = Peripheral chemoreceptors	48	B = Pleural effusion
24	A = Mechanoreceptors	49	A = Chronic obstructive pulmonary disorder
25	A = Sinusitis	50	D = All of the above

Part-07

1. How much blood passed through the kidney daily in a healthy adult
   - (A) 900 gallons
   - (B) 100 gallons
   - (C) 440 gallons
   - (D) 1200 gallons

2. Which organ lies on the posterior abdominal wall, one on each side of the vertebral column, behind the peritoneum and below the diaphragm
   - (A) Brain
   - (B) Tongue
   - (C) Kidney
   - (D) Heart

3. The length of kidney is about
   - (A) 30 – 40 cm
   - (B) 10 – 11 cm
   - (C) 40 – 45 cm
   - (D) 1 – 2 cm

4. Each kidney weighs in male is about
   - (A) 200 gm
   - (B) 400 gm
   - (C) 150 gm
   - (D) 340 gm

5. Each kidney weighs in female is about
   - (A) 135 gm
   - (B) 400 gm
   - (C) 335 gm
   - (D) 225 gm

6. The outer layer made of fibrous connective tissue that fixes the kidney to the abdominal wall and to the surrounding structures
   - (A) Renal pedicle
   - (B) Renal fascia
   - (C) Renal fissure
   - (D) Renal fundus

7. The middle layer of fat that holds the kidneys in the upright position in the abdominal cavity
   - (A) Renal fundus
   - (B) Renal fissures
   - (C) Adipose capsule
   - (D) Renal pedicle

8. The inner layer made of transparent, fibrous connective tissues that enclose the kidneys
   - (A) Renal capsule
   - (B) Renal fissures
   - (C) Renal pedicle
   - (D) Renal fundus

9. Which gland located superior to the kidney
   - (A) Pineal gland
   - (B) Pituitary gland
   - (C) Thyroid gland
   - (D) Adrenal gland

10. The cortex extends into the medulla, dividing it into triangular shapes called

   (A) Renal pyramids
   (B) Renal pentagonal
   (C) Renal hexane
   (D) Renal octan

11. The apex of a renal pyramid is called a

   (A) Renal tails
   (B) Renal crista
   (C) Renal papilla
   (D) Renal fundus

12. Each renal papilla is associated with structure know as

   (A) Minor calyx
   (B) Major crista
   (C) Major cisternae
   (D) Minors' crista

13. How many minor calyx present in each kidney?

   (A) 20 – 30
   (B) 30 – 35
   (C) 8 – 10
   (D) 40 – 45

14. The outer region of kidney is called

   (A) Renal cortex
   (B) Renal medulla
   (C) Renal suture
   (D) Renal fundus

15. The inner region of kidney is called

   (A) Renal medulla
   (B) Renal cortex
   (C) Renal fundus
   (D) Renal suture

16. The renal cortex is subdivided into

   (A) Cortical zone
   (B) Juxtamedullary zone
   (C) Both (A) and (B)
   (D) None of the above

17. The renal pyramids have a broad base towards the cortex and a narrow end called

   (A) Renal papilla
   (B) Renal fundus
   (C) Renal ilium
   (D) Renal sternal

18. The renal cortex extends in between the space of renal pyramids in the form of colums called

   (A) Renal bands
   (B) Renal fundus
   (C) Renal columns
   (D) Renal meatus

19. Renal columns along with the renal pyramid and superimposed area of the renal cortex constituents a

   (A) Renal lobe
   (B) Renal bands
   (C) Renal fundus
   (D) Renal meatus

20. The hilum expands into a cavity within the kidney called
    (A) Renal meatus
    (B) Renal sinus
    (C) Renal cristae
    (D) Renal fundus

21. Sever minor calices merge to form a
    (A) Major crista
    (B) Major calyx
    (C) Minor cisternae
    (D) Minor crista

22. Urine passes through the major calices into the
    (A) Renal pelvis
    (B) Hepatic pelvis
    (C) Pulmonary pelvis
    (D) Tibial pelvis

23. The medial margin of each kidney is marked by a deep fissure known as
    (A) Renal crista
    (B) Renal cisternae
    (C) Renal hilum
    (D) Renal lobules

24. The kidneys are supplied with blood via
    (A) Renal arteries
    (B) Facial arteries
    (C) Tibial arteries
    (D) Pulmonary arteries

25. The functional unit of kidney is
    (A) Nephron
    (B) Neuron
    (C) Fundus
    (D) Pharynx

26. How many nephrons consists in kidney?
    (A) 10 – 20 million
    (B) 20 – 30 million
    (C) 1 – 2 million
    (D) 30 – 40 million

27. How long the nephron is
    (A) 10 cm
    (B) 3 cm
    (C) 20 cm
    (D) 30 cm

28. The kidneys receive cardiac output about
    (A) 90 %
    (B) 60 %
    (C) 20 %
    (D) 80 %

29. Which of the following have their renal corpuscles in the outer cortex of the kidney and have a very short loop of Henle, which penetrates only the outer zone of the medulla?
    (A) Cortical nephrons
    (B) Cuticle nephrons
    (C) Compact nephrons
    (D) Parietal nephrons

30. How many percent comprise the cortical nephrons of the total nephrons in human kidney
    (A) 10 %
    (B) 20 %
    (C) 80 %
    (D) 25 %

31. Which of the following have their corpuscles in the inner cortex near the corticomedullary junction?

    (A) Juxtamedullary nephrons
    (B) Parietal nephrons
    (C) Peritoneum nephrons
    (D) Hepatic nephrons

32. Glomerulus consists of the bunch of fine networks of capillaries called

    (A) Glomerular lobules
    (B) Glomerular capillaries
    (C) Glomerular globules
    (D) Hepatic lobules

33. The glomerular capillaries are made of a single layer of endothelial called that rest on a basement membrane. The endothelial cells have many pores between them called

    (A) Ossification
    (B) Conduction
    (C) Fenestrations
    (D) Alterations

34. The diameter of fenestrae is about

    (A) 300 nm
    (B) 70 nm
    (C) 450 nm
    (D) 190 nm

35. The cup – shaped structure present in the renal cortex that forms the beginning of the nephron

    (A) Bowman's shells
    (B) Bowman's capsule
    (C) Bowman's canal
    (D) Bowman's fundus

36. The bowman's capsule encloses the glomerulus, and it is formed by the layers are

    (A) Visceral layer
    (B) Parietal layer
    (C) Both (A) and (B)
    (D) None of the above

37. The space between the visceral layer and parietal layer is called

    (A) Capsular space
    (B) Hepatic space
    (C) Pulmonary space
    (D) Ventricular space

38. The Bowman's capsule and glomerular together the constitute the

    (A) Hepatic corpuscle
    (B) Pulmonary corpuscle
    (C) Renal corpuscle
    (D) Nervous corpuscle

39. The visceral layer and parietal layer both composed of single layer of

    (A) Cuboidal epithelial cells
    (B) Columnar epithelial cells
    (C) Ciliated epithelial cells
    (D) Squamous epithelial cells

40. The cells of visceral layer are called

    (A) Osteocytes
    (B) Oocytes
    (C) Podocytes
    (D) Osteoblasts

41. The podocytes subdivide into primary secondary and tertiary branches to terminates into
    - (A) Fundus
    - (B) Pedicles
    - (C) Fissures
    - (D) Sutures

42. Pedicles have gaps between them called
    - (A) Filtration slits
    - (B) Excretion bands
    - (C) Digestion slits
    - (D) Respiration tails

43. The coiled tubule arising from the Bowman's capsule and located in the cortex of kidney
    - (A) Proximal convoluted tubule
    - (B) Frontal convoluted tubule
    - (C) Temporal convoluted tubule
    - (D) Sternal convoluted tubule

44. The walls of the proximal convoluted tubule consist of a single layer of
    - (A) Columnar epithelial cells
    - (B) Cuboidal epithelial cells
    - (C) Cardiac intercalated tissue
    - (D) Nervous tissue

45. The proximal convoluted tubule has a high capacity for
    - (A) Digestion
    - (B) Respiration
    - (C) Reabsorption
    - (D) Inhalation

46. The solutes and water move from the PCT to interstitial and then into
    - (A) Peritubular capillaries
    - (B) Ilium capillaries
    - (C) Fundus capillaries
    - (D) Peritoneum capillaries

47. The route transports solutes through a cell
    - (A) Extracellular route
    - (B) Transcellular route
    - (C) Interstitial route
    - (D) Interstitial route

48. The route transports solutes between cells through the intercellular space
    - (A) Interstitial route
    - (B) Extracellular route
    - (C) Paracellular route
    - (D) Interfacial route

49. How many percent of water reabsorbed by proximal tubules?
    - (A) 10 %
    - (B) 14 %
    - (C) 65 %
    - (D) 34 %

50. How many percent of bicarbonate reabsorbed by proximal tubules?
    - (A) 10 – 20 %
    - (B) 20 – 25 %
    - (C) 30 – 35 %
    - (D) 85 – 90 %

Answer Key

Respiratory System and Urinary System (Part-07)

Question	Answer	Question	Answer
01	C = 440 gallons	26	C = 1 – 2 million
02	C = Kidney	27	B = 3 cm
03	B = 10 – 11 cm	28	C = 20 %
04	C = 150 gm	29	A = Cortical nephrons
05	A = 135 gm	30	C = 80 %
06	B = Renal fascia	31	A = Juxtamedullary nephrons
07	C = Adipose capsule	32	B = Glomerular capillaries
08	A = Renal capsule	33	C = Fenestrations
09	D = Adrenal gland	34	B = 70 nm
10	A = Renal pyramids	35	B = Bowman's capsule
11	C = Renal papilla	36	C = Both (A) and (B)
12	A = Minor calyx	37	A = Capsular space
13	C = 8 – 10	38	C = Renal corpuscle
14	A = Renal cortex	39	D = Squamous epithelial cells
15	A = Renal medulla	40	C = Podocytes
16	C = Both (A) and (B)	41	B = Pedicles
17	A = Renal papilla	42	A = Filtration slits
18	C = Renal columns	43	A = Proximal convoluted tubule
19	A = Renal lobe	44	B = Cuboidal epithelial cells
20	B = Renal sinus	45	C = Reabsorption
21	B = Major calyx	46	A = Peritubular capillaries
22	A = Renal pelvis	47	B = Transcellular route
23	C = Renal hilum	48	C = Paracellular route
24	A = Renal arteries	49	C = 65 %
25	A = Nephron	50	D = 85 – 90 %

Part-08

1. The U – shaped segment of nephron that extends into the renal medulla, makes a hairpin turn and then returns to the renal cortex

   (A) Loop of Henle
   (B) Islets of Langerhans
   (C) Cells of Langerhans
   (D) Loop of cystic

2. The loop of Henle is continuous with PCT and has parts

   (A) Descending limb
   (B) Loop
   (C) Ascending limb
   (D) All of the above

3. In final part of the ascending limb, which lies close to the afferent arteriole, the cuboidal cells are closely packed, and this zone is known as

   (A) Tubula band
   (B) Macula densa
   (C) Tubula fundus
   (D) Tibial fissures

4. The loop of Henle absorbed filtered water about

   (A) 89 %
   (B) 67 %
   (C) 15 %
   (D) 79 %

5. The loop of Henle contributes to the absorption of filtered sodium approximately

   (A) 100 %
   (B) 90 %
   (C) 98 %
   (D) 25 %

6. The descending loop of Henle is highly permeable to water and reabsorption occurs via

   (A) AQPI channels
   (B) ARTP channels
   (C) APOT channels
   (D) ASTI channels

7. The wall of afferent arteriole alongside the macula densa is composed of modified smooth muscle fibres called

   (A) Pulmonary cells
   (B) Cystic cells
   (C) Juxtaglomerular cells
   (D) Canaliculi cells

8. The juxtaglomerular cells along with macula densa constituent the

   (A) Juxtaglomerular apparatus
   (B) Canaliculi apparatus
   (C) Cystic apparatus
   (D) Soleus apparatus

9. The tightly coiled and lies in the renal cortex
   - (A) Lateral convoluted tubule
   - (B) Distal convoluted tubule
   - (C) Vertebral convoluted tubule
   - (D) Sternal convoluted tubule

10. A short terminal part of the DCT that collects urine is called the
    - (A) Cystic duct
    - (B) Canaliculi duct
    - (C) Collecting duct
    - (D) Condensed duct

11. The first step in the formation of urine is
    - (A) Hepatic filtration
    - (B) Glomerular filtration
    - (C) Pulmonary filtration
    - (D) Nervous filtration

12. the fluid filtered from the bloodstream into the glomerular capsule is now called
    - (A) Glomerular filtrate
    - (B) Pulmonary filtrate
    - (C) Gastric filtrate
    - (D) Salivary filtrate

13. Glomerular filtrate contains
    - (A) Glucose
    - (B) Amino acids
    - (C) Urea
    - (D) All of the above

14. The volume of filtrate formed by both kidneys each minute is called
    - (A) Lacrimal filtration rate
    - (B) Glomerular filtration rate
    - (C) Pulmonary filtration rate
    - (D) Gastrointestinal filtration rate

15. In healthy adult the glomerular filtration rate is about
    - (A) 300 mL / min
    - (B) 125 mL / min
    - (C) 340 mL / min
    - (D) 450 mL / min

16. How much filtrate are formed each day by the two kidneys
    - (A) 290 litres
    - (B) 400 litres
    - (C) 180 litres
    - (D) 450 litres

17. Glomerular filtration is also called
    - (A) Ultrafiltration
    - (B) Minifiltration
    - (C) Microfiltration
    - (D) Macrofiltration

18. The blood pressure in glomerular capillaries is called
    - (A) Glomerular kinetic blood pressure
    - (B) Glomerular blood hydrostatic pressure
    - (C) Glomerular potential energy pressure
    - (D) Renal mechanical blood pressure

19. Glomerular blood hydrostatic pressure is about
    (A) 120 mmHg
    (B) 300 mmHg
    (C) 60 mmHg
    (D) 340 mmHg

20. The Bowman's capsule pressure is about
    (A) 30 mmHg
    (B) 18 mmHg
    (C) 44 mmHg
    (D) 50 mmHg

21. The pressure is exerted due increased concentration of plasma proteins in the glomerulus during filtration is called
    (A) Glomerular synthetic potential pressure
    (B) Glomerular solution kinetic pressure
    (C) Glomerular colloid osmotic pressure
    (D) Glomerular solution kinetic energy

22. Glomerular colloid osmotic pressure is about
    (A) 32 mmHg
    (B) 55 mmHg
    (C) 88 mmHg
    (D) 90 mmHg

23. The net filtration pressure is about
    (A) 40 mmHg
    (B) 90 mmHg
    (C) 10 mmHg
    (D) 80 mmHg

24. The renal blood flow is maintained at a constant pressure across a wide range of systolic blood pressures around
    (A) 200 – 300 mmHg
    (B) 80 – 200 mmHg
    (C) 340 – 400 mmHg
    (D) 500 – 550 mmHg

25. In severe shock, when the systolic blood pressure falls below
    (A) 80 mmHg
    (B) 190 mmHg
    (C) 290 mmHg
    (D) 160 mmHg

26. The kidneys help maintain a constant renal blood flow and GRF despite normal changes in blood pressure every day. This capability is called
    (A) Autoregulation
    (B) Autogeneration
    (C) Autohydration
    (D) Automaintainence

27. Which refers to the qualitative and quantitative changes in the glomerular filtrate during its passage through the tubular portion of the nephron till the collecting duct
    (A) Fundus reabsorption
    (B) Tubular reabsorption
    (C) Soleus reabsorption
    (D) Pulmonary reabsorption

28. Which involves the movement of molecules against electrochemical gradient. This process needs energy, which is derived from ATP
    - (A) Active reabsorption
    - (B) Passive reabsorption
    - (C) Facilitate reabsorption
    - (D) Conduction reabsorption

29. Which process involves the movement of molecules along the electrochemical gradient. This process does not need energy
    - (A) Conduction reabsorption
    - (B) Passive reabsorption
    - (C) Active reabsorption
    - (D) Diffusion reabsorption

30. The active reabsorption of glucose by sodium – glucose transport and GLUT is about
    - (A) 10 %
    - (B) 14 %
    - (C) 100 %
    - (D) 30 %

31. The active reabsorption of Oligopeptides, proteins and amino acids is about
    - (A) 35 %
    - (B) 45 %
    - (C) 32 %
    - (D) 95 %

32. Oligopeptides, proteins, and amino acids appears in urine is about
    - (A) 40 %
    - (B) 5 %
    - (C) 69 %
    - (D) 60 %

33. The sodium and potassium ions are reabsorbed actively by
    - (A) Na – H antiport
    - (B) Calcium channels
    - (C) Chloride channels
    - (D) Ferric channels

34. Bicarbonate ions are reabsorbed about
    - (A) 10.9 %
    - (B) 20.3 %
    - (C) 99.9 %
    - (D) 59.9 %

35. The DCT and collecting duct actively reabsorb sodium from the filtrate under the influence of the hormone
    - (A) Oxytocin
    - (B) Growth hormone
    - (C) Melanin
    - (D) Aldosterone

36. Which drugs are actively secreted in PCT?
    - (A) Penicillin
    - (B) Aspirin
    - (C) Both (A) and (B)
    - (D) None of the above

37. Carbonic acid is converted to
    - (A) CO_2
    - (B) SO_2
    - (C) Cl_2
    - (D) F_2

38. The specific gravity of urine is between

    (A) 2300 – 2340

    (B) 1020 – 1030

    (C) 2100 – 2150

    (D) 3010 – 3020

39. Which hormone secreted by adrenal cortex and increases the reabsorption of sodium and water and the excretion of potassium

    (A) Oxytocin

    (B) Thyroid

    (C) Aldosterone

    (D) Melatonin

40. The minimum urinary output, i.e. the smallest volume required to excrete body waste product, is about

    (A) 1200 mL per day

    (B) 500 mL per day

    (C) 1340 mL per day

    (D) 1250 mL per day

41. The distal convoluted tubule and collecting duct reabsorbed solutes about

    (A) 30 %

    (B) 45 %

    (C) 7 %

    (D) 77 %

42. Which cells responsible for the resorption of sodium ions and water and secretion of K+ ions

    (A) Principal cells

    (B) Mast cells

    (C) Stem cells

    (D) Sternal cells

43. Which cells containing carbonic anhydrase which involved in acid – base balance

    (A) Mast cells

    (B) Stem cells

    (C) Intercalated cells

    (D) Intervertebral cells

44. The normal pH of urine is

    (A) 2.3 to 3.4

    (B) 4.5 to 8

    (C) 1.2 to 2.1

    (D) 13 to 13.9

45. How many percent of urea present in urine?

    (A) 10 %

    (B) 43 %

    (C) 51 %

    (D) 2 %

46. In the collecting duct, H_2O reabsorption is driven by

    (A) Antidiuretic hormone

    (B) Oxytocin

    (C) Melatonin

    (D) Melanin

47. The transporters that move two molecules in the same direction is called

    (A) Symporters

    (B) Antiporters

    (C) Miniporters

    (D) Macroporters

48. The transporters that move two molecules in the opposite direction is called

    (A) Miniporters   (B) Miniporters

    (C) Antiporters   (D) Symporters

49. The afferent and efferent arterioles enter and exit the glomerulus is called

    (A) Vascular pole   (B) Rugae pole

    (C) Oblique pole   (D) Serosa pole

50. The pole where the ultrafiltrate exits Bowman's space and a proximal convoluted tubule begins

    (A) Cricoid pole   (B) Urinary pole

    (C) Cardia pole   (D) Curvature pole

Answer Key

Respiratory System and Urinary System (Part-08)

Question	Answer	Question	Answer
01	A = Loop of Henle	26	A = Autoregulation
02	D = All of the above	27	B = Tubular reabsorption
03	B = Macula densa	28	A = Active reabsorption
04	C = 15 %	29	B = Passive reabsorption
05	D = 25 %	30	C = 100 %
06	A = AQPI channels	31	D = 95 %
07	C = Juxtaglomerular cells	32	B = 5 %
08	A = Juxtaglomerular apparatus	33	A = Na – H antiport
09	B = Distal convoluted tubule	34	C = 99.9 %
10	C = Collecting duct	35	D = Aldosterone
11	B = Glomerular filtration	36	C = Both (A) and (B)
12	A = Glomerular filtration	37	A = CO_2
13	D = All of the above	38	B = 1020 – 1030
14	B = Glomerular filtration rate	39	C = Aldosterone
15	B = 125 mL / min	40	B = 500 mL per day
16	C = 180 litres	41	C = 7 %
17	A = Ultrafiltration	42	A = Principal cells
18	B = Glomerular blood hydrostatic pressure	43	C = Intercalated cells
19	C = 60 mmHg	44	B = 4.5 to 8
20	B = 18 mmHg	45	D = 2 %
21	C = Glomerular colloid osmotic pressure	46	A = Antidiuretic hormone
22	A = 32 mmHg	47	A = Symporters
23	C = 10 mmHg	48	C = Antiporters
24	B = 80 – 200 mmHg	49	A = Vascular pole
25	A = 80 mmHg	50	B = Urinary pole

Part-09

1. The long tubular structures that extend from the renal pelvis of the kidney to connect to the posterior surface of the urinary bladder
    (A) Oesophagus
    (B) Ureters
    (C) Pharynx
    (D) Bronchus

2. How long each ureter is
    (A) 100 – 200 cm
    (B) 25 – 30 cm
    (C) 50 – 60 cm
    (D) 80 – 90 cm

3. The diameter of ureter is
    (A) 0.3 cm
    (B) 3.0 cm
    (C) 3.2 cm
    (D) 3.9 cm

4. The inner layer is made up of transitional epithelium that can stretch
    (A) Connective tissue
    (B) Mucosa
    (C) Osteoblast
    (D) Parenchyma

5. The middle layer is made up of two layers of smooth muscle
    (A) Meristem layer
    (B) Adipose layer
    (C) Muscular layer
    (D) Cartilage layer

6. The outer layer is made up of fibrous tissue that forms the outer covering of ureters
    (A) Cartilage layer
    (B) Adipose layer
    (C) Neuronal layer
    (D) Fibrous layer

7. Which serve to propel the urine from the kidney into the urinary bladder
    (A) Ureters
    (B) Oesophagus
    (C) Bronchus
    (D) Aorta

8. The lumen of each ureter is lined by a mucosal layer of
    (A) Transitional epithelium
    (B) Areolar tissue
    (C) Hyaline cartilage
    (D) Skeletal tissues

9. The ureter receives parasympathetic supply from the
    (A) Pelvic splanchnic nerves
    (B) Inferior hypogastric plexus
    (C) Both (A) and (B)
    (D) None of the above

10. The peristaltic wave rises in the calyces of the kidney and pass to the urinary bladder about
    (A) 10 – 20 times per minute
    (B) 1 – 5 times per minute
    (C) 20 – 25 times per minute
    (D) 25 – 30 times per minute

11. The hollow, distensible pear-shaped sac located in the lower or pelvic region of the abdominal cavity, just behind the symphysis pubis
    (A) Urinary bladder
    (B) Gall bladder
    (C) Aorta
    (D) Cystic bladder

12. The average capacity of urinary bladder is
    (A) 2000 – 3000 mL
    (B) 700 – 800 mL
    (C) 1500 – 1800 mL
    (D) 2100 – 2500 mL

13. Which layer of urinary bladder composed of transitional epithelium; it consists of rugae that help in the distension of the wall
    (A) Distal layer
    (B) Inner layer
    (C) circular layer
    (D) Oblique layer

14. Which layer of urinary bladder is also called detrusor muscles?
    (A) Middle layer
    (B) Outer layer
    (C) Circular layer
    (D) Oblique layer

15. Which smooth muscle fibres consists in inner layer of detrusor muscles layer of urinary bladder is
    (A) Longitudinal fibres
    (B) Vertical fibres
    (C) Distal fibres
    (D) Oblique fibres

16. Which smooth muscle fibres consists in middle layer of detrusor muscles layer of urinary bladder is
    (A) Oblique fibres
    (B) Circular fibres
    (C) Vertical fibres
    (D) Lateral fibres

17. The contraction of which layer results in the emptying of the urinary bladder
    (A) Soleus muscles
    (B) Pectineus muscles
    (C) Sartorius muscles
    (D) Detrusor muscles

18. The outer layer of urinary bladder is composed of connective tissues contains
    (A) Blood vessels
    (B) Nerves
    (C) Both (A) and (B)
    (D) None of the above

19. How many openings are there in interior of the urinary bladder
   - (A) Six
   - (B) Three
   - (C) Five
   - (D) Seven

20. How many posterior openings are there in urinary bladder?
   - (A) Four
   - (B) Five
   - (C) Two
   - (D) Six

21. The internal urethral sphincter is made up of
   - (A) Detrusor muscle
   - (B) Soleus muscle
   - (C) Sartorius muscle
   - (D) Tibialis posterior

22. The small tubular structure leading from the floor of the urinary bladder to the exterior of the body
   - (A) Oesophagus
   - (B) Urethra
   - (C) Bronchus
   - (D) Intestine

23. How long the urethra in females
   - (A) 7 – 8 cm
   - (B) 20 – 24 cm
   - (C) 3 – 5 cm
   - (D) 30 – 35 cm

24. How long the urethra in males
   - (A) 40 cm
   - (B) 1 cm
   - (C) 20 cm
   - (D) 5 cm

25. In male's urethra carries urine and also carries
   - (A) Saliva
   - (B) Lacrimal fluid
   - (C) Synovial fluid
   - (D) Spermatic fluid

26. The mucosa of the urethra consists of
   - (A) Simple cuboidal epithelium
   - (B) Stratified squamous epithelium
   - (C) Cardiac tissue
   - (D) Simple ciliated epithelium

27. Which layer of urethra consists of the spongy connective tissue that contain blood vessels and nerves
   - (A) Submucosa
   - (B) Tendon
   - (C) Ligament
   - (D) Cartilage

28. Which layer of urethra forms the internal and external urethral sphincter
   - (A) Cartilage layer
   - (B) Ligament layer
   - (C) Muscle layer
   - (D) Tendon layer

29. The internal urethral sphincter composed of
    - (A) Smooth muscle fibres
    - (B) Elastic tissue
    - (C) Both (A) and (B)
    - (D) None of the above

30. Which of the following serves as a channel through which the urine is expelled out of the body?
    - (A) Urethra
    - (B) Intestine
    - (C) Appendix
    - (D) Oesophagus

31. Which part of male urethra begins as a continuation of the bladder neck and passes through the prostate gland
    - (A) Prostate urethra
    - (B) Soleus urethra
    - (C) Deltoid urethra
    - (D) Tibialis urethra

32. Prostate urethra supplied by the
    - (A) Inferior vesical artery
    - (B) Inferior facial artery
    - (C) Superior parietal artery
    - (D) Inferior tibial artery

33. Which part of male urethra receives the ejaculatory ducts and the prostatic ducts
    - (A) Calves' urethra
    - (B) Membranous urethra
    - (C) Pectoralis urethra
    - (D) Tibialis urethra

34. Membranous urethra supplied by the
    - (A) Facial artery
    - (B) Bulbourethral artery
    - (C) Tibial artery
    - (D) Clavicle artery

35. Which part of male urethra passes through the bulb and corpus spongiosum of the penis, ending at the external urethral orifice
    - (A) Tibialis urethra
    - (B) Gracilis urethra
    - (C) Rectus urethra
    - (D) Penile urethra

36. Penile urethra supplied directly by the branches of the
    - (A) Internal pudendal artery
    - (B) Internal facial artery
    - (C) Internal clavicle artery
    - (D) External tibial artery

37. The nerve supply to the female urethra arises from the
    - (A) Pudendal nerve
    - (B) Facial nerve
    - (C) Tibial nerve
    - (D) Clavicle nerve

38. The superolateral aspects of the urinary bladder drains into the
    - (A) External iliac nodes
    - (B) Axillary lymph node
    - (C) Subclavian lymph node
    - (D) Cervical lymph node

39. Lymphatic drainage of the proximal female urethra is to the
    (A) Subclavian lymph node
    (B) Pectoral lymph node
    (C) Internal iliac nodes
    (D) Cervical lymph node

40. The process by which urine is voided from the urinary bladder is called
    (A) Ossification
    (B) Micturition
    (C) Conduction
    (D) Digestion

41. Micturition is also called as
    (A) Digestion
    (B) Respiration
    (C) Urination
    (D) Ossification

42. The impulses that initiate a conscious desire to expel urine by triggering a spinal reflex
    (A) Micturition reflex
    (B) Digestion reflex
    (C) Respiration reflex
    (D) Ossification reflex

43. The reflex starts when the urinary bladder is filled with about
    (A) 1000 – 1200 mL
    (B) 300 – 400 mL
    (C) 900 – 1000 mL
    (D) 1400 – 1500 mL

44. The stretch receptors transmit sensory impulses to the micturition centre located at
    (A) C1 – C2 segments of the cervical spinal cord
    (B) S2 – S3 segments of the sacral spinal cord
    (C) T1 – T5 segments of the thoracic spinal cord
    (D) L1 – L3 segments of the lumbar spinal cord

45. Urine output is less than 400 mL per day is called
    (A) Oliguria
    (B) Polyuria
    (C) Incontinence
    (D) Ketonuria

46. Presence of ketone in urine is called
    (A) Oliguria
    (B) Polyuria
    (C) Ketonuria
    (D) Nocturia

47. Passing urine during the night is called
    (A) Ketonuria
    (B) Nocturia
    (C) Polyuria
    (D) Oliguria

48. Involuntary loss of urine is called
    (A) Incontinence
    (B) Polyuria
    (C) Oliguria
    (D) Ketonuria

49. Absence of urine is called
    (A) Anuria
    (B) Oliguria
    (C) Ketonuria
    (D) Polyuria

50. Passing unusually large amounts of urine is called
    (A) Anuria
    (B) Ketonuria
    (C) Polyuria
    (D) Oliguria

Answer Key

Respiratory System and Urinary System (Part-09)

Question	Answer	Question	Answer
01	B = Ureters	26	B = Stratified squamous epithelium
02	B = 25 – 30 cm	27	A = Submucosa
03	A = 0.3 cm	28	C = Muscle layer
04	B = Mucosa	29	C = Both (A) and (B)
05	C = Muscular layer	30	A = Urethra
06	D = Fibrous layer	31	A = Prostate urethra
07	A = Ureters	32	A = Inferior vesical artery
08	A = Transitional epithelium	33	B = Membranous urethra
09	C = Both (A) and (B)	34	B = Bulbourethral artery
10	B = 1 – 5 times per minute	35	D = Penile urethra
11	A = Urinary bladder	36	A = Internal pudendal artery
12	B = 700 – 800 mL	37	A = Pudendal nerve
13	B = Inner layer	38	A = External iliac nodes
14	A = Middle layer	39	C = Internal iliac nodes
15	A = Longitudinal fibres	40	B = Micturition
16	B = Circular fibres	41	C = Urination
17	D = Detrusor muscles	42	A = Micturition reflex
18	C = Both (A) and (B)	43	B = 300 – 400 mL
19	B = Three	44	B = S2 – S3 segments of the sacral spinal cord
20	C = Two	45	A = Oliguria
21	A = Detrusor muscle	46	C = Ketonuria
22	B = Urethra	47	B = Nocturia
23	C = 3 – 5 cm	48	A = Incontinence
24	C = 20 cm	49	A = Anuria
25	D = Spermatic fluid	50	C = Polyuria

Part-10

1. The microbial infection that are most common in females due to the shorter length of urethra
   - (A) Urinary tract infection
   - (B) Respiratory tract infection
   - (C) Digestive tract infection
   - (D) Oesophagus infection

2. Which of the following does not include UTIs?
   - (A) Urethritis
   - (B) Cystitis
   - (C) Urethritis
   - (D) Bronchitis

3. The microorganism cause UTI
   - (A) E. coli
   - (B) S. Typhi
   - (C) Orbivirus
   - (D) Plasmodium

4. The inflammation of glomerulus is called
   - (A) Bronchitis
   - (B) Glomerulonephritis
   - (C) Hepatitis
   - (D) Arthritis

5. The genetic disorder characterized by the formation of cysts at the junction of the DCT and collecting duct
   - (A) Polycystic disease
   - (B) Pneumonia
   - (C) Typhoid
   - (D) Influenza

6. Which of the following refers to the microbial infection of the renal pelvis of the kidney?
   - (A) Arthritis
   - (B) Pyelonephritis
   - (C) Influenza
   - (D) Typhoid

7. Which of the following refers to the condition in which the kidney is dented reversibly, characterized by decreased glomerular filtration?
   - (A) Acute liver failure
   - (B) Acute lungs failure
   - (C) Acute renal failure
   - (D) Acute pancreas failure

8. The reasons associated with acute renal failure may include
   - (A) Severe shock
   - (B) Tubular necrosis
   - (C) Tumour of uterus
   - (D) All of the above

9. Symptoms of acute renal failure is
   - (A) Oliguria
   - (B) Coughing
   - (C) Sneezing
   - (D) Chest pain

10. The condition in which the kidney is dented irreversibly, characterized by irreversible decline in glomerular filtration rate

    (A) Chronic renal failure   (B) Chronic spleen failure

    (C) Chronic lung failure   (D) Chronic liver failure

11. Patients with end – stage renal failure require

    (A) Incision   (B) Haemodialysis

    (C) Hysteroscopy   (D) Laparoscopy

12. Renal stones are also known as

    (A) Renal calculi   (B) Renal compact

    (C) Renal crista   (D) Renal cisternae

13. The inferior displacement or slipping of the kidney from its normal position

    (A) Hepatosis   (B) Pulmotosis

    (C) Nephroptosis   (D) Pancreotosis

14. Presence of protein in urine is called

    (A) Proteinuria   (B) Alkalinouria

    (C) Ketonuria   (D) Glycosuria

15. Pain on passing urine, often described as a burning sensation is called

    (A) Anuria   (B) Dysuria

    (C) Glycosuria   (D) Ketonuria

16. Presence of sugar glucose in urine is called

    (A) Oliguria   (B) Ketonuria

    (C) Glycosuria   (D) Proteinouria

17. Which stage of kidney disease characterized by mild kidney damage, through its function may still be normal and kidney function is about 90 %

    (A) Stage 7   (B) Stage 6

    (C) Stage 5   (D) Stage 1

18. Which stage of kidney disease means that mild loss of kidney function has started and kidney function is at about 89 – 60 %

    (A) Stage 2   (B) Stage 8

    (C) Stage 6   (D) Stage 5

19. Which stage of kidney disease means that there is mild – to – moderate loss of kidney and kidney function is at 59 – 45 %

    (A) Stage 3d   (B) Stage 3e

    (C) Stage 3a   (D) Stage 4a

20. Which stage of kidney disease means that there is moderate – to –severe loss of kidney and kidney function is at 44 – 30 %
    (A) Stage 5a
    (B) Stage 3b
    (C) Stage 4b
    (D) Stage 4a

21. Which stage of kidney disease characterized by severe loss of kidney function and kidney function is at about 29 – 15 %
    (A) Stage 4
    (B) Stage 6
    (C) Stage 7
    (D) Stage 8

22. Which stage of kidney disease means kidney failure and kidney function is now less than 15 %
    (A) Stage 1
    (B) Stage 2
    (C) Stage 5
    (D) Stage 7

23. Acute kidney injury are classified as
    (A) Prerenal
    (B) Renal
    (C) Postrenal
    (D) All of the above

24. Which acute kidney injury is the result of reduced renal blood flow?
    (A) Prerenal
    (B) Renal
    (C) Hepatic
    (D) Cystic

25. Which acute kidney injury is due to damage to the kidney itself?
    (A) Prerenal
    (B) Renal
    (C) Hepatic
    (D) Cystic

26. Which acute kidney injury arises from obstruction to the outflow of urine
    (A) Hepatic
    (B) Cystic
    (C) Postrenal
    (D) Prerenal

27. Example of prerenal acute kidney injury
    (A) Severe shock
    (B) Tumour of uterus
    (C) Glomerulonephritis
    (D) Hepatitis

28. Example of postrenal acute kidney injury
    (A) Severe shock
    (B) Tumour of uterus or cervix
    (C) Hepatitis
    (D) Arthritis

29. Example of renal acute kidney injury
    (A) Hepatisis
    (B) Arthritis
    (C) Acute tubular necrosis
    (D) Osteomyelitis

30. Which condition is almost always associated with reflux of urine from the bladder to the ureter, allowing spread of infection upwards the kidneys?

    (A) Reflux nephropathy
    (B) Reflux hepatopathy
    (C) Reflux pulmopathy
    (D) Reflex cardiopathy

31. The acute bacterial infection of the renal pelvis and calyces, which spreads to the kidney substance and causing small abscesses

    (A) Acute presbycusis
    (B) Acute pyelonephritis
    (C) Acute presbyopia
    (D) Acute hepatosis

32. The dilation of the renal pelvis and calyces, caused by accumulation of urine above an obstruction in the urinary tract

    (A) Hydronephrosis
    (B) Hydroarthritis
    (C) Hydrobronchitis
    (D) Hydrolactosis

33. Which of the following leads to destruction of the nephrons and fibrosis and atrophy of the kidney?

    (A) Hydrogastritis
    (B) Hydrolactosis
    (C) Hydronephrosis
    (D) Hydrobronchitis

34. When the nerve supply to the bladder is interrupted is called

    (A) Spinal lesions
    (B) Sternal lesions
    (C) Synovial lesions
    (D) Hydration lesions

35. The leakage of urine when intra – abdominal pressure is raised

    (A) Stress incontinence
    (B) Simplex incontinence
    (C) Tension incontinence
    (D) Sternal incontinence

36. Leakage of urine follows a sudden and intense urge to void and there is inability to delay passing urine

    (A) Simplex incontinence
    (B) Urge incontinence
    (C) Visual incontinence
    (D) Sternal incontinence

37. Which of the following occurs when there is chronic overfilling of the bladder and may be caused by retention of urine due to incomplete voiding when there is obstruction of urinary outflow?

    (A) Overload incontinence
    (B) Overflow incontinence
    (C) Tolerate incontinence
    (D) Simplex incontinence

38. The reduction in glomerular filtration, selective reabsorption and secretion by the tubules

    (A) Heart failure due to fluid overload
    (B) Generalised and pulmonary oedema
    (C) Accumulation of urea
    (D) All of the above

39. When death is likely without renal replacement therapy, such as haemodialysis, peritoneal dialysis or a kidney transplant, the condition is referred as

    (A) End – stage renal disease

    (B) Before - stage renal disease

    (C) After - stage renal disease

    (D) Previous - stage renal disease

40. The disease that causes proteins made by your immune system to build up in kidneys and damage the glomeruli is called

    (A) ACE nephropathy

    (B) IgA nephropathy

    (C) ECG nephropathy

    (D) Abd nephropathy

41. There are hard deposits of minerals or salts formed inside the kidneys

    (A) Renal stones

    (B) Hepatic stones

    (C) Gastric stones

    (D) Pulmonary stones

42. The condition in which enlarged prostate and increase the size of the prostate gland

    (A) Blepharitis

    (B) Benign prostatic hyperplasia

    (C) Labyrinthitis

    (D) Meniere's disease

43. Symptoms of urinary disorder include

    (A) Abdominal cramping

    (B) Cloudy urine

    (C) Frequent urination

    (D) All of the above

44. Kidney stone is also called

    (A) Nephrolithiasis

    (B) Arthritis

    (C) Bronchitis

    (D) Meningitis

45. A chronic problem that causes bladder pain and frequent, urgent urination is called

    (A) Interstitial cystitis

    (B) Intramedullary cystitis

    (C) Intraoccular cystitis

    (D) Tubular cystitis

46. A condition in which the bladder squeezes urine out at the wrong time

    (A) Overloaded bladder

    (B) Overactive bladder

    (C) Over sensitive bladder

    (D) Over responding bladder

47. The outward bulge of the inner epithelial lining of the bladder through a defect in its muscular layer

    (A) Bladder diffusion

    (B) Bladder diversion

    (C) Bladder diverticulum

    (D) Bladder differentiation

48. If a child is born with a ureter that does not connect with the bladder, it can drain somewhere outside the bladder

    (A) Ectopic ureter

    (B) Extern ureter

    (C) Interna ureter

    (D) Intropic ureter

49. The ureter that exceeds the upper limits of normal size

    (A) Microureter

    (B) Macroureter

    (C) Megaureter

    (D) Forced ureter

50. When urine flows back from the bladder is called

    (A) Vesicoureteral reflux

    (B) Ventroureter reflex

    (C) Vascular reflex

    (D) Ventral reflux

Answer Key

Respiratory System and Urinary System (Part-10)

Question	Answer	Question	Answer
01	A = Urinary tract infection	26	C = Postrenal
02	D = Bronchitis	27	A = severe shock
03	A = E. coli	28	B = Tumour of uterus or cervix
04	B = Glomerulonephritis	29	C = Acute tubular necrosis
05	A = Polycystic disease	30	A = Reflux nephropathy
06	B = Pyelonephritis	31	B = acute pyelonephritis
07	C = Acute renal failure	32	A = Hydronephrosis
08	D = All of the above	33	C = Hydronephrosis
09	A = Oliguria	34	A = Spinal lesions
10	A = Chronic renal failure	35	A = Stress incontinence
11	B = Haemodialysis	36	B = Urge incontinence
12	A = Renal calculi	37	B = Overflow incontinence
13	C = Nephrotosis	38	D = All of the above
14	A = Proteinuria	39	A = End – stage renal disease
15	B = Dysuria	40	B = IgA nephropathy
16	C = Glycosuria	41	A = Renal stones
17	D = Stage 1	42	B = Benign prostatic hyperplasia
18	A = Stage 2	43	D = All of the above
19	C = Stage 3a	44	A = Nephrolithiasis
20	B = Stage 3b	45	A = Interstitial bladder
21	A = Stage 4	46	B = Overactive bladder
22	C = Stage 5	47	C = Bladder diverticulum
23	D = All of the above	48	A = Ectopic ureter
24	A = Prerenal	49	C = Megaureter
25	B = Renal	50	A = Vesicoureteral reflux

Notes

Unit - X

Reproductive System and Introduction to Genetics

Part-01

1. The organ involved in human reproduction is called
   - (A) Reproductive organs
   - (B) Circulatory organs
   - (C) Respiratory organs
   - (D) Digestive organs
2. The fusion of male gametes and female gametes by a process called
   - (A) Conduction
   - (B) Fertilization
   - (C) Polarization
   - (D) Digestion
3. The male gametes is called
   - (A) Spermatozoa
   - (B) Osteoblast
   - (C) Ova
   - (D) Osteoclast
4. The female gametes is called
   - (A) Osteoclast
   - (B) Ova
   - (C) Spermatozoa
   - (D) Osteoblast
5. The paired oval – shaped glands housed in the scrotum is called
   - (A) Testes
   - (B) Vagina
   - (C) Ovary
   - (D) Cervix
6. The length of testes is about
   - (A) 10 cm
   - (B) 13 cm
   - (C) 5 cm
   - (D) 14 cm
7. The diameter of testes is about
   - (A) 5.5 cm
   - (B) 6.5 cm
   - (C) 7.6 cm
   - (D) 2.5 cm
8. The outer membrane covered the testes is called
   - (A) Tunica vaginalis
   - (B) Tunica basale
   - (C) Tunica corneum
   - (D) Tunica lucideum

9. The layer surrounds the tunica albuginea that shields the seminiferous tubules

(A) Visceral layer

(B) Lateral layer

(C) Medial layer

(D) Circular layer

10. Which layer is an empty space between the visceral layer and the outermost layer of the tunica vaginalis?

(A) Stratum basale

(B) Cavum vaginale

(C) Stratum corneum

(D) Stratum lucideum

11. Which layer is the outermost layer protective layer that surrounds almost the entire testicular structure?

(A) Stratum layer

(B) Basale layer

(C) Parietal layer

(D) Lucideum layer

12. Beneath the tunica vaginalis, there is a layer dense white fibrous connective tissue called

(A) Stratum corneum

(B) Tunica albuginea

(C) Stratum basale

(D) Stratum spinosum

13. The tunica albuginea extends inwards and divides the testis into a number of small, internal compartments known as

(A) Lobules

(B) Globules

(C) Vacuoles

(D) Lysosomes

14. Each of the 200 – 300 lobules contain 1 – 3 tightly coiled tubules, called the

(A) Seminiferous tubules

(B) Proximal convoluted tubules

(C) Distal convoluted tubules

(D) Lateral tubules

15. The seminiferous tubules are lined by

(A) Mast cells

(B) Sertoli cells

(C) Stem cells

(D) Nerve cells

16. Between the seminiferous tubules are groups of interstitial cells that secrete the hormone

(A) Melatonin

(B) Melanin

(C) Testosterone

(D) Thyroid

17. The interstitial cells of seminiferous tubules are also called

(A) Leydig cells

(B) Nerve cells

(C) Stem cells

(D) Mast cells

18. The long, coiled tube that stores sperm and transports it from the testes
    - (A) Epididymis
    - (B) Humerus
    - (C) Femur
    - (D) Glomerulus

19. The length of epididymis is about
    - (A) 20 feet
    - (B) 40 feet
    - (C) 50 feet
    - (D) 70 feet

20. The most proximal part of the epididymis is
    - (A) Band
    - (B) Head
    - (C) Branch
    - (D) Stem

21. Which of the following formed by the heavily coiled duct of the epididymis
    - (A) Body
    - (B) Band
    - (C) Branch
    - (D) Stem

22. The most distal part of the epididymis
    - (A) Band
    - (B) Branch
    - (C) Tail
    - (D) Stem

23. Sperm is produced by the process of
    - (A) Ossification
    - (B) Spermatogenesis
    - (C) Osteogenesis
    - (D) Oogenesis

24. Sperm is produced in the
    - (A) Seminiferous tubules
    - (B) Proximal convoluted tubules
    - (C) Distal convoluted tubules
    - (D) Lateral tubules

25. In human, spermatogenesis takes about
    - (A) 30 – 32 days
    - (B) 40 – 45 days
    - (C) 65 – 75 days
    - (D) 10 – 20 days

26. The sperm production begins in the stem cells called
    - (A) Spermatogonia
    - (B) Spermatogion
    - (C) Spermatonion
    - (D) Spermatolion

27. The spermatogonia undergo mitotic division to produce the daughter cells called
    - (A) Tertiary spermatocytes
    - (B) Primary spermatocytes
    - (C) Quandary spermatocytes
    - (D) Primary osteocytes

28. The primary spermatocytes undergo first meiotic division to form

    (A) Secondary spermatocytes   (B) Tertiary spermatocytes

    (C) Secondary osteocytes   (D) Primary osteocytes

29. The secondary spermatocytes then undergo second meiotic division to fom

    (A) Spermatids   (B) Spermadids

    (C) Spermalits   (D) Spermatoids

30. Each spermatid eventually matures into single sperm / spermatozoa by a process called

    (A) Osteogenesis   (B) Spermiogenesis

    (C) Ossification   (D) Oogenesis

31. Successful spermatogenesis takes place at a temperature about

    (A) 40 °C   (B) 3 °C

    (C) 16°C   (D) 26 °C

32. How many sperm mature each day?

    (A) 1200 million   (B) 1400 million

    (C) 300 million   (D) 900 million

33. Which cells secrete testicular fluid, androgen – binding protein and inhibin hormone

    (A) Mast cells   (B) Sertoli cells

    (C) Stem cells   (D) Nerve cells

34. Sertoli cells developed and mature sperm cells and then released in the lumen of the seminiferous tubule by a process called

    (A) Spermiation   (B) Oomiation

    (C) Lactation   (D) Ossification

35. How long the sperm survive in female reproductive system once ejaculated

    (A) 120 hours   (B) 48 hours

    (C) 72 hours   (D) 108 hours

36. How long the human sperm is

    (A) 20 μm   (B) 10 μm

    (C) 60 μm   (D) 120 μm

37. Which part of sperm contains the nucleus with genetic material and acrosome

    (A) Head   (B) Band

    (C) Tail   (D) Root

38. Acrosome contains enzymes are
    (A) Hyaluronidase
    (B) Proteinase
    (C) Both (A) and (B)
    (D) None of the above

39. Which part of sperm contains spirally arranged mitochondria that produce ATP required for sperm mobility
    (A) Corner piece
    (B) Middle piece
    (C) Side piece
    (D) Front piece

40. Which of the following part of sperm is a typical flagellum?
    (A) Head
    (B) Band
    (C) Middle piece
    (D) Tail

41. Testosterone is converted to more potent dihydrotestosterone by the action of enzyme
    (A) 5 – á – reductase
    (B) 10 – â – reductase
    (C) 29 – ã – synthase
    (D) 50 – â – synthetase

42. Both testosterone and dihydrotestosterone bind to the
    (A) Adrenalin receptors
    (B) Androgen receptors
    (C) Olfactory receptors
    (D) Ach receptors

43. The straight tubules lead to a network of ducts in the testes called the
    (A) Rete testis
    (B) Date testis
    (C) Hydro testis
    (D) Lacto testis

44. The testis and epididymis receive innervation from the
    (A) Pedicular plexus
    (B) Testicular plexus
    (C) Cervical plexus
    (D) Intercostal plexus

45. The main arterial supply to the testes and epididymis is via the paired
    (A) Testicular arteries
    (B) Femoral arteries
    (C) Carotid arteries
    (D) Radial arteries

46. The testis are originally retroperitoneal organs, the lymphatic drainage is to the
    (A) Lumbar nodes
    (B) Para – aortic nodes
    (C) Both (A) and (B)
    (D) None of the above

47. Each spermatic cord contains
    (A) Testicular artery
    (B) Testicular veins
    (C) Lymphatics
    (D) All of the above

48. Deferent duct is also called
  (A) Vas deferens
  (B) Bas deferens
  (C) Mas deferens
  (D) Las deferens

49. How long the vas deferens is
  (A) 90 cm
  (B) 45 cm
  (C) 120 cm
  (D) 130 cm

50. The end of the ductus deferens has a dilated terminal portion known as the
  (A) Ampulla
  (B) Tubula
  (C) Virtula
  (D) Pedicle

Answer Key

Reproductive System and Introduction to Genetics (Part-01)

Question	Answer	Question	Answer
01	A = Reproductive organs	26	A = Spermatogonia
02	B = Fertilization	27	B = Primary spermatocytes
03	A = Spermatozoa	28	A = Secondary spermatocytes
04	B = Ova	29	A = Spermatids
05	A = Testes	30	B = Spermiogenesis
06	C = 5 cm	31	B = 3 °C
07	D = 2.5 cm	32	C = 300 million
08	A = Tunica vaginalis	33	B = Sertoli cells
09	A = Visceral layer	34	A = Spermiation
10	B = Cavum vaginale	35	B = 48 hours
11	C = Parietal layer	36	C = 60 μm
12	B = Tunica albuginea	37	A = Head
13	A = Lobules	38	C = Both (A) and (B)
14	A = Seminiferous tubules	39	B = Middle piece
15	B = Sertoli cells	40	D = Tail
16	C = Testosterone	41	A = 5 – α – reductase
17	A = Leydig cells	42	B = Androgen receptors
18	A = Epididymis	43	A = Rete testis
19	A = 20 feet	44	B = Testicular plexus
20	B = Head	45	A = Testicular arteries
21	A = Body	46	C = Both (A) and (B)
22	C = Tail	47	D = All of the above
23	B = Spermatogenesis	48	A = Vas deferens
24	A = Seminiferous tubules	49	B = 45 cm
25	C = 65 – 75 days	50	A = Ampulla

Part-02

1. The length of each ejaculatory duct is about
   - (A) 5 cm
   - (B) 8 cm
   - (C) 2 cm
   - (D) 10 cm

2. Which duct is formed by the union of the ductus deferens and duct from seminal vesicles?
   - (A) Ejaculatory duct
   - (B) Cystic duct
   - (C) Biliary duct
   - (D) Salivary duct

3. Which duct passes through the prostate gland and ejects sperms into the urethra
   - (A) Salivary duct
   - (B) Ejaculatory duct
   - (C) Cystic duct
   - (D) Salivary duct

4. How many tubes are ejaculatory ducts?
   - (A) Ten
   - (B) Five
   - (C) Two
   - (D) Seven

5. Which of the following serves as a common passageway for both urine coming from the bladder and sperms?
   - (A) Ureter
   - (B) Uterus
   - (C) Urethra
   - (D) Vagina

6. The accessory glands include in reproductive system of male are
   - (A) Seminal vesicles
   - (B) Prostate gland
   - (C) Bulbourethral glands
   - (D) All of the above

7. The length of seminal vesicles is about
   - (A) 14 cm
   - (B) 19 cm
   - (C) 5 cm
   - (D) 32 cm

8. Which of the following located posterior to and at the base of the urinary bladder anterior to the rectum?
   - (A) Seminal vesicles
   - (B) Cystic vesicles
   - (C) Salivary vesicles
   - (D) Pancreatic vesicles

9. Fluid secreted by the seminal vesicles have constituents of the total volume of semen about
   - (A) 10 %
   - (B) 60 %
   - (C) 90 %
   - (D) 30 %

10. A single doughnut – shaped gland that surrounds the prostatic urethra and is located inferior to the urinary bladder
    (A) Prostate gland
    (B) Pineal gland
    (C) Adrenal gland
    (D) Thymus gland

11. The weight of prostate gland in youth is about
    (A) 100 gm
    (B) 8 gm
    (C) 80 gm
    (D) 50 gm

12. The secretion from the prostate gland is acidic in nature and contains various proteolytic enzymes such as
    (A) Pepsinogen
    (B) Amylase
    (C) Lysozyme
    (D) All of the above

13. The secretion from prostate gland has constituents of the total volume of semen about
    (A) 90 %
    (B) 89 %
    (C) 25 %
    (D) 68 %

14. The paired pea – shaped glands present inferior to the prostate on either side of the membranous urethra
    (A) Cowper's gland
    (B) Pineal gland
    (C) Thyroid gland
    (D) Adrenal gland

15. The secretion from Cowper's gland has constituents of the total volume of semen about
    (A) 30 %
    (B) 60 %
    (C) 1 %
    (D) 78 %

16. Seminal fluid is also called
    (A) Serum
    (B) Sebum
    (C) Semen
    (D) Saliva

17. The pH pf semen is
    (A) 13.4 – 13.7
    (B) 1.2 – 2.1
    (C) 12.4 – 12.9
    (D) 7.2 – 7.7

18. The volume of semen per ejaculation is about
    (A) 2.5 – 5 mL
    (B) 10.3 – 15.5 mL
    (C) 2.5 – 5 mL
    (D) 30.4 – 34.4 mL

19. The pendulous structure hanging from the front that functions as a passage for the ejaculation of semen and the excretion of urine
    (A) Penis
    (B) Ilium
    (C) Adrenal gland
    (D) Jejunum

20. Which part of penis composed of three cylindrical masses of erectile tissue and smooth muscle

   (A) Band
   (B) Tail
   (C) Root
   (D) Body

21. The two dorsolateral masses of penis is called

   (A) Corpora cavernosa
   (B) Meissner's corpuscle
   (C) Stratified papilla
   (D) Pacinian corpuscle

22. Which of the following constituents most of the body of the penis and contain spongy urethra that keeps urethra open during ejaculation?

   (A) Pacinian corpuscle
   (B) Corpus spongiosum
   (C) Stratum corneum
   (D) Papilla corpuscle

23. The distal end of corpus spongiosum is slightly enlarge, tapered and expanded into a triangular structure called

   (A) Glans penis
   (B) Bulb penis
   (C) Crista penis
   (D) Labia penis

24. The glans penis is covered by a loose foreskin called

   (A) Papillae
   (B) Pedicle
   (C) Prepuce
   (D) Laminae

25. The surgical removal of the prepuce is called

   (A) Circumcision
   (B) Laparoscopy
   (C) Hysteroscopy
   (D) Endoscopy

26. The root of penis is triradiate in form and consists of

   (A) Bulb of penis
   (B) Crura of penis
   (C) Both (A) and (B)
   (D) None of the above

27. Scrotum appears externally as a single pouch divided into lateral portions by

   (A) Raphe
   (B) Bulb
   (C) Pili
   (D) Scar

28. Scrotum internally divided into two sacs by a

   (A) Stratum corneum
   (B) Scrotal septum
   (C) Stratum basale
   (D) Stratum dermis

29. As the scrotum lies outside the body cavity, the temperature of the scrotum is about

   (A) $20 - 25\ °C$
   (B) $40 - 43\ °C$
   (C) $2 - 3\ °C$
   (D) $18 - 20\ °C$

30. The scrotal septum is composed of
    (A) Dartos muscle
    (B) Soleus muscle
    (C) Pili muscle
    (D) Papilla muscle

31. The two large folds forming the boundary of the vulva is called
    (A) Labia majora
    (B) Labia pili
    (C) Labia fibres
    (D) Labia corneum

32. The two smaller folds of skin between the labia majora containing numerous sebaceous and eccrine sweat glands
    (A) Labia corneum
    (B) Labia minora
    (C) Labia pili
    (D) Labia papilla

33. The cleft between the labia minora is the
    (A) Papilla
    (B) Pacinian
    (C) Vestibule
    (D) Meissner's corpuscle

34. The vagina, urethra and ducts of the greater vestibular glands open into the
    (A) Vallate
    (B) Vestibule
    (C) Filiform
    (D) Fungiform

35. Which of the following corresponds to the penis in the male and contains sensory nerve endings and erectile tissue?
    (A) Clitoris
    (B) Papillae
    (C) Filiform
    (D) Fungiform

36. Which gland are situated one on each side near the vaginal opening?
    (A) Pineal gland
    (B) Adrenal gland
    (C) Thymus gland
    (D) Vestibular gland

37. The roughly triangular area extending from the base of the labia minora to the anal canal
    (A) Perineum
    (B) Palatine
    (C) Filiform
    (D) Fungiform

38. Perineum consists of
    (A) Connective tissue
    (B) Muscle
    (C) Fat
    (D) All of the above

39. Which gives attachment to the muscles of the pelvic floor
    (A) Filiform
    (B) Perineum
    (C) Fungiform
    (D) Vallate

40. Vestibular glands is also called
 (A) Bartholin's glands
 (B) Pineal glands
 (C) Thyroid glands
 (D) Adrenal glands

41. Vestibular glands are size of a small pea and their ducts open into the
 (A) Vallate
 (B) Fungiform
 (C) Vestibule
 (D) Filiform

42. The thin layer of mucous membrane that stretches across the vaginal lumen, just inside the external opening
 (A) Hymen
 (B) Hyaline
 (C) Humas
 (D) Helium

43. The vagina runs obliquely upwards and backwards between the bladder in front and rectum and anus behind at an angle is about
 (A) 100 degrees
 (B) 45 degrees
 (C) 180 degrees
 (D) 90 degrees

44. In adults, the anterior wall of vagina is about
 (A) 1 cm
 (B) 2.3 cm
 (C) 7.5cm
 (D) 12.9 cm

45. In adults, the posterior wall of vagina is about
 (A) 14 cm
 (B) 9 cm
 (C) 19 cm
 (D) 31 cm

46. An arterial plexus is formed round the vagina, derived from the uterine and vaginal arteries, which are branches of the
 (A) Internal iliac arteries
 (B) Inferior thyroid arteries
 (C) Superior thyroid arteries
 (D) Left subclavian arteries

47. An venous plexus situated in the muscular wall of vagina drains into the
 (A) Superior parathyroid veins
 (B) Superior thyroid veins
 (C) Internal iliac veins
 (D) Inferior thyroid veins

48. The paired oval – shaped structures that produce secondary oocyte
 (A) Ovaries
 (B) Cervix
 (C) Clavicle
 (D) Thymus

49. Which of the following present in the upper pelvic cavity, one on each side of the uterus?
 (A) Cervix
 (B) Clavicle
 (C) Ovaries
 (D) Thymus

50. The ovarian ligament attaches ovaries to the upper part of the uterus, and the
 (A) Suspensory ligament
 (B) Medullary ligament
 (C) Sensitive ligament
 (D) Filiform ligament

Answer Key

Reproductive System and Introduction to Genetics (Part-02)

Question	Answer	Question	Answer
01	C = 2 cm	26	C = Both (A) and (B)
02	A = Ejaculatory duct	27	A = Raphe
03	B = Ejaculatory duct	28	B = Scrotal septum
04	C = Two	29	C = 2 – 3 °C
05	C = Urethra	30	A = Dartos muscle
06	D = All of the above	31	A = Labia majora
07	C = 5 cm	32	B = Labia minora
08	A = Seminal vesicles	33	C = Vestibule
09	B = 60 %	34	B = Vestibule
10	A = Prostate gland	35	A = Clitoris
11	B = 8 gm	36	D = Vestibular gland
12	D = All of the above	37	A = Perineum
13	C = 25 %	38	D = All of the above
14	A = Cowper's gland	39	B = Perineum
15	C = 1 %	40	A = Bartholin's glands
16	C = semen	41	C = Vestibule
17	D = 7.2 – 7.7	42	A = Hymen
18	C = 2.5 – 5 mL	43	B = 45 degrees
19	A = Penis	44	C = 7.5 cm
20	D = Body	45	B = 9 cm
21	A = Corpora cavernosa	46	A = Internal iliac arteries
22	B = Corpus spongiosum	47	C = Internal iliac arteries
23	A = Glans penis	48	A = Ovaries
24	C = Prepuce	49	C = Ovaries
25	A = Circumcision	50	A = Suspensory ligament

Part-03

1. The broad ligament of the uterus encloses the ovarian by a double – layered fold of peritoneum called
   - (A) Mesovarium
   - (B) Orthovarium
   - (C) Hydrovarium
   - (D) Paravarium

2. The surface of the ovary is covered by ovarian surface epithelium previously called
   - (A) Intercalated epithelium
   - (B) Intervertebral epithelium
   - (C) Germinal epithelium
   - (D) Medullae epithelium

3. Beneath of germinal epithelium of ovary there is a white capsule of dense irregular connective tissue called
   - (A) Tunica albuginea
   - (B) Tunica basale
   - (C) Filiform papillae
   - (D) Fungiform papillae

4. The ovaries have tissue are
   - (A) Medulla
   - (B) Cortex
   - (C) Both (A) and (B)
   - (D) None of the above

5. The tunica albuginea of ovary encloses an outer area called
   - (A) Ovarian pili
   - (B) Ovarian lobe
   - (C) Ovarian cortex
   - (D) Ovarian pleura

6. Beneath of ovarian cortex is the ovarian medulla that consists of
   - (A) Connective tissue
   - (B) Nerves
   - (C) Lymphatic vessels
   - (D) All of the above

7. Which of the following are the ova and surrounding tissue going through different stages of development?
   - (A) Ovarian follicles
   - (B) Ovarian granules
   - (C) Ovarian packets
   - (D) Ovarian vesicles

8. Each ovarian follicle contains an immature ovum called
   - (A) Secondary follicle
   - (B) Primary follicle
   - (C) Tertiary follicle
   - (D) Quandary follicle

9. As the immature ovum gradually develops, it gains an increase in size and shape and developed a central region filled with fluid called

   (A) Antrum

   (B) Crista

   (C) Cisternae

   (D) Pedicle

10. When the secondary follicle becomes fully matures containing matures ovum, it is called

    (A) Graafian follicle

    (B) Filiform follicle

    (C) Fungiform follicle

    (D) Visceral follicle

11. As a result, the graafian follicle ruptures to release the matures ovum a process called

    (A) Digestion

    (B) Ovulation

    (C) Respiration

    (D) Ossification

12. The process of formation of female gamete in the ovaries called

    (A) Oogenesis

    (B) Osteogenesis

    (C) Spermatogenesis

    (D) Ossification

13. Before birth, the primordial germ cells from the yolk sac migrate towards the ovaries and begin to differentiate within the ovaries to form

    (A) Oogonia

    (B) Oomedia

    (C) Oosonia

    (D) Ooponia

14. The oogonia divide mitotically to form millions of germ cells, few of which deveop into larger cells called

    (A) Primary oocytes

    (B) Secondary oocytes

    (C) Tertiary oocytes

    (D) Quandary oocytes

15. The primary oocyte is surrounded by a single layer of follicular cells and is called

    (A) Primordial follicles

    (B) Fungiform follicles

    (C) Filiform follicles

    (D) Papillae follicles

16. As the primary follicles grow, the follicular cells surrounding the primary oocyte form several layers and are referred to as

    (A) Papillae cells

    (B) Granulosa cells

    (C) Filiform cells

    (D) Intercoastal cells

17. A layer of glycoproteins begins to appear between the granulosa cells and primary oocyte called as

    (A) Zona papillae

    (B) Zone filiform

    (C) Zona pellucida

    (D) Zona crura

18. As the primary follicle continues to grow, a region called
   (A) Theca folliculi
   (B) Theca crura
   (C) Thera dome
   (D) Thera recoils

19. The granulosa cells start secreting the follicular fluid that develops into a cavity at the centre called
   (A) Crura
   (B) Dome
   (C) Antrum
   (D) Recoils

20. Fallopian tube is also called
   (A) Uterine tubes
   (B) Gastric tubes
   (C) Bronchus tubes
   (D) Alveoli

21. How long the fallopian tube is
   (A) 20 cm
   (B) 30 cm
   (C) 40 cm
   (D) 10 cm

22. There is funnel – shaped open of each uterine tube called
   (A) Infundibulum
   (B) Central tendon
   (C) Intercoastal
   (D) Sprung

23. The infundibulum ends with finger – like projections called
   (A) Filiform
   (B) Fungiform
   (C) Fimbriae
   (D) Crura

24. From the infundibulum, the uterine tube medially and them inferiorly to form the longest widest part of the uterine tube called
   (A) Crura
   (B) Ampulla
   (C) Dome
   (D) Sprung

25. From the ampulla, the uterine tube becomes thick and narrow and gets attached to the uterus by a portion called
   (A) Isthmus
   (B) Sprung
   (C) Crura
   (D) Coastal

26. The walls of uterine tube are made of the following layer are
   (A) Mucosa
   (B) Muscularis
   (C) Serosa
   (D) All of the above

27. The inner layer of wall of uterine tube is
   (A) Pedicle
   (B) Serosa
   (C) Muscularis
   (D) Mucosa

28. The middle layer of wall of uterine tube is
    - (A) Serosa
    - (B) Mucosa
    - (C) Muscularis
    - (D) Fundus

29. The outer layer of wall of uterine tube is
    - (A) Fundus
    - (B) Muscularis
    - (C) Serosa
    - (D) Mucosa

30. Which cells help transport the fertilized ovum through uterine tube to uterus
    - (A) Ciliated cells
    - (B) Coastal cells
    - (C) Compact cells
    - (D) Crura cells

31. Which cells having microvilli secrete a fluid that serves to provide nutrition to the fertilized ovum
    - (A) Crura cells
    - (B) Non ciliated cells
    - (C) Sprung cells
    - (D) Sulcus cells

32. The muscularis layer of uterine tube is composed of
    - (A) Inner circular smooth muscles
    - (B) Outer longitudinal smooth muscles
    - (C) Both (A) and (B)
    - (D) None of the above

33. After ovulation fertilization can occur at any time up to
    - (A) 56 hours
    - (B) 24 hours
    - (C) 108 hours
    - (D) 72 hours

34. To reach the uterus the fertilized ovum takes about
    - (A) 10 – 12 days
    - (B) 15 – 20 days
    - (C) 6 – 7 days
    - (D) 20 – 22 days

35. The hollow muscular pear – shaped organ located in the pelvic cavity between the urinary bladder and the rectum is
    - (A) Uterus
    - (B) Stomach
    - (C) Spleen
    - (D) Kidney

36. The dome – shaped part superior to the uterine tube forms the
    - (A) Fissure of the uterus
    - (B) Fundus of the uterus
    - (C) Band of the uterus
    - (D) Tail of the uterus

37. The slightly tapered central portion forms the
    - (A) Tail of the uterus
    - (B) Head of the uterus
    - (C) Body of the uterus
    - (D) Band of the uterus

38. The narrow inferior portion that opens into the vagina is called
    - (A) Ilium
    - (B) Jejunum
    - (C) Cervix
    - (D) Clavicle

39. Between the body of the uterus and the cervix is constricted portion called
    - (A) Ischium
    - (B) Isthmus
    - (C) Ilium
    - (D) Jejunum

40. The interior of the body of the uterus is known as the
    - (A) Uterine cavity
    - (B) Splenic cavity
    - (C) Renal cavity
    - (D) Gastric cavity

41. The interior of the cervix is known as
    - (A) Cervical canal
    - (B) Cervical route
    - (C) Cervical path
    - (D) Cervical band

42. The junction of the uterine cavity with the cervical canal is called the
    - (A) Internal OP
    - (B) Internal OS
    - (C) External OT
    - (D) External OA

43. The opening of the cervix into the vagina is called
    - (A) External OS
    - (B) Internal OP
    - (C) Internal OC
    - (D) Internal OP

44. The highly vascularised innermost layer of uterus is
    - (A) Myocardium
    - (B) Endocardium
    - (C) Endometrium
    - (D) Pericardium

45. Endometria are functionally divided into the layers are
    - (A) Stratum functionalis
    - (B) Stratum basalis
    - (C) Both (A) and (B)
    - (D) None of the above

46. The upper layer that forms the lining of the uterine cavity and this layer is shed during menstruation
    - (A) Stratum functionalis
    - (B) Stratified basale
    - (C) Stratified corneum
    - (D) Stratified sulcus

47. The permanent basal layer and is not lost during menstruation
    - (A) Stratified sulcus
    - (B) Stratum basalis
    - (C) Stratified matter
    - (D) Corpus callosum

48. The thickest and the middle layer of uterus is
    - (A) Myocardium
    - (B) Pericardium
    - (C) Myometrium
    - (D) Endocardium

49. The outermost layer of uterus is
    (A) Perimetrium
    (B) Pericardium
    (C) Endocardium
    (D) Myocardium

50. The perimetrium of the uterus is composed of
    (A) Simple squamous epithelium
    (B) Areolar connective tissue
    (C) Both (A) and (B)
    (D) None of the above

Answer Key

Reproductive System and Introduction to Genetics (Part-03)

Question	Answer	Question	Answer
01	A = Mesovarium	26	D = All of the above
02	C = Germinal epithelium	27	D = Mucosa
03	A = Tunica albuginea	28	C = Muscularis
04	C = Both (A) and (B)	29	C = Serosa
05	C = Ovarian cortex	30	A = Ciliated cells
06	D = All of the above	31	B = Non-ciliated cells
07	A = Ovarian follicles	32	C = Both (A) and (B)
08	B = Primary follicles	33	B = 24 hours
09	A = Antrum	34	C = 6 – 7 days
10	A = Graafian follicle	35	A = Uterus
11	B = Ovulation	36	B = Fundus of the uterus
12	A = Oogenesis	37	C = Body of the uterus
13	A = Oogonia	38	C = Cervix
14	A = Primary oocytes	39	B = Isthmus
15	A = Primordial follicles	40	A = Uterine cavity
16	B = Granulosa cells	41	A = Cervical canal
17	C = Zona pellucida	42	B = Internal os
18	A = Theca folliculi	43	A = External os
19	C = Antrum	44	C = Endometrium
20	A = Uterine tubes	45	C = Both (A) and (B)
21	D = 10 cm	46	A = Stratum functionalis
22	A = Infundibulum	47	B = Stratum basalis
23	C = Fimbriae	48	C = Myometrium
24	B = Ampulla	49	A = Perimetrium
25	A = Isthmus	50	C = Both (A) and (B)

Part-04

1. Anteriorly the perimetrium extends over the fundus and forms a shallow pouch called
   (A) Rectouterine pouch
   (B) Morison's pouch
   (C) Hepatorenal pouch
   (D) Duodenal pouch

2. Posteriorly the perimetrium extends over the fundus, body and cervix and forms a deep pouch called
   (A) Duodenal pouch
   (B) Hepatorenal pouch
   (C) Rectouterine pouch
   (D) Morison's pouch

3. The secretory cells of cervical mucosa secrete
   (A) Cervical mucus
   (B) Clavicle mucus
   (C) Testicular mucus
   (D) Hepatorenal mucus

4. Cervical mucus contains the
   (A) Glycoproteins
   (B) Lipids
   (C) Inorganic salts
   (D) All of the above

5. A cervical mucus is secreted by a woman per day during her reproductive years about
   (A) 100 – 120 mL
   (B) 20 – 60 mL
   (C) 300 – 320 mL
   (D) 200 – 260 mL

6. Which produce serve to produce milk for the nourishment of the infant
   (A) Breast
   (B) Liver
   (C) Kidney
   (D) Heart

7. How many lobes of glandular tissue separated by adipose tissue in each mammary gland
   (A) 100 – 120
   (B) 15 – 20
   (C) 230 – 240
   (D) 150 – 200

8. In each lobe of mammary glands have several smaller compartments called
   (A) Globules
   (B) Packets
   (C) Lobules
   (D) Vacuoles

9. The lobules that contain milk – secreting glands called
   (A) Pineal glands
   (B) Alveoli glands
   (C) Adrenal gland
   (D) Thyroid gland

10. The circular pigmented projection of the breast is called
   (A) Dimple
   (B) Nipple
   (C) Dipple
   (D) Pimple

11. The circular pigmented area around the nipple is known as
   (A) Pedicle
   (B) Fundus
   (C) Areola
   (D) Calyx

12. The breasts are supported by suspensory ligaments of the breast called
   (A) Cooper's ligament
   (B) Goffer's ligament
   (C) Snopper's ligament
   (D) Blower's ligament

13. The mammary glands serve to synthesize, secrete and eject the milk a process called
   (A) Depression
   (B) Lactation
   (C) Digestion
   (D) Respiration

14. Primary female sex hormone is called
   (A) Melatonin
   (B) Oestrogen
   (C) Melanin
   (D) Thyroid

15. Human female contains different oestrogen in significant quantities are
   (A) Estrone
   (B) Estradiol
   (C) Estriol
   (D) All of the above

16. Which hormone promotes the development of breasts and appearance of pubic hair and axillary hair at puberty
   (A) Oestrogen
   (B) Melatonin
   (C) Melanin
   (D) Histamine

17. Which hormone promotes the development and maintenance of female reproductive structures
   (A) Melatonin
   (B) Melanin
   (C) Thyroid
   (D) Oestrogen

18. The important female sex hormone involved in the female menstrual cycle, pregnancy and embryogenesis
   (A) Progesterone
   (B) Melatonin
   (C) Adrenaline
   (D) Melanin

19. Which hormone is also called "hormone of pregnancy"
    (A) Melatonin
    (B) Thyroxin
    (C) Progesterone
    (D) Melanin

20. Which hormone produced during each menstrual cycle by the corpus luteum
    (A) Relaxin
    (B) Melanin
    (C) Histamine
    (D) Thyroxine

21. Which hormone secreted by granulosa cells of the ovarian follicles and by the corpus luteum of the ovary
    (A) Melanin
    (B) Inhibin
    (C) Thyronine
    (D) Melatonin

22. The average duration of menstrual cycle is about
    (A) 39 days
    (B) 28 days
    (C) 48 days
    (D) 58 days

23. The first menstrual cycle of a woman is called
    (A) Menarche
    (B) Denarche
    (C) Penaeche
    (D) Henarche

24. The first menstruation occurs between the age of
    (A) 20 – 22 years
    (B) 19 – 20 years
    (C) 10 – 14 years
    (D) 25 – 30 years

25. The cessation of the menstrual cycle of a woman is called
    (A) Menopause
    (B) Micropause
    (C) Macropause
    (D) Metapause

26. Menopause occurs between the age of
    (A) 20 – 25 years
    (B) 45 – 55 years
    (C) 70 – 75 years
    (D) 30 – 32 years

27. Which of the following responds to changes in the blood levels of oestrogen and progesterone?
    (A) Cerebrum
    (B) Pons
    (C) Meninges
    (D) Hypothalamus

28. In which phase menstrual phase, levels of oestrogen and progesterone are very low because of corpus luteum, which was active during the second half of the previous cycle, has degenerated
    (A) Menstrual phase
    (B) Proliferative phase
    (C) Secondary phase
    (D) Menopause

29. The menstrual fluid contains blood about

    (A) 200 – 300 mL

    (B) 50 – 150 mL

    (C) 400 – 450 mL

    (D) 550 – 600 mL

30. Which phase is the phase between the menstruation and ovulation

    (A) Preovulatory phase

    (B) Precaution phase

    (C) Predominant phase

    (D) Predetermined phase

31. The menstrual phase and the preovulatory phase are collectively termed as

    (A) Testicular phase

    (B) Globular phase

    (C) Follicular phase

    (D) Vascular phase

32. On which day of the 28 – day menstrual cycle the ovulation usually occurs

    (A) 26 days

    (B) 27 days

    (C) 21 days

    (D) 14 days

33. On how many days of the 28 – day menstrual cycle the postovulatory phase occurs

    (A) 15 to 28 days

    (B) 10 to 14 days

    (C) 1 to 3 days

    (D) 4 to 9 days

34. Which phase represents the time between ovulation and beginning of a new menstrual cycle

    (A) Menstrual phase

    (B) Preovulatory phase

    (C) Postovulatory phase

    (D) Ovulation

35. Which hormone stimulates pituitary to secrete FSH and LH above a basal level

    (A) Growth hormone

    (B) GnRH

    (C) Melatonin

    (D) Vasopressin

36. The source of GnRH hormone is

    (A) Hypothalamus

    (B) Stomach

    (C) Kidney

    (D) Liver

37. The source of LH hormone is

    (A) Kidney

    (B) Stomach

    (C) Pituitary

    (D) Intestine

38. Which hormone causes rapid growth of endometrium of uterus

    (A) Melatonin

    (B) Vasopressin

    (C) Adrenaline

    (D) Oestrogen

39. The source of oestrogen hormone is
    (A) Cervix
    (B) Vagina
    (C) Ovary
    (D) Adrenal gland

40. Which of the following act on theca cells to stimulate production and secretion of androgens?
    (A) Growth hormone
    (B) Luteinising hormone
    (C) Vasopressin hormone
    (D) Thyroxine hormone

41. Which hormone causes endometrium to become thick, spongy, glandular, and receptive to a fertilized ovum
    (A) Vasopressin
    (B) Progesterone
    (C) Thyroxine
    (D) Melatonin

42. The source of progesterone hormone is
    (A) Vagina
    (B) Ilium
    (C) Ovary
    (D) Adrenal gland

43. After ovulation, a secondary oocyte is viable for about
    (A) 48 hours
    (B) 24 hours
    (C) 56 hours
    (D) 108 hours

44. As the zygote moves down the uterine tube towards the uterine cavity, it undergoes a aery of rapid mitotic divisions, resulting in a hollow ball – like mass of cells called
    (A) Blastula
    (B) Osteula
    (C) Castula
    (D) Astrocytes

45. The blastocyst has an outer covering of cells called
    (A) Teloblast
    (B) Trophoblast
    (C) Hydroblast
    (D) Mesoblast

46. The blastocyst has an inner cell mass and an internal fluid – filled cavity called the
    (A) Tastocele
    (B) Hydrocele
    (C) Blastocele
    (D) Orthocele

47. The embryo secretes proteases to allow deep invasion into the
    (A) Uterine stroma
    (B) Uterine trauma
    (C) Uterine hydra
    (D) Uterine crista

48. About 6 days after fertilization, the blastocyst attaches to the endometrial lining of the uterus and eventually gets embedded in it, a process called
    (A) Implantation
    (B) Transformation
    (C) Transportation
    (D) Mobilization

49. The first major event of the embryonic periods is the differentiation of the inner cell mass of blastocyst into primary germ layer are

    (A) Ectoderm   (B) Endoderm

    (C) Mesoderm   (D) All of the above

50. The process during embryonic development that changes the embryo from a blastula with a single layer of cells to a gastrula containing multiple layers of cells

    (A) Digestion   (B) Gastrulation

    (C) Respiration   (D) Elimination

Answer Key

Reproductive System and Introduction to Genetics (Part-04)

Question	Answer	Question	Answer
01	A = Vesicouterine pouch	26	B = 45 – 55 years
02	C = Rectouterine pouch	27	D = Hypothalamus
03	A = Cervical mucus	28	A = Menstrual phase
04	D = All of the above	29	B = 50 – 150 mL
05	B = 20 – 60 mL	30	A = Preovulatory phase
06	A = Breast	31	C = Follicular phase
07	B = 15 – 20	32	D = 14 days
08	C = Lobules	33	A = 15 to 28 day
09	B = Alveoli glands	34	C = Postovulatory phase
10	B = Nipple	35	B = GnRH
11	C = Areola	36	A = Hypothalamus
12	A = Cooper's ligament	37	C = Pituitary
13	B = Lactation	38	D = Oestrogen
14	B = Oestrogen	39	C = Ovary
15	D = All of the above	40	B = Luteinising hormone
16	A = Oestrogen	41	B = Progesterone
17	D = Oestrogen	42	C = Ovary
18	A = Progesterone	43	B = 24 hours
19	C = Progesterone	44	A = Blastula
20	A = Relaxin	45	B = Trophoblast
21	B = Inhibin	46	C = Blastocele
22	B = 28 days	47	A = Uterine stroma
23	A = Menarche	48	A = Implantation
24	C = 10 – 14 days	49	D = All of the above
25	A = Menopause	50	B = Gastrulation

Part-05

1. The process by which the fetus is expelled from the uterus through the vagina to the outside is called
   - (A) Labour
   - (B) Defence
   - (C) Fertile
   - (D) Divide

2. Which stage includes rupturing of the amniotic sacs and dilation of the cervix
   - (A) Dilution stage
   - (B) Concentration stage
   - (C) Dilation stage
   - (D) Expansion stage

3. The dilation stage lasts up to
   - (A) 29 hours
   - (B) 12 hours
   - (C) 39 hours
   - (D) 48 hours

4. The stage in which child moves through the cervix and vagina to the outside
   - (A) Expulsion stage
   - (B) Dilution stage
   - (C) Concentration stage
   - (D) Repulsion stage

5. The stage within the 15 minutes after birth, the placenta detaches from the uterus and is expelled by powerful uterine contraction called
   - (A) Expansion stage
   - (B) Repulsion stage
   - (C) Placental stage
   - (D) Dilution stage

6. The condition in which a man is unable to attain or maintain an erection
   - (A) Impotence
   - (B) Renal calculi
   - (C) Nephroptosis
   - (D) Polyuria

7. The condition in which ejaculation occurs too early either during foreplay or shortly after penetration
   - (A) Polyuria
   - (B) Premature ejaculation
   - (C) Pyelitis
   - (D) Uraemia

8. Which refers to the lack of function of the gonads, with regard to either hormones or gamete production
   - (A) Hypogonadism
   - (B) Hyperthyroidism
   - (C) Hypertension
   - (D) Hypotension

9. The cancer of penis is called
   (A) Testicular cancer
   (B) Penile cancer
   (C) Uterine cancer
   (D) Ovarian cancer

10. The cancer of cervix is called
   (A) Penile cancer
   (B) Uterine cancer
   (C) Cervical cancer
   (D) Ovarian cancer

11. The cancer of mammary gland is called
   (A) Breast cancer
   (B) Lung cancer
   (C) Testicular cancer
   (D) Skin cancer

12. The cancer of testicles is called
   (A) Cervical cancer
   (B) Ovarian cancer
   (C) Breast cancer
   (D) Testicular cancer

13. The initial symptoms of ovarian cancer include
   (A) Nausea
   (B) Abdominal discomfort
   (C) Loss of appetite
   (D) All of the above

14. Which disease caused by human immunodeficiency virus
   (A) AIDS
   (B) Typhoid
   (C) Tuberculosis
   (D) Arthritis

15. Full form of AIDS
   (A) Adrenaline immune dilation syndrome
   (B) Acquired immune deficiency syndrome
   (C) Appetite immune dehydration syndrome
   (D) Acquired immune disease stage

16. Which of the following is sexually transmitted disease?
   (A) Herpes simplex
   (B) Typhoid
   (C) Malaria
   (D) Dental carries

17. Herpes simplex is caused by
   (A) Plasmodium
   (B) S. Typhi
   (C) Herpes virus
   (D) Mycobacterium tuberculosis

18. The common sexually transmitted disease caused by bacterium Neisseria gonorrhoeae
   (A) Malaria
   (B) Gonorrhoea
   (C) Typhoid
   (D) Pneumonia

19. The sexually transmitted disease caused by bacterium Treponema pallidum
   - (A) Stye
   - (B) Typhoid
   - (C) Syphilis
   - (D) Peptic ulcer

20. The sexually transmitted infection caused by human papillomavirus
   - (A) Genital warts
   - (B) Pneumonia
   - (C) Bronchitis
   - (D) Tuberculosis

21. The vaginal infection caused by any species of the fungus genus Candida
   - (A) Protozoa infection
   - (B) Yeast infection
   - (C) Typhoid
   - (D) Peptic ulcer

22. The sexually transmitted infection caused by the protozoan parasite Trichomonas vaginalis
   - (A) Trichomoniasis
   - (B) Stye
   - (C) Tuberculosis
   - (D) Pneumonia

23. The absence of one or both testes from the scrotum
   - (A) Polyuria
   - (B) Pyelonephritis
   - (C) Cryptorchidism
   - (D) Uraemia

24. The condition in which a person has genitalia and/or other sexual traits that are not clearly male or female
   - (A) Intersexuality
   - (B) Extra sexuality
   - (C) Tetra sexuality
   - (D) Hydra sexuality

25. The collection of serous fluid in tunica vaginalis of the testis
   - (A) Hydrocele
   - (B) Polyuria
   - (C) Uraemia
   - (D) Pyelitis

26. Hydrocele is caused by inflammation of
   - (A) Vagina
   - (B) Ovary
   - (C) Cervix
   - (D) Epididymis

27. The condition in which scrotum gets swollen
   - (A) Varicocelle
   - (B) Cystitis
   - (C) Renal calculi
   - (D) Polycystic disease

28. The fluid – filled sac in the ovary is called
   - (A) Ovarian crista
   - (B) Ovarian cyst
   - (C) Ovarian cele
   - (D) Ovarian hydra

29. The growth of endometrial tissue outside the uterus called
    (A) Endometriosis
    (B) Exometriosis
    (C) Parametriosis
    (D) Orthometriosis

30. The noncancerous tumours in the uterus composed of muscular and fibrosis tissue
    (A) Fibroids
    (B) Uterus failure
    (C) Nephritis
    (D) Nephroptosis

31. Symptoms of uterine fibroids
    (A) Heavy bleeding
    (B) Frequent urination
    (C) Constipation
    (D) All of the above

32. The whitish vaginal discharge containing mucus and pus cells
    (A) Leukorrhoea
    (B) Nephroptosis
    (C) Floating kidney
    (D) Polycystic disease

33. The condition of painful menstruation is called
    (A) Polycystic disease
    (B) Glomerulonephritis
    (C) Dysmenorrhoea
    (D) UTI

34. The absence of menstruation is called
    (A) Amenorrhoea
    (B) Polycystic disease
    (C) Glomerulonephritis
    (D) Pyelonephritis

35. The condition of pain during sexual intercourse
    (A) Uraemia
    (B) Pyelonephritis
    (C) Typhoid
    (D) Dyspareunia

36. The inflammation of breast tissue due to bacterial infection
    (A) Nephritis
    (B) Arthritis
    (C) Mastitis
    (D) Vaginitis

37. The inflammation of the vagina due to bacterial infection or sexually transmitted infection
    (A) Vaginitis
    (B) Bronchitis
    (C) Mastitis
    (D) Arthritis

38. The symptom of vaginitis is
    (A) Itching
    (B) Vaginal discharge
    (C) Inflammation of genial area
    (D) All of the above

39. The implantation of a fertilised ovum outside the uterus, usually in the uterine tube is called

    (A) Ectopic pregnancy   (B) Erectile pregnancy

    (C) Emergency pregnancy   (D) Engaged pregnancy

40. The inflammation of uterine tube is called

    (A) Arthritis   (B) Bronchitis

    (C) Salpingitis   (D) Nephritis

41. The bacterium Chlamydia trachomatis causes inflammation of the female cervix

    (A) Nephritis   (B) Pneumonia

    (C) Tuberculosis   (D) Chlamydia

42. The inflammation of testis is called

    (A) Orchitis   (B) Otitis

    (C) Arthritis   (D) Nephritis

43. The proliferation of breast tissue in men

    (A) Gynaecomastia   (B) Pyelonephritis

    (C) Nephrotic syndrome   (D) Renal calculi

44. Gynaecomastia is associated with

    (A) Endocrine disorders   (B) Cirrhosis of the liver

    (C) Malnutrition   (D) All of the above

45. The surgical form of contraception is called

    (A) Endoscopy   (B) Microscopy

    (C) Vasectomy   (D) Dialysis

46. A condition in which tight foreskin cannot be pulled back over the head of penis called

    (A) Phimosis   (B) Pyelonephritis

    (C) Pneumonia   (D) Pyelitis

47. Which condition occurs when a testicle rotates, twisting the spermatic cord that brings blood to the scrotum

    (A) Testicular uraemia   (B) Testicular pyelitis

    (C) Testicular torsion   (D) Testicular cystitis

48. Sign and symptoms of testicular torsion

    (A) Swelling of the scrotum   (B) Abdominal pain

    (C) Frequent urination   (D) All of the above

49. The prolonged erection of the penis
    - (A) Priapism
    - (B) Polyurea
    - (C) Pyelonephritis
    - (D) Nephrotic syndrome

50. A hormonal disorder causing enlargement ovaries
    - (A) Polycystic ovary syndrome
    - (B) Polycystic testicles syndrome
    - (C) Polyhydrate ovary disease
    - (D) Polyhydrate scrotum disease

Answer Key

Reproductive System and Introduction to Genetics (Part-05)

Question	Answer	Question	Answer
01	A = Labour	26	D = Epididymis
02	C = Dilation stage	27	A = Varicocelle
03	B = 12 hours	28	B = Ovarian cyst
04	A = Expulsion stage	29	A = Endometriosis
05	C = Placental stage	30	A = Fibroids
06	A = Impotence	31	D = All of the above
07	B = Premature ejaculation	32	A = Leukorrhoea
08	A = Hypogonadism	33	C = Dysmenorrhoea
09	B = Penile cancer	34	A = Amenorrhoea
10	C = Cervical cancer	35	D = Dyspareunia
11	A = Breast cancer	36	C = Mastitis
12	D = Testicular cancer	37	A = Vaginitis
13	D = All of the above	38	D = All of the above
14	A = AIDS	39	A = Ectopic pregnancy
15	B = Acquired immune deficiency syndrome	40	C = Salpingitis
16	A = Herpes simplex	41	D = Chlamydia
17	C = Herpes virus	42	A = Orchitis
18	B = Gonorrhoea	43	A = Gynaecomastia
19	C = Syphilis	44	D = All of the above
20	A = Genital warts	45	C = Vasectomy
21	B = Yeast infection	46	A = Phimosis
22	A = Trichomoniasis	47	C = Testicular torsion
23	C = Cryptorchidism	48	D = All of the above
24	A = Intersexuality	49	A = Priapism
25	A = Hydrocele	50	A = Polycystic ovary syndrome

Part-06

1. Chromosomes are present within the
   - (A) Nucleus
   - (B) Ribosomes
   - (C) Lysosomes
   - (D) Mitochondria
2. Chromosomes are not found in
   - (A) Red blood cells
   - (B) Sex cells
   - (C) Both (A) and (B)
   - (D) None of the above
3. How many pair of chromosomes in human cell?
   - (A) 44 pairs
   - (B) 23 pairs
   - (C) 13 pairs
   - (D) 34 pairs
4. A cell with 23 pairs of chromosomes is termed as
   - (A) Tetraploid
   - (B) Decaploid
   - (C) Diploid
   - (D) Pentaploid
5. Chromosomes belonging to the same pair called
   - (A) Homogenous chromosomes
   - (B) Homologus chromosomes
   - (C) Heterogenous chromosomes
   - (D) Mesogenous chromosomes
6. The first 22 pairs of chromosomes are collectively known as
   - (A) Autosomes
   - (B) Mesosomes
   - (C) Orthosomes
   - (D) Metasomes
7. The chromosome of pair 23 are called
   - (A) Sex chromosome
   - (B) Disc chromosome
   - (C) Tail chromosome
   - (D) Band chromosome
8. Chromosomes are made of a slightly coiled strand of DNA along with supporting protein
   - (A) Histones
   - (B) Pistons
   - (C) Gistones
   - (D) Systone
9. Uncoiled the total length of DNA in each body cell is about
   - (A) 9 metres
   - (B) 2 metres
   - (C) 10 metres
   - (D) 11 metres

10. Each end of the chromosomes is capped with a length of DNA called a
    (A) Helomere
    (B) Phelomere
    (C) Telomere
    (D) Seromere

11. During replication the telomere is shortened, which would damage the chromosome, and so it is repaired with an enzyme called
    (A) Amylase
    (B) Telomerase
    (C) Lipase
    (D) Ligase

12. Which of the following considered as a basic unit of inheritance?
    (A) Tissue
    (B) Organ
    (C) Organ system
    (D) Gene

13. How many genes contain in human genome?
    (A) 20,0000
    (B) 20,5000
    (C) 20,500
    (D) 13,000

14. The DNA – histone material is called
    (A) Chromatin
    (B) Condensed
    (C) Compact
    (D) Conduct

15. How many chains of nucleotides contain in DNA molecule?
    (A) Six
    (B) Ten
    (C) Seven
    (D) Two

16. Nucleotides consist of subunits are
    (A) A sugar
    (B) A phosphate
    (C) A base
    (D) All of the above

17. The nitrogenous base is found in DNA is
    (A) Purines
    (B) Pyrimidines
    (C) Both (A) and (B)
    (D) None of the above

18. Each base along one strand of DNA pairs with a base on the other strand in a precise and predictable way. This is known as
    (A) Complementary base pairing
    (B) Supplementary base repelling
    (C) Intermediatory base repelling
    (D) Intrainhibitory base pairing

19. Which of the following is purine?
    (A) Adenine
    (B) Thymine
    (C) Cytosine
    (D) Cytonine

20. Which of the following is pyrimidine?
    (A) Thymine
    (B) Adenine
    (C) Guanine
    (D) Glycosine

21. Adenine always pair with
    (A) Cytosine
    (B) Guanine
    (C) Thymine
    (D) Thyronine

22. Cytosine always together with
    (A) Guanine
    (B) Thymine
    (C) Adenine
    (D) Thyronine

23. The bases on opposite strands run down the middle of the helix and bind to one another with
    (A) Chloride bond
    (B) Fluorine bond
    (C) Hydrogen bond
    (D) Sodium bond

24. Each body cell has on average mitochondria
    (A) 10000
    (B) 5000
    (C) 30000
    (D) 45000

25. One turn of the helix measures about
    (A) 3.4 nm
    (B) 5.5 nm
    (C) 8.5 nm
    (D) 9.3 nm

26. One turn of the helix contains nucleotides are
    (A) 30
    (B) 10
    (C) 43
    (D) 36

27. The distance between adjacent nucleotides is
    (A) 4.4 nm
    (B) 5.2 nm
    (C) 0.34 nm
    (D) 6.1 nm

28. The diameter of helix of DNA is
    (A) 2 nm
    (B) 5 nm
    (C) 9 nm
    (D) 10 nm

29. Who give X – ray diffraction method, proposed a double helical model of DNA to explain their molecular structure?
    (A) Louis Pasteur
    (B) Watson and Crick
    (C) Charles Darwin
    (D) Carolus Linnaeus

30. Watson and crick model of DNA got Nobel prize in
    (A) 1921
    (B) 1931
    (C) 1962
    (D) 1992

31. The RNA involved in protein synthesis is

   (A) mRNA
   (B) tRNA
   (C) rRNA
   (D) All of the above

32. The process by which the information in a strand of DNA is copied into a new molecule of mRNA

   (A) Transcription
   (B) Conduction
   (C) Polarization
   (D) Depolarization

33. Transcription is carried out by an enzyme called

   (A) RNA hydroxylase
   (B) RNA polymerase
   (C) RNA lipase
   (D) RNA amylase

34. Only one strand of DNA copied during the process of transcription known as the template strand and RNA formed is called

   (A) pRNA
   (B) nRNA
   (C) mRNA
   (D) eRNA

35. in which step the RNA polymerase attaches to the DNA molecule and moves along the DNA strand until it recognises a promoter sequence

   (A) Initiation
   (B) Inhibition
   (C) Conduction
   (D) Polarization

36. In which step the ribonucleotides are added tothe template strand that enables the growth of mRNA growth

   (A) Elimination
   (B) Elongation
   (C) Conduction
   (D) Filtration

37. A methylated guanine cap is added to protect the mRNA is called

   (A) Chipping
   (B) Conduction
   (C) Capping
   (D) Hydration

38. The poly – A tail also protects the mRNA from degradation is called

   (A) Polymerization
   (B) Hyperpolarization
   (C) Depolarization
   (D) Polyadenylation

39. Within all cells, the translation machinery resides within a specialized organelle called

   (A) Lysosome
   (B) Ribosome
   (C) Mitochondria
   (D) Cytoplasm

40. The ribosome is composed of subunit are

   (A) 30S subunit
   (B) 50S subunit
   (C) Both (A) and (B)
   (D) None of the above

41. Sudden inheritable changes in the genetic material are called
   (A) Mutation
   (B) Conduction
   (C) Dehydration
   (D) Polymerization

42. The mutation occur without any cause is called
   (A) Conduction mutation
   (B) Spontaneous mutation
   (C) Simultaneous mutation
   (D) Diffraction mutation

43. The mutation resulting from the exposure of organisms to mutagenic agents
   (A) Diffraction mutation
   (B) Simultaneous mutation
   (C) Induced mutation
   (D) Conduction mutation

44. The disorder in which three copies of chromosome 21, meaning that an extra chromosome is present
   (A) Down's syndrome
   (B) Blue baby syndrome
   (C) Cushing syndrome
   (D) Cervical syndrome

45. Which syndrome is caused when part of chromosome 5 is missing?
   (A) Cri – du – chat syndrome
   (B) Cushing syndrome
   (C) Central syndrome
   (D) Dysplastic nevus syndrome

46. Which of the following usually associated with having only one sex chromosome, an X, as well as 22 normal pairs of autosomes?
   (A) Central syndrome
   (B) Grey baby syndrome
   (C) Turner's syndrome
   (D) Cushing syndrome

47. The human genome project was an international collaboration completed in
   (A) 2009
   (B) 1998
   (C) 1990
   (D) 2003

48. The example of autosomal dominant disorders is
   (A) Huntington's disease
   (B) Marfan syndrome
   (C) Both (A) and (B)
   (D) None of the above

49. The example of autosomal recessive is
   (A) Typhoid
   (B) Malaria
   (C) Sickle cells anaemia
   (D) Pneumonia

50. Collectively, all genetic material in a cell is called its
   (A) Genome
   (B) Organ
   (C) Tissue
   (D) Organ system

Answer Key

Reproductive System and Introduction to Genetics (Part-06)

Question	Answer	Question	Answer
01	A = Nucleus	26	B = 10
02	C = Both (A) and (B)	27	C = 0.34 nm
03	B = 23 pairs	28	A = 2 cm
04	C = Diploid	29	B = Watson and crick
05	B = Homologous chromosome	30	C = 1962
06	A = Autosomes	31	D = All of the above
07	A = Sex chromosome	32	A = Transcription
08	A = Histone	33	B = RNA polymerase
09	B = 2 metres	34	C = mRNA
10	C = Telomere	35	A = Initiation
11	B = Telomerase	36	B = Elongation
12	D = Gene	37	C = Capping
13	C = 20,500	38	D = Polyadenylation
14	A = Chromatin	39	B = Ribosome
15	D = Two	40	C = Both (A) and (B)
16	D = All of the above	41	A = Mutation
17	C = Both (A) and (B)	42	B = Spontaneous mutation
18	A = Complementary base pairing	43	C = Induced mutation
19	A = Adenine	44	A = Down's syndrome
20	A = Thymine	45	A = Cri – du – chat syndrome
21	C = Thymine	46	C = Turner's syndrome
22	A = Guanine	47	D = 2003
23	C = Hydrogen bond	48	C = Both (A) and (B)
24	B = 5000	49	C = Sickle cells anaemia
25	A = 3.4 nm	50	A = Genome

www.ingramcontent.com/pod-product-compliance
Lightning Source LLC
Chambersburg PA
CBHW050744150726
48196CB00003B/351